W0050174

Health Informatics

Margunn Aanestad · Miria Grisot
Ole Hanseth · Polyxeni Vassilakopoulou
Editors

Information Infrastructures within European Health Care

Working with the Installed Base

OPEN

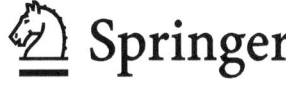 Springer

Editors

Margunn Aanestad
University of Oslo
Oslo
Norway

Miria Grisot
University of Oslo
Oslo
Norway

Ole Hanseth
University of Oslo
Oslo
Norway

Polyxeni Vassilakopoulou
University of Oslo
Oslo
Norway

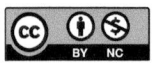

ISSN 1431-1917   ISSN 2197-3741   (electronic)
Health Informatics
ISBN 978-3-319-51018-7   ISBN 978-3-319-51020-0   (eBook)
DOI 10.1007/978-3-319-51020-0

Library of Congress Control Number: 2017933448

© The Editor(s) (if applicable) and The Author(s) 2017. This book is an open access publication.
Open Access This book is distributed under the terms of the Creative Commons Attribution-NonCommercial 2.5 International License (http://creativecommons.org/licenses/by-nc/2.5/), which permits any noncommercial use, duplication, adaptation, distribution and reproduction in any medium or format, as long as you give appropriate credit to the original author(s) and the source, provide a link to the Creative Commons license and indicate if changes were made.
The images or other third party material in this book are included in the book's Creative Commons license, unless indicated otherwise in the credit line; if such material is not included in the book's Creative Commons license and the respective action is not permitted by statutory regulation, users will need to obtain permission from the license holder to duplicate, adapt or reproduce the material.
This work is subject to copyright. All *commercial* rights are reserved by the Publisher, whether the whole or part of the material is concerned, specifically the rights of translation, reprinting, reuse of illustrations, recitation, broadcasting, reproduction on microfilms or in any other physical way, and transmission or information storage and retrieval, electronic adaptation, computer software, or by similar or dissimilar methodology now known or hereafter developed.
The use of general descriptive names, registered names, trademarks, service marks, etc. in this publication does not imply, even in the absence of a specific statement, that such names are exempt from the relevant protective laws and regulations and therefore free for general use.
The publisher, the authors and the editors are safe to assume that the advice and information in this book are believed to be true and accurate at the date of publication. Neither the publisher nor the authors or the editors give a warranty, express or implied, with respect to the material contained herein or for any errors or omissions that may have been made. The publisher remains neutral with regard to jurisdictional claims in published maps and institutional affiliations.

Printed on acid-free paper

This Springer imprint is published by Springer Nature
The registered company is Springer International Publishing AG
The registered company address is: Gewerbestrasse 11, 6330 Cham, Switzerland

Contents

Introduction

Margunn Aanestad, Miria Grisot, Ole Hanseth,
and Polyxeni Vassilakopoulou

1.1   Background and Aim of the Book

Confronting quality-of-care problems and achieving cost containment in healthcare delivery is one of the greatest challenges for the twenty-first century. Realising the promise of eHealth for ensuring sustainability of Europe's healthcare systems is becoming urgent. When seen in a context of increasing needs for health personnel, growth in chronic disease, an ageing population and a consequential expected rise in public health expenditures, the successful utilisation of information and communication technologies becomes crucial. The eHealth Strategies Report prepared on behalf of the European Commission, Directorate General Information Society and Media, in 2011, points to implementation as a key challenge: "Reaching agreement about eHealth strategies and, even more so, implementing them has almost everywhere proven to be considerable more complex and time-consuming than initially anticipated. The complexity of eHealth as a management challenge was vastly underestimated." (Stroetmann et al. 2011). If we want substantial advancements in healthcare information infrastructures, we need knowledge on actual experiences, and the contributions in this book aim to give the readers a better grip on what facilitates and hinders successful implementation and utilization.

M. Aanestad (✉)
University of Oslo & UIT The Arctic University of Norway,
P.O. Box 1080 Blindern, N-0316 Oslo, Norway
e-mail: margunn@ifi.uio.no

M. Grisot • O. Hanseth
University of Oslo, P.O. Box 1080 Blindern, N-0316 Oslo, Norway
e-mail: miriag@ifi.uio.no; oleha@ifi.uio.no

P. Vassilakopoulou
University of Agder & University of Oslo, P.O. Box 422, N-4604 Kristiansand, Norway
e-mail: polyxenv@uia.no

© The Author(s) 2017
M. Aanestad et al. (eds.), *Information Infrastructures within European Health Care*, Health Informatics, DOI 10.1007/978-3-319-51020-0_1

Currently, European countries have reached a level of technological maturity where most healthcare organisations (both within hospitals and within primary care) have impressive systems to support their day to day operations (European Commission DG Communications Networks Content & Technology 2013; European Commission Joint Research Centre Institute for Prospective Technological Studies (JRC-IPTS) 2014). But, the systems tend not to talk to each other: if a patient has a blood test at a primary care outlet, then a treatment at a specialist hospital, and then an operation in a different hospital, it may take weeks for the electronic records to reflect comprehensively all encounters. Information flows that cross organisational boundaries are still a major issue for healthcare.

Within European healthcare, the problem that we now have to address is how to introduce new technological capabilities that link and leverage what is already in place, blending in the already densely populated health technology landscapes. In the extant literature on health informatics the relationship between novel systems and pre-existing infrastructural resources has been mostly addressed as an issue of connectivity or interoperability (from a technical point of view) or technology acceptance/appropriation (from an organizational point of view). Novelty is viewed as something distinct from what is already in place and the main concern is how the new and the old can be fitted together. In this book we propose an alternative way to understand and approach the challenges of implementation. The central theme here is how change initiatives encounter the pre-existing health technology landscape. The overall aim of the book is to provide insights on the role of existing elements as resources for new development, the conducts through which they contribute to the composition of novelty and the modes through which the pre-existing technological and institutional resources are mobilized, recombined, or obliterated. We explore this issue by analysing cases of inter-organizational information systems where a multitude of pre-existing infrastructural elements exist.

Specifically, the book includes a number of case studies on the design and implementation of systems that span organisational boundaries in different healthcare settings across Europe. The two types of systems covered are: e-prescription and governmental patient-oriented web platforms. The case descriptions go beyond the trajectories of design and development to include experiences of reworking and reconfiguration during and after deployment as this has proved to be pivotal for systems' evolution. We have selected the two specific types of systems not only because they are widespread around Europe and allow comparisons but also because they are exemplary of two different types of grand aims. E-prescription initiatives are usually seen as opportunities to improve health care delivery by systematic and not dramatic change (controlling the ever-increasing medication costs, improving patient safety and providing rich information for performance management). Governmental patient-oriented web platforms are seen as opportunities to pursue wider and more radical innovation, aiming to strengthen the patients' role and to facilitate a shift from provider-centred health care towards patient-centeredness.

The empirical material from the different cases is analysed through the information infrastructure perspective (Star and Ruhleder 1996; Hanseth and Lundberg 2001; Hanseth and Lyytinen 2010). Information Infrastructures go beyond self-contained IT applications as they span localities and temporal scales. Information infrastructures are sociotechnical bases to build upon implying that they cannot be defined through a distinct set of functions, or strict boundaries. Infrastructures are never built "de novo"; they develop amidst a stream of technical antecedents, social conventions and professional rules and have to be adaptive to the developments of practice. At the same time, they have to be stable enough to reliably support activities that make use of them: "only a stable installed base allows new connections to be created" (Tilson et al. 2010). Working with infrastructures within healthcare is especially challenging because novelty has to link to complex conventions of practice and to technologically congested landscapes that have gradually matured during several decades. Taking an infrastructural perspective does not only orient attention to interconnections and relationships but also to issues of durability, permanence and strategies for effectively managing future evolution (Ribes and Finholt 2009; Karasti et al. 2010).

The chapters of the book present rich empirical cases analysed through a specific theoretical lens. Therefore, we offer a book where theoretical insights and practical experiences are tightly connected. The contributions to the book are sourced from a network of academics that have been working on the topic for years, have previously collaborated and share a common understanding of the challenges entailed in expanding information infrastructures within health care.

The book aims to to respond to the needs of different audiences:

- Academic researchers from different disciplines including: information systems research, health care management, innovation studies
- Practitioners involved in the design and development of information systems within health care, policy makers and ordering organizations
- Students in information systems, technology management and health care management programs.

1.2   Outline of the Book

The book is organized in three sections. In section A we present the empirical domain of the book, the context of eHealth infrastructures, the core theoretical concepts, and the cross-case analysis of the cases. This is followed by eleven chapters analysing various European experiences with putting in place eHealth infrastructures. Section B includes empirical chapters on e-prescription from Spain, Norway, Greece, the UK and Germany. Section C includes empirical chapters on governmental platforms for patient-oriented eHealth services from Spain, Norway, Denmark, Sweden and Italy.

1.2.1   Section A: Information Infrastructures in Healthcare

The first chapter in this section provides an introductory overview of the eHealth landscape, and then a more detailed discussion of e-prescription solutions and governmental patient-oriented web platforms and their drivers. E-prescription initiatives are driven by concerns to monitor and control prescriptions not only for ensuring healthcare quality but also for reasons of cost control. Patient platforms seek to realize visions of patient-centered care, but are also driven by needs to improve the efficiency of healthcare provision, such as overcoming existing communication barriers and mobilizing citizens towards self-care and proactive disease prevention. We argue that eHealth infrastructures have a dual character. They have a transformative orientation and are expected to instigate the reshaping of core roles and relationships within the healthcare systems. However, they also leverage and need to fit to, existing services, capabilities, institutions, data sources, systems, and communication channels.

Then, in the second chapter of the section, we give an account of the theoretical lens used in this book, the information infrastructure perspective, with a special emphasis on the notion of "installed base", which is central to the empirical chapters´ analyses. The installed base, we argue, serves as the foundation for any change and development, and can be both enabling and constraining. New developments need to fit and make use of existing arrangements and at the same time transform them. This paradoxical relationship is illuminated through the book's empirical investigations of how new eHealth initiatives make use of existing arrangements and at the same time transform them.

The last chapter in this section presents a cross-case analysis of the eleven empirical chapters of the book. We discuss the six e-prescription cases and the five patient-oriented eHealth cases in terms of the initiatives' scope, starting point, motivation, and then, we turn to observed strategies towards the installed base for the two types of infrastructures. The e-prescription cases illustrate a variety of approaches towards the installed base, and we identify what we call installed base-friendly, installed base-hostile and installed base-ignorant approaches. The cases of patient-oriented eHealth initiatives illustrate a variety of approaches for the coordination of multiple involved actors, for handling technical heterogeneity, for addressing uncertainty and for supporting transformations. We conclude by pointing to the importance of taking an installed base perspective.

1.2.2   Section B: E-Prescription Infrastructures

In this section, the first chapter is written by Joan Rodon Modol and presents the genesis and evolution of the public ePrescription information infrastructure of Catalonia, Spain from 2000 to 2013. The implementation of this solution required a transition from a mainly paper-based and asynchronous prescription model to a digital and synchronous one, and required changes in the practices, systems and roles of the Catalan Health Service, doctors and health providers, pharmacists and Colleges of Pharmacists, and ultimately patients. The chapter shows how the pre-existing technological and institutional resources of professionals shaped the design, and evolution of the infrastructure. The narrative traces events from the perspective of pharmacists, and shows how the exploitation and expansion of the installed base of pharmacists helped maintain the existing pharmacy model.

The second chapter, written by Ole Hanseth and Bendik Bygstad presents the Norwegian experience. While early attempts to put in place an e-prescription solution in Norway failed, the current solution is widely adopted and considered a great success. The chapter analyses the approaches for coping with the existing installed base and how they played a major role in the initiative. A combination of changes in the strategy towards the installed base (i.e. loose coupling and flexibility in integration between EPR systems and the prescribing module); in the development approach (from specification driven to a prototyping/evolutionary approach); and in the organizing and governance structures is seen as key to the (final) success of the Norwegian ePrescription initiative.

In the third chapter, Polyxeni Vassilakopoulou and Nicolas Marmaras examine the surprisingly swift deployment of a national e-prescription service in Greece. The analysis identifies how a series of pragmatic decisions allowed building upon a "good-enough" installed base by exploiting its latent potential without perpetuating all of its weaknesses, and by being responsive to exogenous shifts. These tactical decisions, were supported by an enabling combination of novel technological capabilities, standards and architectural arrangements that allowed connections, extensions and continuous adaptations to exogenous shifts in the installed base.

In the fourth chapter, written by Ralph Hibberd, Tony Cornford, Valentina Lichtner, Will Venters and Nick Barber, the development of the Electronic Prescription Service (EPS), adopted by the English NHS for primary care is presented. The analysis illustrates how EPS has been assembled within a rich institutional and organizational context including causal pasts, contemporary practices and policy visions. This process of assembly is traced using three perspectives: as the realization and negotiation of constraints found in the wider NHS context, as a response to inertia arising from limited resources and weak incentive structures, and as a purposive fidelity to the existing institutional cultures of the NHS.

The fifth chapter, by Hajar Mozaffar, Robin Williams, Kathrin M. Cresswell, Neil Pollock, Zoe Morrison and Aziz Sheikh, describes a second case from the UK about the Hospital Electronic Prescribing and Medicine Administration (HEPMA) systems and their difficult implementation processes. The chapter analyses how the implementation of Commercial-Off-The-Shelf (COTS) solutions resulted in systems with limited configurability, poorly matched to the needs and practices of English hospitals. The analysis reflects on the case by recollecting a similar experience with Enterprise Resource Planning systems in the 1980s/1990s when immature, often unfinished, products went into the market. An analysis of the installed base influence on information infrastructures illuminates how the evolution of COTS solutions is conditioned by the structure of adopter and vendor 'communities'.

Finally, the sixth chapter by Stefan Klein and Stefan Schellhammer presents the experience with ePrescription in Germany. The narrative focuses on a specific initiative on medication management for polypharmacy patients, and traces the associated discourse over the last 10 years. The difficulties faced, which ultimately led to the termination of the initiative are analysed with the notion of "installed base of opposition".

1.2.3   Section C: Governmental Patient-Oriented eHealth Infrastructures

In the first chapter of this section, Joan Rodon Modol describes the genesis and evolution of the public patient portal called Carpeta Personal de Salut (CPS) of Catalonia, Spain from 2008 to 2015. The CPS started as a web-browser viewer of a subset of citizens' health data stored in the systems of the public health system, and has gradually turned into an information infrastructure as new relations with other systems, services, actors, regulations, practices have been established. This chapter suggests how in order to cope with the conditions of indeterminacy and uncertainty characterizing the building of patient-oriented information infrastructures, designs must always be open and connectable so as to be able to respond to new possibilities.

The second chapter by Miria Grisot, Polyxeni Vassilakopoulou and Margunn Aanestad, describes the conceptualization process, early stage development, and incremental changes in the creation of the Norwegian eHealth platform for patient-oriented services. The platform was launched in 2011 and was gradually developed into a complex platform enabling several eHealth services. The narrative focuses on how some of these services required the linking and reuse of existing components and resources, while other required the creation of novel parts. Three strategies of dealing with the installed base are identified as complementing, creating substitutions, and expanding the installed base.

In the third chapter, Tina Blegind Jensen and Anne Asmyr Thorseng present the experience of another Scandinavian country, Denmark. The chapter describes the evolution of the Danish national e-health portal, sundhed.dk, which has been a frontrunner and reference case for other countries. The initiation phase was characterized by broad engagement and mobilization of core stakeholder in the Danish healthcare sector. Due to the broad buy-in and consensus, sundhed.dk was able to establish itself as an early and comprehensive portal, through assembling existing information resources directly, as well as repurposing and enhancing available information resources. However, the story of sundhed.dk also shows that this mode of working comes with challenges for the further pursuit of innovation.

The fourth chapter by Nina Sellberg and Johan Eltes, describes the evolution of the Swedish patient portal together with the definition of the eHealth architecture and the overall national eHealth infrastructure. The case narrative illustrates the central role played by the national reference architecture. The analysis illustrates how infrastructure evolvement results from the complex interplay between many different actors intertwined in a step-by-step cultivation process.

Finally, in the fifth chapter by Andrea Resca and Mauro Moruzzi a case from Italy is examined. This case is probably the first example of an e-booking system in Europe. The chapter traces the genesis of a booking services put in place in the Municipality of Bologna for accessing specialized care. The narrative focuses on the role played by institutional components as obstacle to the innovation process, and on the mobilization of political, organizational, and technological resources.

The main message coming out of the empirical cases presented in the book, is that the successful development and implementation of initiatives for eHealth infrastructures require much more than creating a clear description of the goal and having in place the necessary technological capabilities and human skills. It also requires a discerning and knowledgeable engagement with the particularities of the situation and an informed and conscious approach for working with the installed base.

References

European Commission DG Communications Networks Content & Technology. Benchmarking deployment of eHealth among general practitioners (2013) – final report. Luxembourg: Publications Office of the European Union; 2013.

European Commission Joint Research Centre Institute for Prospective Technological Studies (JRC-IPTS). European hospital survey: benchmarking deployment of eHealth services (2012–2013). Luxembourg: Publications Office of the European Union; 2014.

Hanseth O, Lundberg N. Designing work oriented infrastructures. Compu Supported Coop Work (CSCW). 2001;10:347–72.

Hanseth O, Lyytinen K. Design theory for dynamic complexity in information infrastructures: the case of building internet. J Inf Technol. 2010;25:1–19.

Karasti H, Baker KS, Millerand F. Infrastructure time: long-term matters in collaborative development. Comput Supported Coop Work (CSCW). 2010;19:377–415.

Ribes D, Finholt TA. The long now of technology infrastructure: articulating tensions in development. J Assoc Inf Syst. 2009;10:375–98.

Star SL, Ruhleder K. Steps toward an ecology of infrastructure: design and access for large information spaces. Inf Syst Res. 1996;7:111–34.

Stroetmann KA, Artmann JH, Stroetmann VN. European countries on their journey towards national eHealth infrastructures. Luxembourg: Office for Official Publications of the European Communities; 2011.

Tilson D, Lyytinen K, Sørensen C. Digital Infrastructures: The Missing IS Research Agenda. Inf Syst Res. 2010;21:748–59.

Open Access This chapter is distributed under the terms of the Creative Commons Attribution-NonCommercial 2.5 International License (http://creativecommons.org/licenses/by-nc/2.5/), which permits any noncommercial use, duplication, adaptation, distribution and reproduction in any medium or format, as long as you give appropriate credit to the original author(s) and the source, provide a link to the Creative Commons license and indicate if changes were made.

The images or other third party material in this chapter are included in the chapter's Creative Commons license, unless indicated otherwise in a credit line to the material. If material is not included in the chapter's Creative Commons license and your intended use is not permitted by statutory regulation or exceeds the permitted use, you will need to obtain permission directly from the copyright holder.

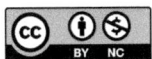

Part I

Information Infrastructures in Healthcare

Margunn Aanestad, Miria Grisot, Ole Hanseth,
and Polyxeni Vassilakopoulou

2.1   Introduction

This chapter provides an introductory overview of healthcare information systems, followed by a more detailed discussion of e-prescription and governmental patient-oriented platforms. We use the umbrella term "eHealth" (also written e-health) that encompasses all health-related digital information systems including clinical, administrative, and research-oriented ones. Specifically, we adopt the eHealth definition introduced by the World Health Organization (WHO). According to this definition, eHealth is "the use of information and communication technologies (ICT) for health; examples include treating patients, conducting research, educating the health workforce, tracking diseases and monitoring public health" (World Health Organisation 2016b). Similarly, the European Commission defines eHealth as: "the use of modern information and communication technologies to meet needs of citizens, patients, healthcare professionals, healthcare providers, as well as policy makers" (European Commission 2003). eHealth is considered pivotal for improving the quality and efficiency of healthcare (Hillestad et al. 2005; Kellermann and Jones 2013), for improving the patient experience of care, and for the eventual revolutionization of healthcare (Drucker 2007).

M. Aanestad (✉)
University of Oslo & UIT The Arctic University of Norway,
P.O. Box 1080 Blindern, N-0316 Oslo, Norway
e-mail: margunn@ifi.uio.no

M. Grisot • O. Hanseth
University of Oslo, P.O. Box 1080 Blindern, N-0316 Oslo, Norway
e-mail: miriag@ifi.uio.no; oleha@ifi.uio.no

P. Vassilakopoulou
University of Agder & University of Oslo, P.O. Box 422, N-4604 Kristiansand, Norway
e-mail: polyxenv@uia.no

© The Author(s) 2017   11
M. Aanestad et al. (eds.), *Information Infrastructures within European Health Care*, Health Informatics, DOI 10.1007/978-3-319-51020-0_2

Strong expectations linked to eHealth are present in policy and advisory documents prepared around the globe. For instance, the introductory passage of a report by the Institute of Medicine of the National Academies (US) states: "Health and health care are going digital. As multiple intersecting platforms evolve to form a novel operational foundation for health and health care the stage is set for fundamental and unprecedented transformation." (Institute of Medicine 2011). In Europe, eHealth has been a major component of the European Commission's eEurope action plan which was endorsed at the Feira European Council in June 2000. In 2004, the Commission also set in place an eHealth map to develop targeted policy initiatives aimed at fostering widespread adoption of eHealth technologies across the EU (eHealth Action Plan). The latest eHealth Action Plan for 2012–2020 states that the promise of eHealth "remains largely unfulfilled" and the vision of a unified, interoperable eHealth Infrastructure in Europe is still not realised. Although the potential of eHealth is being discussed globally since the 1990s it remains a work in progress.

Countries around Europe have already experienced notable successes and some highly publicised costly delays and failures. These have brought attention to the complexity of dealing with a multiplicity of involved parties with diverging interests and agendas, existing fragmented systems' landscape, rapid technological advancements and regulative perplexities. In most European countries, healthcare is predominantly public and public agencies have a central role for stimulating and orchestrating eHealth efforts. In many countries, the driving force for ICT in health care has been the trend toward a better coordination of care (Winter et al. 2011). This means a change of focus for eHealth from self-contained processes within single healthcare institutions to overall care processes spreading across institutional boundaries.

The remainder of this chapter is structured as follows. In the next section we give an overview of the eHealth landscape. Then, in Sects. 2.3 and 2.4 we focus on the two types of infrastructures examined in this book: e-prescription and governmental patient-oriented platforms. Finally, Sect. 2.4 concludes the chapter with a discussion on the transformative potential of the two types of eHealth infrastructures.

2.2   The eHealth Landscape

To provide the necessary background for the reader, we initially describe information systems that support healthcare-related work within specific organizational settings (e.g. laboratories, medical imaging departments, general practitioner offices). Next, we move beyond these systems, and we present systems that have more generic character and are common enabling components for eHealth.

2.2.1   Core Information Systems in Healthcare Organizations

There is a multitude of systems that support healthcare provision ranging from more generic systems to the ones that offer specialised functionalities for specific domains. Among the specialized, for example there are Picture archiving and communication systems (PACS) which support storage, retrieval, management, distribution and presentation of medical images, and RIS (Radiology Information Systems) which support patient administration, referrals, reports, and work lists for the medical imaging labs. Computerized physician order entry (CPOE), medication management and vital signs monitoring systems are other examples of special-purpose systems. Of more generic use are Patient Administrative Systems (PAS), also called Admission-Discharge-Transfer (ADT) systems that support registration, scheduling and logistics and Electronic Health Record systems (EHRs). EHRs play a central role in health institutions. An EHR is envisioned as a "repository of information regarding the health of a subject of care in computer processable form, stored and transmitted securely, and accessible by multiple authorised users. It has a commonly agreed logical information model which is independent of EHR systems. Its primary purpose is the support of continuing, efficient and quality integrated health care and it contains information which is retrospective, concurrent and prospective" (ISO/TR 20514 2005). EHRs organize information related to specific patients and may cover several encounters and episodes of care, possibly from birth to death. The information within an EHR may be generated during patient encounters (e.g. diagnoses, lab results, radiology scan reports, etc.) and may also come from the patients (e.g. off-the-shelf medicine, home measurements etc.). This information may be contained in multiple (discrete or interconnected) systems and repositories, each of which will hold and manage specific types of data (Winter et al. 2011). In addition to the systems that directly support healthcare provision, there is also a multitude of systems that support management functions (e.g. systems for management reporting, systems for reimbursement handling, etc.) and research activities (e.g. advanced computational tools for genetic data). There are also systems that support generic, but indispensable services such as user authentication and authorisation services.

2.2.2 Information Systems Beyond the Healthcare Organization

Beyond the spectrum of systems supporting work within the boundaries of a specific healthcare organization, there is also a class of systems and technological capabilities that are more generic, over-arching and serve as common enabling components for a wider eHealth infrastructure. Inter-organizational networks and messaging services for instance, facilitate information flow between organizations (e.g. message exchange between different healthcare providers) and across different levels within the healthcare system (e.g. reporting activities to health authorities and clinical information to health registries). These require the existence of shared infrastructural services like address registries, broadband networks and security infrastructures. In addition, information needs to be shared along a patient's trajectory if it involves diagnosis and treatment in multiple different localities and organizations. To enable easy access to relevant information about a patient, governments have sought to build cross-cutting systems such as e-prescription systems and shared EHRs (often in the form of summary or emergency care record systems). Standards, both interoperability standards and terminology and nomenclature standards are crucial components in facilitating eHealth infrastructures that go beyond organizational boundaries.

Such inter-organizational eHealth information infrastructures are important for multiple users in different organizational settings: clinical and administrative healthcare professionals, health researchers, public health authorities, health insurance companies and various other involved actors. Furthermore, a continuously growing number of eHealth systems are covering the interaction between patients and healthcare providers, or peer-to-peer communication between patients or health professionals. In this book, we explore infrastructures for e-prescription and patient-oriented platforms. Both of them are inter-organizational and have been a strategic priority for several countries recently.

2.3   E-Prescription

E-prescription solutions support the electronic flow of information related to prescribed medications. Most European countries have taken steps for implementing e-prescription solutions while the aim of the European Union is to have a cross-border electronic system which will enable patients to retrieve electronic prescriptions anywhere in Europe (World Health Organisation 2016a). Nevertheless, there are different degrees of maturity and coverage of e-prescription solutions in the different European countries. In some countries, e-prescribing is used routinely while in other countries there are only some early-stage initiatives.

2.3.1   Prescriptions and e-Prescribing

Modern medicine relies heavily on the use of medication. The production, distribution and use of medication is regulated by longstanding institutions. Over-the-counter medication can be purchased freely and used by anybody without medical supervision. If a medication is not available over-the-counter it can only be dispensed when a prescription is provided, to ensure that its use happens within a care scheme approved by a healthcare professional. National regulations govern who can issue a prescription. In general, doctors have the broadest prescriptive authority and are the main prescribers everywhere in the world. Additionally, other healthcare professionals (for instance: dentists, midwives, pharmacists) may also have the right to prescribe medications related to their area of practice; this varies from country to country.

A prescription may be handwritten on a clean sheet of paper or on pre-printed forms, or typed and printed, or transmitted electronically to pharmacies for dispensing. The content of a prescription includes information about both the patient and

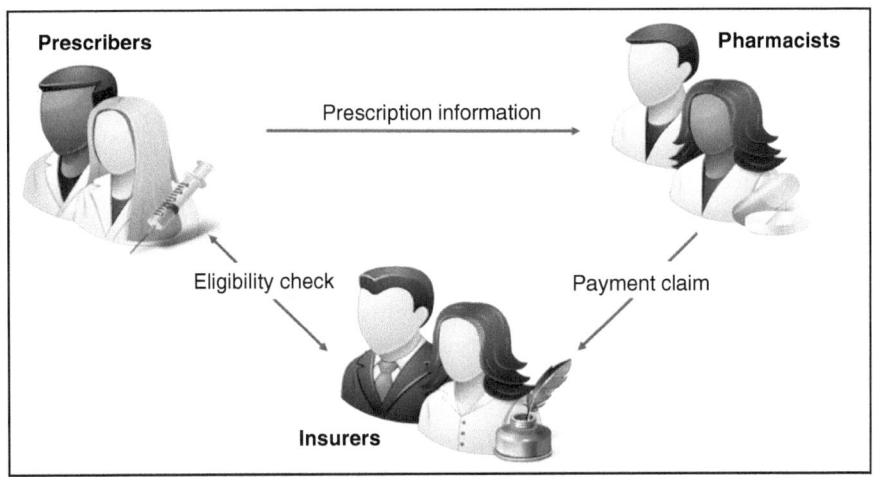

Fig. 2.1 Information flows between prescribers, pharmacists and insurers

the prescriber, the medication specifications (type, quantity) and directions for the patient to follow. Prescribed medication can be partially or fully reimbursed by healthcare insurers (public or private), hence, prescription information is also needed by insurers.

Health authorities around the world support the adoption of electronic prescription systems (e-prescription). E-prescription solutions capture and circulate prescription information between prescribers, pharmacies and insurers that handle related payments (Fig. 2.1) expediting flows and eliminating legibility issues (frequently faced when using handwritten prescriptions). Such solutions can support aims for cost containment, enhancement of patient safety, control over doctors' prescription patterns and process quality assurance. Overall, putting e-prescription in place entails working with multiple and diverse sociotechnical components, finding ways to link and organise them (Rodon and Silva 2015).

Beyond the traditional use of prescriptions in primary care, in hospital settings and in nursing homes, prescription information is needed by nurses that are administering medications. Furthermore, prescription information may be collected and processed by health policy institutions for planning and monitoring purposes. Overall, medication prescriptions and dispense data are monitored for various reasons, for instance, public health authorities may monitor and regulate the use of antibiotics, may monitor and exercise health control over the use of reimbursable drugs, may monitor and supervise imports and distribution. Therefore, most countries have an information infrastructure around the medical prescription. These information infrastructures can be paper-based or digital or in hybrid form and typically link multiple Health Record Systems, Pharmacy Systems, Drug Registries and Health Insurance Systems (electronic or not).

2.3.2 Key Parts of e-Prescription and Variations

It is common to distinguish between three parts of e-prescription infrastructures:

eCapture: support in producing notes for prescribed medication. This can be a simple tool for registering electronically medication information (ensuring quick transmission and elimination of illegibility issues) or more elaborate arrangements that include decision support functionalities such as automatic checking of drug interactions (based on other information from the patient record), automatic retrieval of commercially available drugs and package sizes, support for the selection of drugs with the use of protocols based on the diagnosis descriptions.

eTransfer: transfer of the prescription information. Both electronically generated prescriptions and paper prescriptions filled by hand and scanned can be transferred digitally. Various models are adopted, for instance, the prescription can go from the prescriber to a specific pharmacy, or it can be deposited to a central repository accessible by all pharmacies (allowing the patient to choose where to go at a later stage). With electronic transfers the information flows can be expedited and also, it is possible to better control the duration of prescription's validity (for instance, the message or the information content can expire after a set date). Furthermore, the electronic transfer of prescriptions can allow secondary uses of the data (e.g. facilitating the checking and payment of pharmacy claims and the accumulation of information to support quality healthcare and effective cost management).

eDispensing: support in producing records of the actual medication dispensing. This can be a simple note on the date and place of dispensing or can include complete medication packaging information allowing full traceability and control of drugs.

The coverage of e-prescription projects varies in terms of:

- Actors: the e-prescription infrastructure must cover at least pharmacies and prescribers. In many cases e-prescription is covering only key prescribers (e.g. General Practitioners in primary care). In other cases it includes also hospitals, or even, other prescribers depending on national regulations (e.g. dentists, midwives, pharmacists). Furthermore, most e-prescription systems cover also information flows to insurers.
- Functionality: basic or advanced support for eCapture (e.g. might include decision support for prescribers), eTransmission (can be fully digital or quasi-digital e.g. paper with barcodes), eDispensing (registration of extended or limited information upon dispensing). Additional functionality may include facilities for patients to trigger prescription refills, full integration with Electronic Health Record Systems (EHRs), repository management facilities.
- Access: rules for data access can vary depending on national regulations and on designers´ choices. Actors that can access personalised medication lists may

include prescribing healthcare professionals, other healthcare professionals that provide services to the patient, pharmacists, public authorities, private insurers and patients.

There are variations among countries with different health systems. Variations relate to: what constitutes prescriptions drugs, who can issue a prescription, what is the minimum required content of a prescription, who can dispense a prescription, how medications are reimbursed. There are also legal differences: is electronic transmission of prescriptions legal? Are digital signatures accepted? Does the patient need to consent? Should the patient be able to request a paper copy? Is counselling compulsory before prescriptions are written? In Europe, each country has some particularities, for example: in UK there is some authority transferred to community pharmacies, in Norway nurses can prescribe some drugs (e.g. contraceptives), in Greece and Italy there is control over the physical medication packages that have unique identification numbers. Also, there are differences on insurance schemes for medication reimbursement. For example, in some countries (e.g. Norway) public insurance is unified while in other countries (e.g. Germany and Greece), there are multiple insurance institutions or social security funds.

2.3.3 Drivers for e-Prescription Projects

Expenses for medications contribute significantly to total healthcare expenditures. The expenditure on medications as a share of overall health expenditure varies throughout Europe ranging from 6 % (Denmark, Norway) up to 29 % (Greece), furthermore, the public share of this medication expenditure can range from less than 50 % (Denmark, Finland) up to around 70 % (Germany, Greece) (OECD 2013; World Health Organisation 2014). Therefore, it is seen as critical for governmental authorities to monitor and control prescriptions not only for ensuring healthcare quality but also for reasons of cost control. The expectations for better cost control fuelled the interest for e-prescription systems in European countries during the past decade. Sixteen of the member states of the EU included e-Prescription in their national strategies or eHealth implementation plans already in 2006; in 2011 this number was raised to 22 (Stroetmann et al. 2012). Still, in 2011, only Denmark, Estonia, Iceland and Sweden had in place a full, national e-Prescription solution while at the same time, there were partial implementations in the UK and the Netherlands, regional implementations in Spain, and several initiatives including pilots in Portugal, Czech Republic, Finland, Italy, Norway, Greece and Poland (Kierkegaard 2013; Stroetmann et al. 2011).

With the introduction of e-prescription the collaboration between physicians and pharmacists is mediated by technologies. E-prescription reduces the risks associated with traditional prescription-writing, and has the potential of bringing different benefits to different stakeholders, especially if implemented at scale (Cornford et al. 2014). At the same time, the inscription of rules to the system can be a powerful control mechanism for prescribers and dispensing pharmacists. In this respect, e-prescription has a dual role: it is not only a tool introduced to everyday work to improve healthcare delivery but also, a governance mechanism for regulating, controlling and monitoring a large array of dispersed temporally and geographically professional tasks (Vassilakopoulou et al. 2012).

In the chapters included in the e-prescription section of this book we present the experiences of different European countries that implemented e-prescription during the past decade. The different cases illustrate different strategies for linking pre-existing infrastructural arrangements (the installed base) to new technological solutions and for extending and renewing the overall prescription related infrastructures. The cases are linked to each country context, the specific characteristics of health systems, the technological maturity of the healthcare environment and the different institutional actors. The cross-examination of the cases can bring a number of insights about different implementation approaches and overall, about the dynamics of infrastructural evolution.

2.4   E-Services for Patients and Citizens

The development of patient-oriented eHealth services is recent. Traditionally, healthcare information systems were developed for clinical and administrative use of health personnel in the context of healthcare organizations. However, recently several countries have initiated projects for establishing patient- or citizen-oriented eHealth solutions and infrastructures. Overall, the aim of these initiatives is to put in place secure and reliable technologies allowing patients to access general and personalised health information and providing electronic services for communication, self-management, and administrative tasks.

2.4.1   Patient-Oriented eHealth Services

Patient-oriented eHealth services are diverse (Fig. 2.2). Some services are mainly information-oriented. For instance, many governmental eHealth websites, but also hospital websites provide citizens with updated and quality-assured information about symptoms and treatment options. These services respond to the increasing interest for using the Internet as a source for health information, and to the problem of the variable quality of information available. Other services are set up to offer access to personal health data that healthcare institutions have registered about individuals, e.g. in the patient record systems, laboratory and imaging systems etc. To support the collation and use of personal health data, various specialised solutions for Personal Health Records (PHR) have been developed. PHRs are in some cases standalone patient-controlled solutions, while in other cases as "tethered" to institutional EHRs.

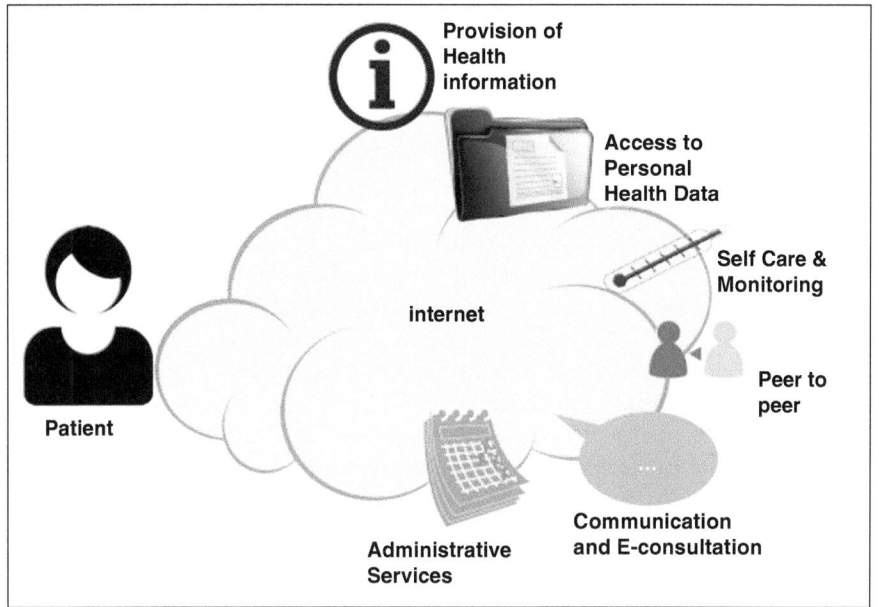

Fig. 2.2 Patient-oriented eHealth services

Additionally, a range of services for self-monitoring and self-care are made available to patients. Some of these services do not entail any involvement of healthcare practitioners while others are linked to healthcare providers that take responsibility for care plans and may assess the information collected. Furthermore, patient-oriented eHealth services may also support peer-to-peer patient networks and forums and in some cases, connections to social media platforms.

Patients and citizens are also offered administrative eHealth services. For instance, many countries offer to patients the possibility to choose among health care service providers, check waiting times, and book appointments. Additionally, solutions for e-consultation services and more generally, electronically sup-ported patient-healthcare provider communications are also in place, often by GP offices in primary care. With these solutions patients are given secure electronic channels for online communication. E-consultation services are mostly used for asking follow up questions after a consultation, asking about medication use and passing on to healthcare providers health related data from self-monitoring practices.

Many European countries have established governmental eHealth patient portals with the aim of offering to citizens one single entry point to the various patient-oriented eHealth services offered in the public health sector.

2.4.2 Drivers for Patient-Oriented eHealth Projects

Many health strategies and policies contain visions of more patient-centric healthcare systems (Klecun 2016). Several countries initiated the development of patient-oriented eHealth solutions seeking to realize visions for patient-centeredness. The informed and empowered patient is prominent in the visions. Within medicine, the formulation of "patient-centered care", as articulated nearly a century ago (Peabody 1927) promotes a model of care that entails keeping patients informed, involving them in decisions and self-care management activities, and acknowledging their experience of illness and psychosocial context. In the seminal "Crossing the Quality Chasm" report (Institute of Medicine 2001) patient-centred care was defined as: "providing care that is respectful of and responsive to individual patient preferences, needs, and values, and ensuring that patient values guide all clinical decisions". Patients are seen as integral part of the care team and responsibilities of care-taking and monitoring are partially transferred to patients. Empowerment, transparency and individualization of treatments are emphasized. To realize these visions, new information and communication solutions need to be provided for both patients (enabling them to contribute meaningfully in decision-taking) and providers (providing them better insight on patient circumstances). Such eHealth solutions can support communications, information sharing and distributed data management. Hence, eHealth is seen as a core mechanism for reorienting healthcare towards patient-centeredness.

Another driver for patient-oriented eHealth is a more managerial vision to improve the efficiency of healthcare provision. Organizing shared care solutions around individual patients is expected to help overcome existing communication barriers between institutions and across administrative levels. For instance, a shared patient record system, may help to bridge unconnected "islands" and allow a more efficient overall utilization of resources (Ball et al. 2007; Piras and Zanutto 2010). Furthermore, providing patients with solutions that will allow them to make informed choices can put them in a quasi-customer role. This new patient role is expected to to incentivize a stronger focus on quality and efficiency within the sector. For instance, new patient-oriented services that provide comprehensive information on performance indexes for particular health providers (such as waiting times or treatment-related infection rates) aim to facilitate the patient as a 'customer' to make choices that may create a better working healthcare sector.

Another discourse related to patient-oriented eHealth is the one that emphasizes prevention and the responsibility of each individual to conduct responsible health choices. As such, the scope of attention is expanded from "patients" towards "citizens", i.e. healthy members of the society. This discourse therefore, is not only about disease and treatment, but also, about health and wellness related activities, products, and services that address lifestyle, nutrition and exercise. Currently, information from the mobile applications and devices for self-monitoring used by healthy persons are rarely transferred to the wider institutionalised health system. However, there are initiatives for the provision of eHealth services that can enable the fusion of such privately collected information with medical records. Wellness and health related technologies also enable service models that involve cross-border movement and globalization of health service provision. Furthermore, the spread of medical surveillance of patients living at home (including telemedicine solution and welfare technologies) also produces new data streams, with new potentials for analysis and use, and new requirements for infrastructures. Awareness is arising of the need to provide platforms that are able to receive and integrate data of this kind, often coming through "third-party" or non-health related solutions.

Finally, eHealth services may also seek to support peer-to-peer patient networks or more flexibly organized health communities (Eysenbach 2008; Spagnoletti et al. 2015). Peer networks may help patients cope with handling their disease, help navigating the health system or contribute to political work such as awareness and attention to specific patient groups. Based on collecting patient data that are shared in such peer networks, new types of research are becoming now feasible, sometimes organized and coordinated by the patient collectives themselves (Kallinikos and Tempini 2014).

Conclusion

E-prescription and patient-oriented eHealth services respond to different needs of citizens and healthcare providers and have different roles within European health systems. Overall, e-prescription is more well-defined than patient-oriented services in terms of functionality and in many cases is deeply embedded within pre-existing applications and prescribing tools. Nevertheless, both e-prescription and patient-oriented services have the potential (and frequently the explicit aim) to transform healthcare delivery. E-prescription initiatives are usually seen as opportunities to improve healthcare delivery by systematic and not dramatic change (controlling the ever-increasing medication costs, improving patient safety and providing rich information for performance management). Patient-oriented eHealth services are usually seen as opportunities to pursue wider and more radical innovation, aiming to strengthen the patients' role and to facilitate a shift from provider-centred healthcare towards patient-centeredness.

eHealth infrastructures are expected to instigate the reshaping of core roles and relationships within the healthcare systems (Vikkelsø 2010). Therefore, eHealth is not just about more effective 'tools' for addressing particular problems, but needs to be seen as part of longer and more transformative processes of 'digitalization' (Tilson et al. 2010). Digitalization will transform the existing relationships and institutions in healthcare. For example, electronic tools are changing the clinical encounter between a healthcare professional and a patient (May 2007; Winthereik 2008).

Despite having such a transformative orientation, the novel eHealth infrastructures typically leverage existing services, capabilities, institutions, data sources, systems, and communication channels. These sometimes exist within the healthcare providers' organization, and sometimes they can be built upon applications that are not part of the official healthcare system. The eHealth infrastructures can be part of nationally governed initiatives, or initiatives growing out of local action, e.g. from hospitals or health plan providers.

Expectations are that eHealth infrastructures will help governments improve the quality and efficiency of healthcare and achieve better coordination of care. However, the introduction of novel technologies will not in itself bring into these changes into effect. The underlying premise for this book is the recognition that technology is not an invariant in a transformation process – rather we may expect that any solution will be contested and that it will change shape during realization, implementation and usage. Both technology and institutional transformations trigger complex change processes (Agarwal et al. 2010, Davidson and Chismar 2007) with a reciprocal interaction between technologies and organizations. The stories of building eHealth infrastructures included in this book illustrate several aspects of such complex, interactive transformation processes.

References

Agarwal R, Gao GG, Desroches C, Jha AK. Research commentary—the digital transformation of healthcare: current status and the road ahead. Inf Syst Res. 2010;21:796–809.

Ball M, Carla Smith N, Bakalar R. Personal health records: empowering consumers. J Healthc Inf Manag. 2007;21:77.

Cornford T, Hibberd R, Barber N. The evaluation of the electronic prescription service in primary care: final report on the findings from the evaluation in early implementer sites. London: University College London; 2014.

Davidson E, Chismar W. The interaction of institutionally triggered and technology-triggered social structure change: an investigation of computerized physician order entry. MIS Q. 2007;31:739–58.

Drucker PF. Management challenges for the 21st century. New York and Oxon: Routledge; 2007.

European Commission. Ministerial Declaration [Online]. Brussels. 2003. Available: http://ec. europa.eu/information_society/eeurope/ehealth/conference/2003/doc/min_dec_22_may_03. pdf.

Eysenbach G. Medicine 2.0: social networking, collaboration, participation, apomediation, and openness. J Med Internet Res. 2008;10:e22.

Hillestad R, Bigelow J, Bower A, Girosi F, Meili R, Scoville R, Taylor R. Can electronic medical record systems transform health care? Potential health benefits, savings, and costs. Health Aff. 2005;24:1103–17.

Institute of Medicine. Committee on Quality of Health Care in America. Crossing the quality chasm: A new health system for the 21st century. Washington: National Academies Press. 2001.

Institute of Medicine. Digital infrastructure for the learning health system: the foundation for continuous improvement in health and health care: workshop series summary. Washington: National Academies Press. 2011.

ISO/TR 20514. Health informatics—Electronic health record—Definition, scope and context. In: Technical Committee ISO/TC 215, H. I. (ed.) ISO. Geneva. 2005.

Kallinikos J, Tempini N. Patient data as medical facts: social media practices as a foundation for medical knowledge creation. Inf Syst Res. 2014;25:817–33.

Kellermann A, Jones S. What it will take to achieve the as-yet-unfulfilled promises of health information technology. Health Aff. 2013;32:63–8.

Kierkegaard P. E-prescription across Europe. Heal Technol. 2013;3:205–19.

Klecun E. Transforming healthcare: policy discourses of IT and patient-centred care. Eur J Inf Syst. 2016;25:64–76.

May C. The clinical encounter and the problem of context. Sociology. 2007;41:29–45.

OECD. Health statistics (year of reference: 2011) [Online]. 2013. Available: http://www.oecd-ilibrary.org/social-issues-migration-health/data/oecd-health-statistics_health-data-en.

Peabody FW. The care of the patient. J Am Med Assoc. 1927;88:877–82.

Piras EM, Zanutto A. Prescriptions, x-rays and grocery lists. Designing a Personal Health Record to support (the invisible work of) health information management in the household. Comput Supported Coop Work (CSCW). 2010;19:585–613.

Rodon J, Silva L. Exploring the formation of a healthcare information infrastructure: hierarchy or meshwork? J Assoc Inf Syst. 2015;16:394.

Spagnoletti P, Resca A, Sæbø Ø. Design for social media engagement: insights from elderly care assistance. J Strateg Inf Syst. 2015;24:128–45.

Stroetmann K, Artmann J, Stroetmann V, Protti D, Dumortier J, Giest S, Walossek U, Whitehouse D. European countries on their journey towards national eHealth infrastructures. Luxembourg: Office for Official Publications of the European Communities; 2011.

Stroetmann K, Artmann J, Dumortier J, Verhenneman G. United in diversity: legal challenges on the road towards interoperable eHealth solutions in Europe. Eur J Biomed Inform. 2012;8:3–10.

Tilson D, Lyytinen K, Sorensen C. Digital infrastructures: the missing IS research agenda. Inf Syst Res. 2010;21:748–59.

Vassilakopoulou P, Tsagkas V, Marmaras N. From "rules to interpret" to "rules to follow": ePrescription in Greece. Electron J e-Gov. 2012;10:147–55.

Vikkelsø S. Mobilizing information infrastructure, shaping patient-centred care. Int J Public Sect Manag. 2010;23:340–52.

Winter A, Haux R, Ammenwerth E, Brigl B, Hellrung N, Jahn F. Health information systems: architectures and strategies. Health information systems. London Dordrecht Heidelberg New York: Springer. 2011.

Winthereik B. Shared care and boundaries: lessons from an online maternity record. J Health Organ Manag. 2008;22:416.

World Health Organisation. WHO Global Health Expenditure Database (reference year 2011) [Online]. 2014. Available: http://apps.who.int/nha/database.

World Health Organisation. From innovation to implementation. Copenhagen: WHO Regional Office for Europe; 2016a.

World Health Organisation. Health topics: eHealth [Online]. 2016b. Available: http://www.who.int/topics/ehealth/en/. Accessed 25 June 2016.

Open Access This chapter is distributed under the terms of the Creative Commons Attribution-NonCommercial 2.5 International License (http://creativecommons.org/licenses/by-nc/2.5/), which permits any noncommercial use, duplication, adaptation, distribution and reproduction in any medium or format, as long as you give appropriate credit to the original author(s) and the source, provide a link to the Creative Commons license and indicate if changes were made.

The images or other third party material in this chapter are included in the chapter's Creative Commons license, unless indicated otherwise in a credit line to the material. If material is not included in the chapter's Creative Commons license and your intended use is not permitted by statutory regulation or exceeds the permitted use, you will need to obtain permission directly from the copyright holder.

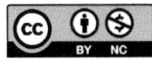

Margunn Aanestad, Miria Grisot, Ole Hanseth, and Polyxeni Vassilakopoulou

3.1   Introduction

In this chapter we present the core theoretical concepts underlying the research included in the book. The empirical cases concern inter-organizational information systems, specifically e-prescription and governmental patient-oriented eHealth platforms. These systems span organizational boundaries and comprise multiple local systems as well as shared system components. Such interconnected networks of systems can be conceptualized in different ways. In software engineering, notions like "system-of-systems" (Maier 1998), "ultra-large scale systems" (Feiler et al. 2006) or "coalitions of systems" (Sommerville et al. 2012) are employed to draw attention to the specific characteristics and challenges that such systems pose.

We employ a perspective that denotes these interconnected, distributed collections of systems as "information infrastructures". This perspective emerges from a different, disciplinary diverse background. It stems from Information Systems studies, Science Technology and Society studies, and Innovation studies; i.e. disciplinary domains that have a dual focus that covers both technology and human/societal aspects (Monteiro and Hanseth 1995). In the next section we present this overall perspective. We then zoom in on one of the core notions of the information

M. Aanestad (✉)
University of Oslo & UIT The Arctic University of Norway,
P.O. Box 1080 Blindern, N-0316 Oslo, Norway
e-mail: margunn@ifi.uio.no

M. Grisot • O. Hanseth
University of Oslo, P.O. Box 1080 Blindern, N-0316 Oslo, Norway
e-mail: miriag@ifi.uio.no; oleha@ifi.uio.no

P. Vassilakopoulou
University of Agder & University of Oslo, P.O. Box 422, N-4604 Kristiansand, Norway
e-mail: polyxenv@uia.no

© The Author(s) 2017   25
M. Aanestad et al. (eds.), *Information Infrastructures within European Health Care*, Health Informatics, DOI 10.1007/978-3-319-51020-0_3

infrastructure perspective – the installed base. This notion helps us examine the trajectories of evolution for the e-prescription solutions and patient platforms.

3.2   Information Infrastructures

Some informatics researchers seek to understand technologies from a socio-technical perspective, i.e. to include the organizational and social context of its design and use. The fields of Information Systems (IS) research, Computer-Supported Collaborative Work (CSCW) and Human Computer Interaction (HCI) have this orientation to actual use situations and real users. Here it has emerged a body of research based on ethnographic studies of how people work with technologies. The recognition of how technology is intimately intertwined with organizational structure, procedures and work practices is a fundamental insight from this stream. For instance, Winthereik and Berg (2003) describe the historical evolution of the patient record over the last century as related to the organizational development of hospitals and the professional development of the medical and other health professions. Technologies for documentation and coordination of work have co-evolved together with the organizational structure, the personnel's skills and the work routines. The resulting collection of paper-based tools (forms, records, binders, tables, shelves etc.) and organizational routines comprise a complex information infrastructure that supports medical work (Berg 1999; Berg and Goorman 1999). This is often taken for granted, and its crucial role is often only realized when disturbances occur, e.g. when a digitization project is initiated (Vikkelsø 2005). For instance, the consequences of replacing a paper form with a digital version may not be fully realized unless one sees the paper form as not just being an information carrier but also a 'signalling device' for the coordination of work. The underlying, supporting and often invisible role of this set of technological components and organizational routines is one reason to call this an "information infrastructure". An organization-wide information infrastructure that is deeply embedded into work routines across several departments will be difficult to change, however, careful analysis of all its aspects can inform change strategies (Hanseth and Lundberg 2001; Ellingsen and Monteiro 2003; Silsand and Ellingsen 2014; Petrakaki et al. 2016).

This underlying and invisible role caused by technology's embeddedness within a work and organizational context is not the only reason to use the label of "information infrastructure". The IT systems implemented in healthcare are usually intended to connect multiple sites, either within an organization or beyond it. An information infrastructure that is non-local and distributed will encompass multiple actors that may have different needs and interests that may not be aligned. For an information infrastructure to work, some working resolution between the multiple local interests and the over-arching or "global" interests of the network as a whole, needs to be found (Star and Ruhleder 1996).

Understanding the complexities and mechanisms involved is a core ambition of information infrastructure studies. Earlier studies on the historical evolution of large-scale technical systems, for instance the emergence of electric power grids

(Hughes 1987), have drawn attention to the contests among the actors and their strategies for promoting their own solutions or interests. From such studies comes a set of concepts that help us understand the role of network effects, which are the mechanisms at play in interconnected setting with a large number of actors with different agendas and interests (Arthur 1989, 1990; David 1985). For instance, recognising that value is generated by the network, not the parts in isolation, and that initial moves in a particular direction encourage further moves along the same path, is crucial. While in early stages in the evolution of systems the path is relatively open, at later stages it becomes more bounded or may create lock-in situations.

Earlier research has illuminated what we may call on the one hand socio-technical complexity (caused by technologies being deeply embedded into organizations, and organizations being deeply embedded into technologies, see e.g. Leonardi 2011) and on the other hand network-related complexity (caused by the unpredictable dynamics between a large number of connected actors without central control, see e.g. Williams 2016). Based on these insights, IS researchers have attempted to formulate different ways to think about and deal with large-scale, complex and interconnected information infrastructures – approaches that are sensitive to the presence of complexity. Based on a number of in-depth case studies in global organizations, Ciborra et al. (2000) challenge traditional management approaches based on a control paradigm and advocates more humble, iterative and incremental managerial strategies. "Cultivation" is a metaphor that serves to characterize this alternative approach, in contrast to the prevalent "construction" mode based on detailed pre-planning and tight control. A cultivation approach would prefer monitoring and intervention activities over strict control and ongoing adjustments over rigid pre-planning. The evolution of the Internet is a paradigmatic example of technology development that has not followed the traditional managerial top-down approach. Hanseth and Lyytinen (2010) uses this case to derive design principles that are sensitive to (and exploit) the network effects that are a core defining feature of information infrastructures.

To build (or grow) infrastructures is a challenging endeavour for several reasons: information infrastructures expand through integrating previously separate systems, however, integration is not only a technical concern of achieving interoperability, rather a process embedding political and institutional interests. For instance, in the context of national or regional e-health infrastructures, a large number of heterogeneous actors, including developers and users' organizations, are involved with diverging interests, which requires ongoing political negotiations (Sahay et al. 2009). In addition, large-scale infrastructural projects require adequate coordination mechanisms. Infrastructure development is characterized by uncertainty. It is basically an open process due to the many interdependencies that need to be dealt with. Furthermore, unintended side effects and the participating actors' reflexivity can add to the complexity (Hanseth and Ciborra 2007; Hanseth et al. 2006). Moreover, infrastructure development is a visionary and political process with a moving target. It deals with an extended time span, as infrastructures are designed today to address future and unknown needs of users.

With this book we aim to contribute to the emerging body of literature that apply the information infrastructure perspective to study eHealth infrastructures.[1] Specifically, this book focuses on the process of evolution of various cases of information infrastructures in the health sector. The information infrastructure perspective encourages such a temporally extended process view, and the "installed base" concept is central in such analyses.

3.3   Installed Base

One of the core messages of the information infrastructure body of research has been to draw the attention to the role of the pre-existing, built environment, which is often overlooked by other conceptualizations of large, complex systems. Studies of information infrastructures emphasize the durability and central role of existing practices, conventions, tools and systems, and this "installed base" is seen to fundamentally impact the evolution of information infrastructures. This perspective emphasizes that "infrastructure does not grow de novo: it wrestles with the "inertia of the installed base" and inherits strengths and limitations from that base." (Star and Ruhleder 1996, p. 113).

Among practitioners the challenges posed by the installed base are well known. For instance, a corporations' huge and messy portfolio of IT systems from different technical generations that have accumulated throughout the years may significantly impacts the corporation's freedom to improve and innovate, for both technical and financial reasons. The metaphors of 'greenfield' versus 'brownfield' projects, imported to systems development discourse from the building industry, signify the same practical recognition of the power of the installed base. While a greenfield site has no prior installations, in a brownfield site there may be existing installations, other buildings, pipes and cables in the ground, or contaminated soil. Changes and innovations happen in that constrained space between what is already there and what can become realized in an already populated landscape.

The notion of installed base refers in general to the number of installations or products sold. The size of the installed base and existence of complementary products may, through self-reinforcing growth mechanisms, determine success or failure in the market (see e.g. Farrell and Saloner 1986; Schilling 1999). However, in Information Infrastructure studies the notion of installed base has a broader meaning. It was initially used in the context of a discussion on standardization and communication protocols, where it was commented that "a fundamental problem with OSI is that it is "installed base hostile" (Hanseth and Monteiro 1998b). The notion was later used in an extended way to encompass "all that is there", including the existing work practices with their tools and established

---

[1]See e.g.: Aanestad and Jensen 2011; Jensen 2013; Schellhammer et al. 2013; Grisot and Vassilakopoulou 2013; Rodon and Chekanov 2014; Grisot et al. 2014; Johnson et al. 2014; Rodon and Silva 2015; Thorseng and Jensen 2015; Hanseth and Bygstad 2015; Vassilakopoulou et al. 2016; Williams 2016.

division of labour, the legal and professional regulations in place, and so on (see e.g. Hanseth and Monteiro 1998a). The main argument is that information infrastructures are never designed from scratch, but they develop through the evolution of an installed base. Hanseth and Lyytinen (2010) define an installed base as the existing "set of ICT capabilities and their users, operations and design communities", and it also encompasses existing institutional and organizational components (Lanzara 2014). In the health sector for example an installed base may encompass patient record systems, medical departments, various groups of professionals as users (nurses, clinicians), dispensing practices, regulations etc. Accordingly, the main argument put forward in this book is that projects for the creation of large-scale health information infrastructures are shaped by the existing installed base: the organizational, institutional, regulatory, sociotechnical arrangements that are already in place.

We should keep in mind that an installed base is not a given 'thing', it is rather a conceptual tool. This conceptual tool can help us to capture the continuities and discontinuities in infrastructure evolution. It becomes observable and visible when analyzing plans and interventions acting upon the existing infrastructural arrangements. Rather than asking "what is the installed base" we should ask "when is an installed base"? In other words, rather than pointing to specific elements, we need to ask when and how some element of an existing reality becomes significant, for whom, with what effects? In what way do the different elements become significant, are they working as triggers, as resources, as competitors, as alternatives? For instance, will a particular feature of the organizational culture serve to facilitate or hinder change? The concept of installed base is a sense-making tool to examine and reflect on the challenges faced in the development of infrastructures. It implies a process-oriented understanding where it becomes crucial to trace and analyse the historical sequence of events and decisions that shape the forming of infrastructures.

The generic change strategy of the information infrastructure perspective – "cultivation of the installed base" – denotes a strategy that starts from what already exists (the installed base). This implies a re-conceptualization of the very notion of design of information infrastructure. Rather than design in the conventional sense, dealing with the evolution of infrastructures requires strategies to intervene and influence ongoing processes. The Information Infrastructure evolution process is best captured by the notion of 'growing' (instead of e.g. 'building' or 'constructing') since it gives a "sense of an organic unfolding within an existing (and changing) environment" where there is a "recurring issue of adjustment in which infrastructures adapt to, reshape, or even internalize elements of their environment in the process of growth and entrenchment" (Edwards et al. 2007, p. 369). These processes of infrastructure evolution happen along multiple temporal scales (Edwards et al. 2009; Ribes and Finholt 2009; Karasti et al. 2010). In this perspective, we approach the cases by paying attention to the strategies enacted in order to deal with the installed base, and examine how developing infrastructures entails engagement in processes of extension, recombination, substitution of parts and arrangements that already exist. In this view, new information technologies should never be seen as isolated and univocal, but embedded in an intricate web of technologies, practices, routines to which they relate in specific ways. The pre-existing systems may serve as a foundation for a new system, components from the previous information infrastructure may be reused in the new, and other components me be redefined or removed. The challenges associated with this is the topic of the next section.

3.4   Challenges of Installed Base Cultivation

Infrastructures are never built "de novo" – they develop amidst a stream of technical antecedents, social conventions and professional rules and have to be adaptive to the developments of work practice. As these elements are changing, the information infrastructures are continuously evolving. At the same time, they have to be stable enough to reliably support activities that make use of them: "only a stable installed base allows new connections to be created" (Tilson et al. 2010). Taking an infrastructural perspective reorients our attention to interconnections and relationships as well as to issues of durability and permanence. The challenge is then to devise strategies for effectively managing future evolution (Ribes and Finholt 2009; Karasti et al. 2010). The installed base is both enabling and constraining infrastructure evolution (Hanseth et al. 1996; Hanseth and Aanestad 2003), it can be "a resource for creative design and innovation or a trap from which it is difficult to escape" (Lanzara 2014 p. 19). To manage the further evolution of the installed base is challenging, as it entails building on the installed base and transforming it at the same time. This creates a paradox: new developments need to fit and make use of existing arrangements and at the same time transform them. Overfitting on the existing installed base may strengthen its irreversibility and hinder change, disregarding it may limit the initial utility of any initiative and impede growth (Henningsson and Hanseth 2011). The paradoxical relationship between the installed base and infrastructural development initiatives cannot be resolved with simplistic approaches e.g. the old obliteration dogma of Business Process Reengineering or naive digitization ("putting electricity on paper"). Rather our argument is that the installed base matters in each case in a specific and contingent way.

This book aims to bring empirically based and theoretically informed insights into how the installed base matters. The book's empirical analyses investigate the various strategies in which infrastructure "builders" engage with (or disregard) the installed base. The stories describe how initiatives are shaped and paced by decisions on how to relate with the installed base, or alternatively, how they are shaped by the insensitivity to what is already in place. The two categories of cases, e-prescription infrastructures and governmental patient-oriented eHealth platforms are differently positioned with respect to the installed base. E-prescription initiatives are typically oriented to digitize an already present paper-based and analogue information infrastructure. The governmental patient-oriented web platforms are typically expected to allow more radical innovation, including new interaction patterns, roles and responsibilities for both patients and healthcare personnel. Overall, e-prescription initiatives are usually aiming to improve healthcare delivery by systematic change, building in an orderly way upon the existing arrangements, while initiatives for patient-oriented eHealth platforms are usually seen as opportunities to pursue wider and more radical innovation (dramatic change) (Huy and Mintzberg 2003). Nevertheless, in any of the two types, pre-existing arrangements need to be taken into account, after all, these pre-existing arrangements are providing the contextual meaning of change. Hence, change has to be managed with a profound appreciation of the installed base.

The book chapters go beyond the initial design and development of each case and include experiences of reworking and reconfiguration during and after deployment as this has proved to be pivotal for systems' evolution. The narratives of each case bring forwards the paradoxical relationship between new eHealth initiatives that need to fit and make use of existing arrangements and at the same time transform them. The accounts of actual trajectories may not necessarily be neat "rollouts"; detours and plan changes are part of the stories. Nevertheless, all cases are about large-scale planned and professionally managed initiatives with specific goals. The book is about this type of initiatives and aims to provide insights on how strategies can be specific to each context. Going beyond universal best practices that can be deadening and unresponsive to the actual challenges requires developing an awareness of the installed base. This awareness means being able to discern what is relevant and needs to be foregrounded and acted upon from what can be handled as mere background. In other words, the aim with the book is to help create an "installed base sensitivity" in decision-making both at the policy/strategic level and at the concrete e-health design level.

References

Aanestad M, Jensen TB. Building nation-wide information infrastructures in healthcare through modular implementation strategies. J Strateg Inf Syst. 2011;20(2):161–76.

Arthur B. Competing technologies, increasing returns, and lock-in by historical events. Econ J. 1989;99:116–31.

Arthur B. Positive feedbacks in the economy. Sci Am. 1990;262(2):92–9.

Berg M. Accumulating and coordinating: occasions for information technologies in medical work. Comput Supported Coop Work. 1999;8(4):373–401.

Berg M, Goorman E. The contextual nature of medical information. Int J Med Inform. 1999;56(1–3):51–60.

Ciborra C, Braa K, Cordella A, Dahlbom B, Failla A, Hanseth O, Hepsø V, Ljungberg J, Monteiro E, Simon KA. From control to drift. The dynamics of corporate information infrastructures. Oxford: Oxford University Press; 2000.

David P. Clio and the economics of QWERTY. Am Econ Rev. 1985;75:332–7.

Edwards PN, Jackson SJ, Bowker GC, Knobel CP. Understanding infrastructure: dynamics, tensions, and design. Report of a workshop on "History & Theory of Infrastructure: Lessons for New Scientific Cyberinfrastructures". Ann Arbor: Deep Blue ; 2007.URL: http://hdl.handle.net/2027.42/49353.

Edwards P, Bowker G, Jackson JS, Williams R. Introduction: an agenda for infrastructure studies. J Assoc Inf Syst (JAIS). 2009;10(5):364–74.

Ellingsen G, Monteiro E. A patchwork planet: integration and cooperation in hospitals. Comput Supported Coop Work. 2003;12(1):71–95.

Farrell J, Saloner G. Installed base and compatibility: innovation, product preannouncements, and predation. Am Econ Rev. 1986;76(5):940–55.

Feiler PH, Sullivan K, Wallnau KC, Gabriel RP, Goodenough JB, Linger RC, Loingstaff TA, Kazman R, Klein MH, Northrop L, Schmidt D. Ultra-large-scale systems: the software challenge of the future. Pittsburgh: Software Engineering Institute, Carnegie Mellon University; 2006.

Grisot M, Vassilakopoulou P. Infrastructures in healthcare: the interplay between generativity and standardization. Int J Med Inform. 2013;82(5):e170–9.

Grisot M, Hanseth O, Thorseng AA. Innovation of, in, on infrastructures: articulating the role of architecture in information infrastructure evolution. J AIS. 2014;15(4):197–219.

Hanseth O, Aanestad M. Design as bootstrapping. On the evolution of ICT network in healthcare. Methods Inf Med. 2003;42(4):385–91.

Hanseth O, Bygstad B. Flexible generification. ICT standardization strategies and service innovation in health care. Eur J Inf Syst. 2015;24(6):645–63.

Hanseth O, Ciborra C, editors. Risk, complexity and ICT. Cheltenham: Edward Elgar Publishing; 2007.

Hanseth O, Lundberg N. Designing work oriented infrastructures. Comput Supported Coop Work. 2001;10(3–4):347–72.

Hanseth O, Lyytinen K. Design theory for dynamic complexity in information infrastructures: the case of building internet. J Inf Technol. 2010;25(1):1–19.

Hanseth O, Monteiro E, Hatling M. Developing information infrastructure: The tension between standardization and flexibility. Science, technology & human values. 1996;21(4):407–26.

Hanseth O, Monteiro E. Changing irreversible networks. In: Baets WRJ, editors. Proceedings from 6th European Conference on Information Systems, p. 1123–39. 1998a.

Hanseth O, Monteiro E. Understanding information infrastructure. Unpublished Manuscript. 1998b. Available at http://heim.ifi.uio.no/~oleha/Publications/bok.pdf.

Hanseth O, Jacucci E, Grisot M, Aanestad M. Reflexive standardization: side effects and complexity in standard making. MIS Q. 2006;30:563–81.

Henningsson S, Hanseth O. The essential dynamics of information infrastructures. In: Proceedings of the 32 International Conference on Information Systems (ICIS), Shanghai, 2011, Paper 14. 2011.

Hughes TP. The evolution of large technological systems. In: Bijker WE, Hughes TP, Pinch TJ, editors. The social construction of technological systems: new directions in the sociology and history of technology. Cambridge, MA: MIT Press; 1987. p. 51–82.

Huy QN, Mintzberg H. The rhythm of change. MIT Sloan Manag Rev. 2003;44:79–84.

Jensen TB. Design principles for achieving integrated healthcare information systems. Health Inform J. 2013;19(1):29–45.

Johnson M, Mozaffar H, Campagnolo GM, Hyysalo S, Pollock N, Williams R. The managed prosumer: evolving knowledge strategies in the design of information infrastructures. Inf Commun Soc. 2014;17(7):795–813.

Karasti H, Baker SB, Millerand F. Infrastructure time: long-term matters in collaborative development. Comput Support Cooperat Work (CSCW). 2010;19(3):377–415.

Lanzara GF. The circulation of agency in judicial proceedings: Designing for interoperability and complexity. In: Contini F, Lanzara GF. The circulation of agency in E-justice. Interoperability and Infrastructures for European Transborder Judicial Proceedings, pp. 3–32. Law, Governance and Technology series, vol. 13 2014. Netherlands: Springer; 2014.

Leonardi PM. When flexible routines meet flexible technologies: affordance, constraint, and the imbrication of human and material agencies. MIS Q. 2011;35(1):147–67.

Maier MW. Architecting principles for systems-of-systems. Syst Eng. 1998;1(4):267–84.

Monteiro E, Hanseth O. Social shaping of information infrastructure: on being specific about the technology. In: Orlikowski WJ, Walsham G, Jones MR, DeGross JI, editors. Information technology and changes in organisational work. London: Chapman & Hall; 1995. p. 325–43.

Petrakaki D, Klecun E, Cornford T. Changes in healthcare professional work afforded by technology: the introduction of a national electronic patient record in an English hospital. Organization. 2016;23(2):206–26.

Ribes D, Finholt TA. The long now of technology infrastructures: articulating tensions in development. J Assoc Inf Syst. 2009;10(5):375–98.

Rodon J, Chekanov A. Architectural constraints on the bootstrapping of a personal health record. Scand J Inf Syst. 2014;26(2):53–78.

Rodon J, Silva L. Exploring the formation of a healthcare information infrastructure: hierarchy or meshwork? J Assoc Inf Syst. 2015;16(5):394–417.

Sahay S, Monteiro E, Aanestad M. Configurable politics and asymmetric integration: health e-infrastructures in India. J Assoc Inf Syst. 2009;10(5):399–414.

Schellhammer S, Reimers K, Klein S. Emergence of information infrastructures: a tale of two islands. Int J Biomed Eng Technol. 2013;11(3):231–51.

Schilling M. Winning the standards race: building installed base and the availability of complementary goods. Eur Manag J. 1999;17(3):265–74.

Silsand L, Ellingsen G. Generification by translation: designing generic systems in context of the local. J Assoc Inf Syst. 2014;15(4):177.

Sommerville I, Cliff D, Kalinescu R, Keen J, Kelly T, Kwiatkowska M, Mcdermid J, Paige R. Large-scale complex IT systems. Commun ACM. 2012;55(7):71–7.

Star SL, Ruhleder K. Steps toward an ecology of infrastructure: design and access for large information spaces. Inf Syst Res. 1996;7(1):111–34.

Thorseng A, Jensen TB. National infrastructures for patient-centred digital services. In: 23rd European Conference on Information Systems (ECIS) 2015.

Tilson D, Lyytinen K, Sørensen C. Digital infrastructures: the missing IS research agenda. Inf Syst Res. 2010;21(4):748–59.

Vassilakopoulou P, Grisot M, Aanestad M. Enabling Electronic Interactions between Patients and Healthcare Providers: a service design perspective. Scand J Inf Syst. 2016;28(1):71–90.

Vikkelsø S. Subtle redistribution of work, attention and risks: electronic patient records and organisational consequences. Scand J Inf Syst. 2005;17(1):3–30.

Williams R. Why is it difficult to achieve e-health systems at scale? Inf Commun Soc. 2016;19(4):540–50.

Winthereik BR, Berg M. Waiting for godot. Episodes from the history of patient records. Chapter 2 in Berg (ed.) Health information management. Integrating information and communication technology in health care work. Routledge. 2003.

Open Access This chapter is distributed under the terms of the Creative Commons Attribution-NonCommercial 2.5 International License (http://creativecommons.org/licenses/by-nc/2.5/), which permits any noncommercial use, duplication, adaptation, distribution and reproduction in any medium or format, as long as you give appropriate credit to the original author(s) and the source, provide a link to the Creative Commons license and indicate if changes were made.

The images or other third party material in this chapter are included in the chapter's Creative Commons license, unless indicated otherwise in a credit line to the material. If material is not included in the chapter's Creative Commons license and your intended use is not permitted by statutory regulation or exceeds the permitted use, you will need to obtain permission directly from the copyright holder.

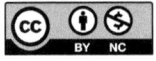

Strategies for Building eHealth Infrastructures

Margunn Aanestad, Miria Grisot, Ole Hanseth, and Polyxeni Vassilakopoulou

4.1 Introduction

This chapter presents a cross-case analysis of the different strategies for dealing with the installed base in the 11 empirical chapters of this book. The empirical chapters are organised in two sections. One focused on cases of design and development of e-prescription and one focused on patient-oriented eHealth platforms. Both e-prescription and patient-oriented eHealth initiatives have a transformative role, but they are differently positioned within the eHealth landscape. Overall, e-prescription is more well-defined in terms of functionality than patient-oriented services. Furthermore, there are clear interdependencies between e-prescription and specific existing healthcare applications (e.g. Electronic Health Record systems and Pharmacy systems) and also with well-established work practices (for prescribing, drug dispensing and reimbursements) and tools (the installed base). Compared with e-prescription initiatives, the initiatives to build patient-oriented eHealth platforms are more open in scope, the functionalities to be included are frequently decided after an exploratory process, and the needs for linkages to existing systems and practices are concretised only after the specifics of functionalities are defined. Overall, e-prescription initiatives are usually seen as opportunities to improve

M. Aanestad (✉)
University of Oslo & UIT The Arctic University of Norway,
P.O. Box 1080 Blindern, N-0316 Oslo, Norway
e-mail: margunn@ifi.uio.no

M. Grisot • O. Hanseth
University of Oslo, P.O. Box 1080 Blindern, N-0316 Oslo, Norway
e-mail: miriag@ifi.uio.no; oleha@ifi.uio.no

P. Vassilakopoulou
University of Agder & University of Oslo, P.O. Box 422, N-4604 Kristiansand, Norway
e-mail: polyxenv@uia.no

© The Author(s) 2017
M. Aanestad et al. (eds.), *Information Infrastructures within European Health Care*, Health Informatics, DOI 10.1007/978-3-319-51020-0_4

healthcare delivery by systematic and not dramatic change while patient-oriented eHealth services are usually seen as opportunities to pursue wider and more radical innovation.

In the sections that follow, we unpack these aspects drawing from the six prescription cases and the five patient-oriented eHealth cases included in this book. Specifically, we present the actual scope of the different initiatives (i.e. the actual services included), their starting points and their motivations. We then, compare the different cases in terms of the observed strategies towards the installed base. We conclude the chapter with some reflections on the importance of a conscious and well-informed strategy towards the installed base for addressing the challenges of putting in place eHealth infrastructures.

4.2   E-Prescription

4.2.1   Overview of the Case Studies on E-Prescription: Services Offered, Starting Points, Motivation

The six case studies on e-prescription show similarities and differences with respect to the *functionality domains* covered, their *starting points* and their *motivations*. These are described in the following subsections.

Functionality Domains Covered and Starting Points

The projects cover a variety of processes related to prescribing and medication management. The projects in Norway, Catalonia, England, and Greece started with a broad aim and national scope (in the Catalan case the scope covered the semi-autonomous Catalonia region), and with a focus on the *transmission of prescription information* from the prescribing doctor to the pharmacies. Most of these projects did not only support prescribing of drugs by General Practitioners (GPs), but also the prescribing at hospital's outpatient clinics and hospital prescribing for patients that are about to be discharged from the hospital.

The case from Germany and the case on UK hospital prescribing are significantly different from the other cases. The project reported in the case from Germany is not a national e-prescription project, but a project which started with the specific aim to improve medication compliance for polypharmacy patients by providing patient-specific medication packs that could function as dose administration aids. In order to implement this, the electronic transmission of prescriptions was required. The project's starting point was related to the needs of a specific category of patients and to the possibilities offered by a specific way of drug delivery (medication packs). In addition, this project was one of many other initiatives promoting the dispensing of packaged medications in Germany. The case on e-prescription in the UK hospitals is about the implementation of various different Hospital Electronic Prescribing and Medicine Administration (HEPMA) systems in NHS England. The systems' functionality and implementation efforts described in this case are specific to hospital contexts and do not cover any primary care activities.

Motivations

Regarding motivations behind the initiatives and expected benefits and outcomes, the cases have a lot in common. Firstly, they all aimed for *cost containment*, partly through automating parts of the overall process, but also through enhanced monitoring of drugs' expenditures and physicians' prescribing practices; also, they aimed for *improving patient safety* and for *improving the overall quality* of the service delivered to patients. There was, however, also some variety across the projects regarding motivation.

In two cases the interests of *pharmaceutical actors* played a major role. In Germany, the project on the medication packs was initiated and managed by a representative of the pharmaceutical industry with business interests to expand its market presence and promote a specific type of solution (blistering). Also in the Catalan case, although the project was initiated by the health authorities, the pharmacies and their association played a central role in defining its aims. The project got a strong focus on improving the practices in the pharmacies, and the pharmacy association managed to get a key role in the process. This key role was secured by establishing an overall architecture that allowed the pharmacy side infrastructure to be as autonomous as possible from the rest of the e-prescription infrastructure.

In Greece, the e-prescription initiative was motivated by some of the common arguments found in other cases: to enhance control over pharmaceutical expenditure, to improve doctor-pharmacy collaboration and patient safety and to capture data required for evidence-based policy development. However, the economic situation of the country played a role in pushing the project forward. The project was run during a difficult period for the Greek economy, and this accelerated the introduction of new electronic tools to reform the healthcare sector. In Norway, the project was initially triggered by the Office of the Auditor General's critique of inadequate monitoring and control of costs related to drug use. However, in order to ensure physicians' buy-in, the focus of the project changed early on from monitoring, control, and cost containment, towards improving patient safety.

Finally, in the case for establishing e-prescription in UK hospitals, the interests of *the vendors* played a significant role. Vendors of HEPMA applications were investing in expanding their market base internationally and in England, and for this purpose they adopted diverse strategies. Overall, this case brings forward the interests that shape the market within the domain of systems for hospital electronic prescribing and medicine administration.

4.2.2 Strategies Towards the Installed Base

In this section we will compare and contrast the six e-prescription cases regarding their strategies for how to relate to the existing installed base, and how to further develop it.

In section "Strategies for Dealing with Existing Practices and Technologies" we will look more carefully at how the different projects related to their respective installed bases. We will consider the installed base in terms of both existing user practices and technological systems. The different projects under study have followed approaches that were: *installed base-friendly*, *installed base-ignorant* and *installed base-hostile*. The installed base-friendly approach seems to be the one with higher chances to establish a new infrastructure and reach a stage where the adoption and use of the infrastructure get momentum. This approach implies that the new infrastructure first of all supports and aligns with existing work practices, second, that the new technological solution is as simple as possible, third, that it is built upon existing technologies when possible, and, finally, that it requires as few changes to the technological installed base as possible. However, once the infrastructure is established, it remains to see if it will lead to a lock-in process where existing practices are embedded into more complex and hard to change technological structures, or if it may enable future changes and improvement of the actual practices.

Thus, in section "Strategies for Further Development" we will turn our attention to projects' *strategies for enabling future changes* by modifying and extending the infrastructure after it is established, i.e. strategies for how to *"cultivate" the new installed base* built. Across all cases studied, once the initial arrangements for e-prescription were put in place and adopted in practice, a series of modifications and additions followed. These further developments to the e-prescription infrastructures were driven by stakeholders´ interests and were the outcome of case-specific strategies for forward-looking development.

Strategies for Dealing with Existing Practices and Technologies

As described in the introductory chapter on "Information Infrastructures for eHealth", e-prescription is relatively well-defined in terms of functionality and is built upon pre-existing applications and prescribing tools. Accordingly, the Catalan, Norwegian, English and Greek projects started out with *a focus on paper prescriptions* and aimed at first to digitalize the paper-based prescribing processes. They started out with the (implicit) strategy of replicating existing paper-based practices and then, to a varying degree, enriching these with additional functions for detection of medication errors and decision support that would improve patient safety. Such projects can, then, be said to be *"installed base friendly"*. As explained in the analysis of the case on e-prescription in England, new developments show some *fidelity* to established structures, practices and professional roles within the healthcare system. For instance, in the e-prescription project in England, elements of the old paper prescription form were retained and used also for the electronic solution ensuring a better 'fit' of the new prescription service to the wider healthcare context, both conceptually and practically. However, these four projects while trying to stay close to the existing practices, had to find appropriate strategies for actually building e-prescription upon the installed base and faced different challenges.

The Norwegian and Greek projects employed almost opposite strategies for dealing with the existing technological installed base. In the Norwegian case, the strategy chosen was to *integrate tightly* the e-prescription modules implementing the new functionality with existing systems, in particular Electronic Patient Record and Pharmacy Management systems. Due to the comprehensive functionality specified, this implied that the project required extensive work from the vendors' side. The vendors had to develop new and quite complex software components, modify their existing solutions, and integrate them. This resulted in a situation where the overall Norwegian project became heavily dependent not only to the activities of the vendors directly involved in the e-prescription project, but also to the overall situation within the vendor organizations. For instance, the project was slowed down by one vendor's delayed development of a new product.

Differently from the Norwegian project, the Greek one developed first a simple solution based on easily available and straightforward web technologies *without pursuing integration* with the Electronic Patient Record and Pharmacy Management systems that were already in place. These integrations were made possible at a later stage, after the initial launch of the simple solution. Due to economic and political commitments, the initial solution was developed within a very tight timeline and was launched within less than a year from the moment that development started. This is in huge contrast to the Norwegian solution in terms of both complexity and time. The "rollout" of the solution in Norway started 7–8 years after the project was established.

In the English case, the e-prescription solutions for doctors and pharmacists were developed by software vendors according to a set of output-based specifications describing how to manage and process electronic prescriptions. These solutions were built upon the technological installed base which included agreed national informatics standards and common supporting components such as a data centre and communications backbone (the Spine) which enables the transfer of data between computer systems in the NHS. In the Catalan case, the technological installed base included Pharmacy Management Systems, but lacked a national secure health network. This secure network had to be built before the project proceeded.

Differently from the other four cases, the UK hospital case and the German case started from *available technological capabilities*, rather than the existing work practices. E-prescription in hospitals in England was based on Commercial Off-The-Shelf (COTS) 'packaged' software systems that were used for various purposes different from medication management, rather than existing work practices. The vendors of the systems tried to adapt them to support and improve the activities related to medication management. However, in many cases the COTS systems had non-clinical origins and were 'foreign', lacking alignment with UK hospitals' internal processes and needs, and the diversity of practices across hospitals, department, and specialties. In this case, the approach followed in the project could be said to be "*installed base ignorant*" as the existing practices were not taken into consideration in the process of infrastructure development. This resulted in requests to adapt the systems to local practices and preferences, which forced vendors to perform multiple cycles of modification to their products. However, the process turned out to be complex and slow, resulting in the current uneven growth and variable success of HEPMA systems in England.

Similarly, the German project started with a technological vantage point and the ambition to change existing practices. The project promoted the dispensing of packaged medications in blisters, with a specific process flow around it, and a controlled medication lists. However, the innovative blistering practice and the infrastructure supporting it, were seen as a controversial by key actors. Blistering practices would require the *transformation and extension of various existing practices* such as: medication management and related information sharing practices, practices of distributing medication and practices of invoicing and reimbursing medication. In this case new technologies designed for Multi-Dose (or Automatic Dose) Dispensing were not adapted to what was already in place. In addition, core infrastructural components were questioned and opposed. For instance, the assortment of 400 medicines for blistering was perceived as controlling medication practices. Overall, the relation to the installed base in the German case can be seen as 'hostile' for various reasons. From the perspective of the project, the innovative blistering project met an *'installed base of opposition'* as many key actors critiqued and strongly opposed the project. This eventually ended the project. From the perspective of the existing practices and technologies, the project's approach can be said to be "*installed base hostile*" considering the mismatch between the novelty of the blistering project, and the existing arrangements in the surrounding environment.

Overall, all the six cases had to deal with what we have described as the '*paradox*' of the installed base in the chapter on "Information Infrastructures and the challenge of the Installed Base". This paradox is about aiming for developments that need to fit and make use of existing arrangements *and* at the same time transform them. This specific need to be both fitted and transformative can explain why cases that initially adopted *installed base-friendly* approaches may at a later point become more *installed base-hostile*. For instance, in the Norwegian case, the project aimed initially to establish stronger control of public expenses related to drugs, which implied closer monitoring and control of physicians' work practices. The project owners realised that physicians might be unwilling to adopt a technological solution aimed just at such monitoring. Accordingly, it was decided to add functionality to the solution specification to make the solution more aligned with physicians´ work practices. This move however, made the technological solution more complex and more "*installed base hostile*" regarding technology.

Strategies for Further Development

In this section we turn our attention to the different cases' *strategies for enabling forward looking changes* by modifying and extending the infrastructure after it was established. Of the six cases examined, three have enough similarities for being cross-analysed. Specifically, the Catalan, Greek, and Norwegian cases covered similar functionalities, started all with installed base-friendly approaches and were pursued to a great extent through centrally decided and implemented development plans. Those information infrastructures evolved more or less continuously after they were put in place according to different strategies. These three projects illustrate three different ways in which the continuous modification and enhancement of an already established and adopted infrastructure can be facilitated, i.e. how an installed base can be "cultivated."

In Catalonia, the infrastructure was continuously changed and a range of new services have been introduced. Key elements in this process were the architectural changes which turned the SIFARE server into *a platform that could be accessed through an API and web services.* Over the years the API and the web services have been extended and modified to provide a vast range of services. These services offered Pharmacy Management System vendors (14 in total) possibilities for developing new services supporting and improving the work practices of their customers. Over the years the vendors have been innovative and added many new services to their products based on the SIFARE platform. Partly the vendors have innovated and developed new services individually, partly this has happened through coordinated initiatives like the "Paperless Pharmacy" project.

The Greek solution was first extended by developing and providing APIs that the vendors of Pharmacy Management and Electronic Patient Record systems could use to integrate their solutions with the infrastructure. Then, various new functions were added such as the electronic implementation of therapeutic prescribing protocols, and diagnostic tests' ordering. These changes were implemented in short time and at low cost. This was possible because the new infrastructure was based on *an expandable component-based architecture.* In addition, the initiative was run and maintained by a small centralized organization that had flexibility in modifying the solution. Overall, multiple changes have taken place as a sequence of small steps.

The Norwegian infrastructure is significantly more complex than the Greek one. Furthermore, the Norwegian case was the only one of the three that expanded beyond the traditional prescription areas. Specifically, the Norwegian case expanded into medication management of chronically ill patients at home and in nursing homes through the development of new functionalities for supporting Multi-Dose Dispensing. The hospitals in Norway have also expressed interest in integrating the e-prescription solution with their Chart and Medication Systems. For all major changes in this complex infrastructure *the application independent GPM module played an important role.* The central project organization used this module to develop the new functionalities in an experimental fashion being able to test prototypes and the launch pilots without involving application vendors. After having successfully established a number of pilots, the specifications for the extended functionality could be frozen and then implemented as extension to vendor applications if the vendors wanted to.

Due to these improvements and modifications of the e-prescription infrastructures the installed bases of technologies and user practices also changed. Actually, in all cases work practices evolved as the infrastructures were modified and extended.

4.3   Patient-Oriented eHealth Platforms

4.3.1   Overview of the Case Studies on Patient-Oriented eHealth: Services Offered, Starting Points, Motivations

The five case studies on patient-oriented eHealth platforms tell different stories about strategies towards the installed base. This is not unexpected as each case has a different starting point and is related to different sociotechnical settings. Furthermore, the locus of each initiative is different: the case from Italy describes an initiative that started from one *municipality* growing to the region level, the case from Sweden is about multiple parallel *county-level* initiatives under national coordination, the other two cases from Scandinavia are about initiatives taken at the *national level* (Denmark, Norway) while the case from Spain is about an initiative taken centrally at the level of the *semiautonomous region* of Catalonia. The cases offer a good variety of scenarios in which patient oriented services have been successfully developed.

Services Offered and Starting Points

The types of services offered through the platforms cover the whole spectrum described in the second chapter of this book (on Information Infrastructures for eHealth). The three Scandinavian platforms (Denmark, Norway, Sweden) and the Catalan one include an impressive *range of offerings*: quality checked information on health and disease, information on the performance of different health institutions, access to personal health data stored in medical records across the health sector, administrative services (e.g. GP change, tracking of referrals, claims or requests), booking services, patient-provider message exchange and e-consultation. Some of these platforms also include tools for disease-specific self-monitoring and self-care and links to patients' social media platforms or facilities for peer-to-peer networking. There are plans for expanding towards these directions for the platforms that do not yet include such functionalities. The case from Italy is different from the other four as it has a specific focus on booking services, which emerged as an initial service in what later grew to a larger citizens' platform. The Italian case is very interesting as it offers an account of the evolution of (probably) the first e-booking system in Europe.

Interestingly, the initial offerings for the four platforms that are now broad and all-inclusive, were different. In Catalonia, the platform started as an *access point for personal health data* from the Shared Electronic Medical Record of Catalonia that was newly established when the initiative started (started in 2008, first pilot in 2009). In Sweden, it started from a Stockholm County Council initiative to provide a *"secure message feature"* between patients and healthcare providers (initiated in 2000, first pilots in 2002 with a limited number of patient-provider interactions such as requests for appointment scheduling and prescription renewal). In both Denmark and Norway, the starting point was to provide *quality assured but non-personalised information*. In Norway, the platform started by offering consistent and quality-assured definitions of illnesses and treatments in information pages (started in 2010, launched in 2011); personalised services (that required patient authentication) were added in 2013. In Denmark, the national platform started by offering quality-assured medical information for both citizens and healthcare providers and soon after that, information about waiting lists (the initiative started in 2001, launched in 2003); services that required authentication were added in 2004. The differences in the initial offerings relate both to the different initial motivations for putting in place the patient platforms and also, to the different possibilities offered by the installed base in each country during the early development phases.

In the Italian case, the focus is on one specific type of electronic service (booking of appointments) but as the case narrative starts in 1990, it is interesting to observe the *evolution of channels* used throughout the years for providing access to patients. The new electronic service was initially (in 1990) offered through 25 e-booking centres (including hospitals, health centres and department stores). In 1996, e-booking was also offered through pharmacies. In 2000, a call centre was added as an additional channel. In 2003, a website for changes, cancellations and bookings for limited types of appointments was made available. In 2013, a comprehensive regional e-booking website was launched. The different access options provided are directly linked to the characteristics of the installed base throughout the years. In the era before widespread home computer use and network access, it was important to link to the available installed base of patient-provider interfaces (e.g. by including service counters in health facilities and enrolling pharmacies) and by leveraging telephony (through the call centre).

Motivations

The five initiatives are also different in terms of the motivations that ignited them. In the Danish case, a key motivation was to support *better coordination* across healthcare services by providing a government-controlled entry to health information across a relatively decentralized healthcare system. At a strategic level, the ambition was to encourage a common strategy, and to align investments and solutions. In Sweden, the main motivation was to promote the *responsibility and participation of citizens* in matters of their own health. This was very similar to the motivation for the Norwegian initiative which was centred around the need to promote a more active patient role and to *facilitate the engagement* of citizens by offering a national-level, comprehensive platform and *facilitating access to the fragmented eHealth landscape* of many patient-oriented initiatives and webpages related to health. In Catalonia, there was a multifaceted motivation that included *both a new vision for the role of the citizens in healthcare and an aim to improve efficiency*. The patient oriented eHealth initiative was taken to to promote responsibility and participation of citizens in matters of their own health and to improve the health care quality and coordination between different care areas, levels and professionals. Finally, in Italy, the motivation was to facilitate a *transition from a hospital-centred model* towards a new healthcare model that would be better aligned to the demand from citizens and regions. Improving citizens' access to healthcare was an element of this reform and the new electronic booking service aimed to provide remedies for long waiting lists, fragmented offerings and a lack of transparency.

In the section that follows we turn to the specific strategies towards the installed base.

4.3.2   Strategies Towards the Installed Base

Patient-oriented eHealth initiatives require good *coordination* across multiple different actors that are already present in the domain as parts of the installed base (central and local government, healthcare providers in primary care and in the specialist sector including hospitals, software vendors, patient associations).

Furthermore, patient-oriented eHealth initiatives need to be built upon a technical installed base characterised by great *heterogeneity*: multiple different technologies are already part of the healthcare technical landscape and need to be taken into account (health record systems, healthcare organisations' administrative systems, data repositories, citizen registries, healthcare personnel registries, messaging standards, data structuring standards, networks). This heterogeneity is a key challenge for all initiatives of this type.

Additionally, as the patient-oriented eHealth platforms have an open scope and are not confined to a specific type of functionalities and settings of use, all initiatives of this type have to address the challenge of *uncertainty* i.e. the challenge of being able to evolve in many different directions. This requirement is shaping the relationship with the installed base as it creates the need for organising responsiveness to evolving needs.

Finally, as all the cases are about governmental platforms, there is a need to entrench all new developments into the wider health system arrangements and ensure that they will trigger wider changes in the sector. In other words, there is the challenge of being *transformative* i.e. the challenge of becoming embedded into the installed base while reshaping it. The new platforms need to find ways of being patient-oriented in a traditionally provider-centric system.

In the following subsections we identify the different strategies employed for addressing these four key challenges for the relationship with the installed base.

Strategies for Coordination

Different strategies have been employed in the different cases to address the challenge of coordinating the work of development and implementation across multiple different actors. In some cases, there was one core leading entity that had both control and ownership of the core services (Norway, Italy), in other cases, the leading entity was exercising control without owning all services (Catalonia, Denmark) while in one of the cases (Sweden), both the control and the ownership were distributed and coordinated through a common framework. In the next paragraphs we go through these in detail.

In Denmark, *a political governing body* which included the municipalities, the regions, and the Ministry of Health was put in place. This arrangement allowed *wide representation* of interested actors in decision making processes. Since the organisational entity that ran the platform did not have any specific strategic mandate or responsibility, the role of this governing body was significant and promoted up to today a collective and consensual work mode. The challenge now is to maintain this model while keeping pace with the increasing needs of different actors and aligning with changes that happen elsewhere within healthcare.

In Sweden, patient-oriented e-health services evolved in a complex landscape of *multiple authorities with overlapping jurisdictions* that operate under an *overarching set of rules*, the National Architecture Framework for e-Health services, which has been implemented since 2007. This allowed different actors to pursue their own developments in parallel. The different actors include the 21 county councils, Inera (an organisation funded by the counties to coordinate and support their shared e-health services) and Vinnova (the innovation agency in Sweden). The Framework includes service contracts, legal agreement templates, procurement templates, interoperability standards, procedures for tests and certification and a reference architecture which applies to nationally as well as regionally funded e-health projects. The Swedish experience shows that there are potentially positive consequences of heterogeneity within the installed base (both technical and institutional) if an effective mechanism for coordination is in place. For example, the county councils of Uppsala and Stockholm developed competing viewers of health records for patients – both with national ambitions. At the end of 2015 the Uppsala solution had significantly larger number of users, so Stockholm county council decided to decommission their viewer in favour of the Uppsala one. Nevertheless, the backend of the Stockholm solution was retained and used as a national level component. Hence, the solution eventually used is a combination of Uppsala frontend and Stockholm backend. Furthermore, since 2013, the overall Swedish e-health architecture includes a component which facilitates the engagement of external actors with the installed base. This new component is the Health Innovation Platform (HIP) and includes a software development kit, several APIs and methods, guidelines and program code to support the development of e-health services by freelance developers, designers and software companies, both within and outside the healthcare industry.

In Norway and in Catalonia, the governmental patient-oriented eHealth platforms were developed under the leadership of *strong, centrally positioned actors*. In the case of Norway, the central actor was the Health Directorate and in the case of Catalonia, the Department of Health. In both cases the central agencies orchestrated activities that included multiple actors. In the case of Norway, the Health Directorate *managed the evolution of the platform by setting priorities and keeping the ownership of the services*. The Directorate ensured the reuse of public information resources and the enrolment of private software vendors for the development of links to the information systems in use within the health sector. Furthermore, the Directorate established close collaboration with the Norwegian National ICT (NICT) which is the interest body for information and communication technologies in the specialist healthcare sector formed by the four Regional Health Authorities.

In Catalonia, the Department of Health started the initiative similarly to Norway but soon, opened up to include third-party services aiming to leverage existing services offered by health providers, software vendors and pharmaceutical companies. An *interoperability framework* defined the conditions for including third-party devices, systems and services. With the introduction of this framework, the *ownership and control of the services started to separate*. The Department gave up the ownership of the new services but not their control (kept the right to decide which new services would be offered). Since 2015, an *accreditation process* for mobile phone apps was also put in place, aimed at generating trustworthy apps through a quality certificate. Furthermore, apps (and later wearables and medical devices) that are accredited will be allowed to store and/or retrieve information from a governmental repository for patient-generated health data which allows interoperability with both the patient-oriented eHealth services and the health information systems of health providers.

In Italy, the development of e-booking services was owned and managed by a specialised unit created within the Health Department of the municipality of Bologna, the Single Booking Centre (CUP: Centro Unificato di Prenotazione). CUP was an inter-institutional office that included personnel from the three local health units and was *led by the city councillor* in charge of the department. After the launching of the service an improvement process was also launched involving all the main actors, the Health Department, the three health units, ITALSIEL (the state-owned software company that developed the solution which was at that time the largest software company in Italy) and SYNWARE (which employed the workers that staffed the 25 e-booking centres). The Health Department and specifically the CUP directorate led the process. With the advent of the e-booking project, control moved to the CUP directorate, not only for the technical infrastructure, but also for the non-technical parts of the service offering. This involved lengthy negotiations with hospitals to increase the extent of services to be offered on the centralized booking system. In the Italian case, the Health Department, represented by the city councillor, was the main protagonist and played a leadership role in both the design and realization of the project. The leadership orientation was strongly influenced by the political positioning of the city councillor and also by the specific academic background of the councillor (sociology of healthcare). The support of a well-known academic figure in the field helped to legitimize the city councillor's position in health management. Although the booking project was strongly contested by many of the participants (most notably the health units' boards of medical directors and head physicians) it was successfully carried out due to the strong political support.

Strategies for Addressing Heterogeneity in Technical Components

The strategies for addressing the challenge of technical heterogeneity were also diverse. In the case of Sweden, technological heterogeneity was embraced, but a uniform user experience was ensured. Similarly, in Denmark, a uniform user experience was pursued for accessing data from different underlying sources. Still, in the Danish case, the portal included links to external services for information exchange with GP offices that did not have a uniform user interface. In Norway, this was avoided by developing new links to existing GP office health systems. The case from Italy is dissimilar to the other four cases because it started during an earlier technological era. Being a first-mover meant that there were no similar solutions already in the field. In the following paragraphs we go through the different strategies for addressing technical heterogeneity in detail.

In Denmark, the portal solution became part of an eHealth landscape where it was already possible for different technological solutions to "work together" as communication standards for information flows between medical practices, hospitals, and pharmacies were in place. The Danish solution embraced heterogeneity to a great extent. For example, the portal *directs patients to the GP websites* (provided by various vendors) to initiate booking of appointments and conducting email consultations. Overall, health data and services provided through the portal are based on *displaying already existing data* from various heterogeneous sources. In some cases, data are extracted from their sources (such as hospital systems, GP systems, prescription databases) and then presented through the portal's presentation layer. In other cases, services are "framed" to achieve a consistent 'look and feel' although the service is located and run somewhere else.

In Norway, the existing heterogeneous technical components were addressed by a series of decisions. One important decision was to not link the platform with the existing private eHealth portals used by several GP offices for communicating with patients. So, differently to the approach followed in Denmark, the platform that was put in place *does not redirect users to private portals.* Instead, new links with the existing GP office EPR systems were developed in collaboration with the EPR vendors. The main reasons for this decision, were to ensure a uniform user experience and to control the level of security offered. Although the private portals were not linked to the platform, *several components of the public eHealth infrastructures were linked.* These components include the pre-existing national services for changing GPs and for accessing vaccination history. Furthermore, the platform provided access to prescriptions (leveraging the national e-prescription project) and to summary care records (leveraging the national Summary Care Record project). The platform did not only embrace national-level eHealth initiatives, but also regional ones that were aligned with the platform's strategy and had the potential to be scaled to a national level. One such initiative provides access to medical records and another one supports message exchange between hospitals and patients. Overall, the aim was to homogenise the quality levels and user experience for services offered nationally.

In Sweden, heterogeneity is embraced as long as a uniform user experience is ensured. For example, it is possible to allow e-services to be developed and deployed outside of the portal platform itself but this should be accomplished in a way that independently deployed e-services would bring the same user experience as that of an e-service developed and deployed using the tools and infrastructure of the core portal. This allows the development of national e-services using the development and deployment infrastructure of choice. This is aligned with one of the national reference architectural principles which stipulates that integrations shall be loosely coupled and reusable for many purposes.

In Catalonia, the strategy was to embrace multiple different solutions including services offered by health providers, software vendors and pharmaceutical companies. Furthermore, an accreditation process for mobile phone apps was also put in place. Practically, the Catalonian portal *provides an additional channel to access selected applications,* but does not replace the direct access links provided by the service owners. Although this strategy does not ensure a uniform user-experience, it does ensure uniform high levels of quality. As several of the external solutions linked to the portal were developed abroad, keeping pace with the new releases of the APIs proved to be challenging. The experiences from this case study bring forward the complexity of embracing such a wide variety of solutions.

The Italian initiative started during an earlier technological era (the service was launched at the end of January 1990), when many of the currently available technological possibilities for loosely connecting heterogeneous components were not available. Furthermore, the e-booking services were innovative for that era. Being a first mover meant that initiative *did not encounter a landscape filled with alternative solutions*. The main technological concern was to develop a stable and satisfactorily performing solution given the time constraints (the centralized booking system had to be deployable within 6 months).

Strategies of Addressing Uncertainty by Organising Responsiveness to Evolving Needs

Uncertainty was another major challenge for all cases. It was important for all initiatives to put in place organisational and technological strategies that would allow responsiveness to new needs. There were two main types of strategies followed in the cases studied. In Denmark, Norway and Italy, the initiatives were organised towards *fully pre-planned change*. In all three cases, an organised process for collecting needs, prioritising them and planning new development was put in place. The cases of Catalonia and Sweden were different to the other three cases in the sense that allowed more organic change to happen with the contribution of multiple distributed actors. In the paragraphs that follow we go through the different strategies towards uncertainty.

In Denmark, development projects were *prioritised in collaboration with multiple partners* as the organisational entity that ran the platform did not have any specific strategic mandate or responsibility. This was a lengthy process and in some cases the priorities of the partners would shift after certain tasks had been initiated (for example, a new urgent need for adding functionality to register citizens' wishes for organ donation popped up and had to be accommodated). After the decision to handle most development of services in-house (as opposed to development by external consultants), it *became a challenge to keep up with the pace of demands*. Furthermore, the partners started being inpatient with the need to constantly discuss prioritizing services. While the portal was very visionary at the beginning, it could easily get behind regarding current trends in a fast moving sector of digital health services where there always new needs for linking up with new data sources and providers. To ensure responsiveness to needs, a re-organisation took place recently to increase delivery capacity and strengthen portfolio management. The future focus is on being proactive and assist the partners in developing and maturing new service concepts.

In Norway, a similar process of *collecting needs and prioritising development was put in place*. During the early stages of development, a number of studies were prepared with the contribution of multiple stakeholders to plan the services to be developed over time. In 2014, the Health Directorate that has ownership and control over the platform, collaborated with the Norwegian National ICT (NICT) which is the interest body for information and communication technologies in the specialist healthcare sector formed by the four Regional Health Authorities. The collaboration aimed to identify citizens' needs for digital services in specialized care to obtain insights for further developing the platform. The result was an extensive mapping and analysis of users' needs involving health personnel, citizens and management bodies of the health regions. The analysis ended up with the identification of priority service areas, informed the formulation of a strategy for digital specialist health services, and led to the formation of a specific project on digital citizen services for the specialist sector.

In Italy, an *improvement process* was put in place right after launching the e-booking service. The process *involved all the main protagonists*, the Health Department, the three health units, ITALSIEL and SYNWARE. The Health Department, specifically *the CUP directorate, led this process*. Overall, also in this case, organisational processes for planning and controlling changes were implemented.

In Sweden the principle of *local contribution* to the national ecosystem was formalised and became one of the six architecture principles of the national reference architecture. In the cases of local and regional needs that are not aligned with national prioritizations, a group of county councils, municipalities and solution vendors have been able to join forces to develop solutions on their own for more local and regional use. The principles of national functional scope secure that the solution can grow to a national scale in the future. As time passes by, county councils, municipalities and solution vendors continuously negotiate to bring their local or regional solution to a national level, sharing the solution with all publicly funded care in Sweden.

In Catalonia, the new patient-oriented eHealth services had to face uncertainty and multiple possible alternatives. Since many of the services could not be specified in advance, decisions and choices had to be *exploratory and adaptable*. At the beginning of the project, the sponsors of the portal tied the development to the Public Shared Electronic Medical Record. So, the portal started simple, without a big architectural blueprint and complex anticipatory design. A catalyst for further growth has been the decision to put in place the means for connecting to existing applications and *stimulating the development of new ones by third parties*. The interoperability framework and the app accreditation process were critical for this.

Strategies Towards Transformation

In all cases, the new platforms were developed with the aim of achieving a patient-orientation within an overall traditionally provider-centric system. In other words, they had to face the challenge of becoming embedded to the installed base while transforming it. In the cases from Denmark, Norway, Sweden and Catalonia the strategies followed were overall "*installed base friendly*" in the sense, that, all developments were based on wide consensus and transformations were attempted in small steps. The case from Italy stands out as a clearly *disruptive* strategy was followed. In the next paragraphs we elaborate on each case.

In Denmark, there has been *broad support* from relevant players in the Danish healthcare arena. Especially the initial phase can be characterized as a political showcase for regional collaboration with solid political unity and common ambition. During this phase, there was little disagreement concerning what should be offered to citizens and healthcare providers. The political unity and broad collaboration of stakeholders were described as key reasons for the success of the portal.

Similarly, in Norway, the views and needs of the health sector and also of the technology providers were taken into account and multiple processes for "*anchoring*" the initiative within the sector were taken. These anchoring processes allowed stakeholders to voice their concerns and shape the initiative, while at the same time the designers of the new services were able to expose their plans and explain their rationales. The Norwegian platform was expanded by orientating towards the satisfaction of concrete needs expressed by potential users while the overall evolution has been incremental and gradual.

In Sweden, the e-services offered were not perceived as controversial since they *did not entail profound changes* in the role and relationships between doctors and patients, and between doctors themselves. Instead early on results showed increased work processes effectiveness and less need for accessing healthcare centres by phone for renewal of prescriptions or bookings.

In Catalonia, the underlying vision for the new eHealth services has been the idea of self-care and preventive care – i.e., that citizens become more autonomous, responsible and participative in matters concerning their own health. The realization of this vision requires *reconfiguring multiple of the existing relationships* and the creation of new ones. For instance, since patients have more information about their own health, their relation with professionals, who are used to have control over the access to the patients' data, will probably change; the responsibility boundaries among professionals will most likely shift; and since the portal is becoming a new channel for the provision of health services, the public administration will have to reconsider the payment criteria for those services to health professionals and providers. Nevertheless, as the *changes are paced* there has been no major opposition from the wider sector.

Finally, the Italian case is the one where disruptive changes were pursued (and actually implemented). Improving citizens' access to healthcare was an element of the National Health Service reform, especially relevant in Bologna where long waiting lists, fragmented offerings and a lack of transparency characterized access to secondary care. The municipality of Bologna addressed these issues by leveraging new technological capabilities that allowed bookings to be performed without being controlled by the healthcare institutions. This created tensions and strong opposition by key actors from the medical establishment. The institutional components of the installed base revealed themselves as obstacles for achieving innovation and only the large mobilization of political, organizational, and technological resources made it possible.

4.4 Working with the Installed Base for Building eHealth Infrastructures

The cross-case analysis presented in the previous sections should be read together with the rich descriptions and analysis provided in the chapters that relate to each case. The cross-case analysis offers an entry point to the cases and a possible orientation for making sense of the different ways of working with the installed base for building eHealth infrastructures. The perspective taken in this book is that the installed base is the point of departure for change processes. The notion of installed base is a conceptual tool, not a name for some independently existing reality. The notion helps us to 'look for' something particular: by focusing on the installed base, attention is directed towards the links with existing arrangements and the evolutionary processes of the new eHealth infrastructure.

All initiatives aiming for novelty in healthcare delivery will entail planning for the existing elements that need to be retained and reused, and the elements that need to be eliminated or replaced. This act of distinguishing between elements to be reused or discarded identifies the relevant installed base for the initiative. In every change process there are aspects of both continuity and discontinuity. The relevant questions then become: What is continued and what is discontinued? In what sequence are the discontinuities introduced? What is the required work to achieve a certain transformation? How to engage with the existing situation – in a confrontational or cautious way? The questions address how initiatives relate to and deal with the installed base.

The main message of the cross-case analysis is that the successful development and implementation of initiatives for eHealth infrastructures require much more than creating a clear description of the goal, and having in place the necessary technological capabilities and human skills. It also requires a discerning and knowledgeable engagement with the particularities of the situation and an informed and conscious approach for working with the installed base.

Open Access This chapter is distributed under the terms of the Creative Commons Attribution-NonCommercial 2.5 International License (http://creativecommons.org/licenses/by-nc/2.5/), which permits any noncommercial use, duplication, adaptation, distribution and reproduction in any medium or format, as long as you give appropriate credit to the original author(s) and the source, provide a link to the Creative Commons license and indicate if changes were made.

The images or other third party material in this chapter are included in the chapter's Creative Commons license, unless indicated otherwise in a credit line to the material. If material is not included in the chapter's Creative Commons license and your intended use is not permitted by statutory regulation or exceeds the permitted use, you will need to obtain permission directly from the copyright holder.

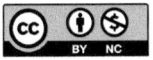

Part II
E-Prescription Infrastructures

Maintaining the Pharmacy Model: The Catalan Electronic Prescription Infrastructure

5

Joan Rodon Modol

5.1 Introduction

This chapter presents the genesis and evolution of the public e-prescription information infrastructure (EPI) of Catalonia, Spain from 2000 to 2013. The implementation of the EPI required a transition from a mainly paper-based and asynchronous prescription model to a digital and synchronous one. This transition involved doing changes into the practices, systems and roles of the CatSalut (the Catalan Health Service), doctors and health providers, pharmacists and Colleges of Pharmacists, and ultimately patients. Our narrative extols those changes and how the pre-existing technological and institutional resources of professionals shaped the design, and evolution of the infrastructure. Our narrative traces those events from the perspective of pharmacists and shows how the installed base of pharmacists was used and extended in a way that maintained and strengthened the pharmacy model.

The reminder of the chapter is structured as follows. In the next section, we present the Catalan model of community pharmacies (see the Chap. 11 for a description of the overall Catalan health system). This section is followed by our narrative of the case. Next we analyze and discuss the implications of our results.

5.2 Site: The Catalan Model of Community Pharmacies

The model of pharmacies in Spain compromises multiple components operating at different levels. At the lower level, there is the pharmacist, a health agent who exercises its professional practice in community pharmacies or hospital

J.R. Modol
ESADE Ramon Llull University, Av. Torreblanca 59, 08172 Sant Cugat del Vallès, Spain
e-mail: joan.rodon@esade.edu

© The Author(s) 2017
M. Aanestad et al. (eds.), *Information Infrastructures within European Health Care*, Health Informatics, DOI 10.1007/978-3-319-51020-0_5

pharmacies by dispensing drugs, producing patient-specific preparations, and other pharmaceutical care tasks (e.g. health promotion, tracking patients' medication record, checking drug interactions, etc.). In order to practice pharmacists must be registered in the College of Pharmacy of the province where they practice.

Community pharmacies are private health facilities of public interest. Pharmacies are the only health establishments authorized to dispense prescription-only medicines and over-the-counter medicines to the general public. Medicines in Spain are publicly funded. Until 2012 medicines were provided to pensioners for free; working age people paid 40% and those suffering from chronic illnesses paid 10% of the cost of medicines. From 2012 several copayment reforms at the regional and national level were approved that ended with this scenario (Puig-Junoy et al. 2014). First, a national coinsurance rate of 10% for retirees with a monthly income-related cap. Second, Catalonia charged temporally a linear one-euro copayment per prescription with a monthly cap. Third, a national reform stopped funding a long list of medicines indicated for minor symptoms.

The ownership of community pharmacies is limited to pharmacists (trained professionals); pharmacy chains are not allowed forms of ownership. One pharmacist or a group of pharmacists can own only one pharmacy. The establishment of pharmacies is regulated responding to demographic and geographic criteria in order to guarantee a homogeneous access of the services to citizens (99% of Spaniards have a community pharmacy in their municipality). On average a community pharmacy serves approximately 2,000 citizens. Regulations are defined at the national and the autonomous region levels. While the central government is in charge of the general coordination of pharmaceutical care and of matter related to pharmaceuticals such as registration, each autonomous region organizes the planning of the pharmacy system.

In the autonomous region of Catalonia, the main actors that constitute the field are: CatSalut (the Catalan Health Service), the Catalan Council of Pharmacists (CCP), the four Colleges of Pharmacists (which coalesce into the CCP), the community pharmacies, pharmacists, and business organization of pharmacies.[1] CatSalut is the public insurer that is responsible for planning, purchasing, and assessing health services according to the needs of the population. The CCP is a corporate and public legal entity that represents the interests of all pharmacists in Catalonia, as well as the interests of community pharmacy owners and ensures that regulations are respected.

A core component of the model of pharmacies is the agreement initially signed by the CatSalut and the CCP on January 31st 1995 that regulates the conditions by which pharmacists provide pharmaceutical care, invoice according to the contract economic regulations, temporary fund the dispensed drugs and health products,

---

[1] The FEFAC (www.fefac.cat) is the business organization of Catalan pharmacies. The FEFAC is non-profit federation that aims to defend the interests of pharmacy owners who voluntary enroll it. In 2015 there were about 1,600 (of the 3,000) pharmacies enrolled.

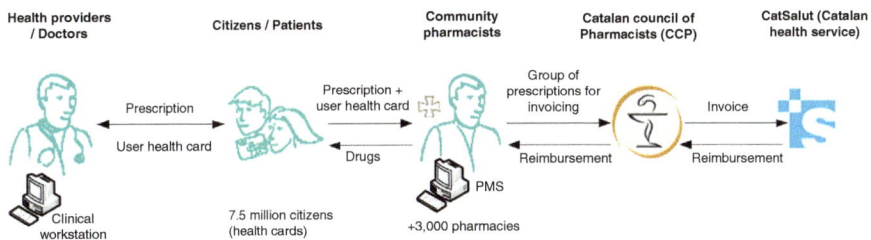

Fig. 5.1   Flows involved in the paper-based prescribing, dispensing and invoicing

continuously deliver health care information to the CatSalut, do health promotion and disease prevention, and perform pharmaceutical surveillance and security alert management of drugs and health products to the population served by the CatSalut. The agreement is continually renegotiated according to changes in the legislation, the profession, and society.

5.2.1   The Installed Base of Pharmacies

A core practice of pharmacists is the dispensing of drugs which interacts with other practices (e.g., prescribing, invoicing) and actors (e.g., doctors, patients, CCP, CatSalut), and involves flows of information, patients, money, and so on. Before the implementation of EPI, the flows were as follows (see Fig. 5.1). Once the doctor had decided the drug treatment for a patient the latter was given a paper prescription. Doctors used clinical workstations to generate the prescriptions and print them. The patient took the prescription and her health card[2] to the community pharmacy, where the drug was dispensed. Then pharmacists stored and signed those paper based prescriptions. Pharmacists used a pharmacy management system (PMS) for tasks such as the management of sales, inventory, or purchasing orders. In 2004, when the EPI project was to start, there were about 35 different types of PMS. Those PMS were developed by pharmaceutical wholesalers, software vendors or individual developers. Periodically, pharmacies grouped the paper-based prescriptions they had dispensed in a given period of time and sent them to the CCP. The CCP then checked all those prescriptions, scanned them, forwarded the scanned and paper prescriptions to the CatSalut, and handled the invoicing for pharmacies. In particular, the CCP submitted a single invoice to the CatSalut. So, the CCP, not pharmacists, was the one in charge of invoicing the CatSalut. The CatSalut reimbursed that invoice to the CCP who checked for errors and finally paid pharmacies according to the signed prescriptions they had previously sent.

---

[2] The individual health card has a magnetic stripe containing data fields such as the code of the insured (the citizen), the name and surname, her number of social security affiliation, type of insured (level of coverage), and the expiration data.

Method

Data was collected from three main sources: semi-structured face-to-face in-depth interviews (20 interviews), participant observation (workshop attendance; informal conversations; direct on-site observation), and archival data (more than 500 press documents, reports, meeting minutes, and videos), aiming at data triangulation (Yin 2003). Data collection has taken place in three intensive period May – August 2008, January – May 2010, and February – May 2013. We identified interviewees by referral from other subjects. All the interviews were recorded and immediately transcribed and analyzed next two the archival data and other observations. In that sense, data collection and analysis took place iteratively.

With all the data gathered, we constructed an initial timeline of events for the genesis and evolution of the EPI. We then wrote a rich chronological case story that put at the forefront the role of the installed base. We organized the case narrative into four stages covering the period 2000–2013.

5.3   Case Narrative

5.3.1   Phase 1: Genesis of the e-Prescription Infrastructure in Catalonia (2000–Mid-2004)

In 2000, the Spanish Ministry of Science and Technology in collaboration with governments of the autonomous regions and the representatives of the diverse professionals involved in prescribing and dispensing – that is, the Colleges of Doctors and the Councils of Pharmacists – started working on the foundations for a common Spanish reference model for e-prescription.

Meanwhile, in 2001 the Catalan Council of Pharmacists (CCP) and the College of Doctors led a successful first pilot of e-prescription in Barcelona for private health involving a hundred private doctors and 25 pharmacies. The CCP proposed the CatSalut to bring that pilot to the public health, but the CatSalut refused it arguing that they were involved in the Spanish project and should wait until it ended. Moreover, as an outcome of this pilot of e-prescription, the CCP and the College of Doctors created Firma Profesional,[3] a Certification Authority that issued digital certificates for those pharmacists and doctors involved in the pilot (Cordobés 2002b). Meanwhile, from October 1st 2001, the citizens insured by the CatSalut had to bring their individual health card at pharmacies in order to pick up the drugs prescribed at the public health system (Gilabert-Perramon and Prat 2001). During the dispensing process pharmacies had to check whether the individual health card matched the patient data that appeared in the paper-based prescription, and store the data of the patient, the code of the prescription and the dispensed drug. From 2003 those data had to be electronically submitted to the CatSalut (Gilabert-Perramon et al. 2010).

---

[3] www.firmaprofesional.com

In short, these events became catalysts for the computerization of all the Catalan pharmacies.

The first draft of the model for the Spanish e-prescription was released in 2002. The model comprised a single central database that would be used by both pharmacists and doctors for prescribing and dispensing respectively. That model dissatisfied the Council of Pharmacists who perceived and argued that the main goal of the central government was to control their practice and to reduce public expenditure on drugs, rather than the use of IT for pharmaceutical care (Cordobés 2002a). Finally, in 2004 in accordance with the decentralized health system of Spain and with the Spanish law for the cohesion and quality of the national health system (CohesionAct 2003) diverse autonomous regions started their own e-prescription projects.

It was in mid-2004 when the CatSalut set the foundations for the building of e-prescription infrastructure (EPI) in Catalonia involving all health agents (e.g., health providers, college of doctors, Catalan Council of Pharmacists). With EPI, the CatSalut sought to improve the efficiency of the health system by streamlining patients' access, containing drug expenditures, and reducing prescription and dispensation errors due to lack of coordination between the agents involved in those processes (Gilabert and Cubi 2009; Gilabert-Perramon et al. 2010). To achieve those goals, the CatSalut proposed doing changes to existing practices. For instance, doctors would not make individual prescriptions anymore but medication plans[4] (see Fig. 5.2) that would last up to 1 year; that in turn, would eliminate the need for co-presence of patients and doctors in the prescribing process and would reduce the number of patient appointments with primary care. Patients would pick up medicines at any pharmacy according to a concrete temporal window thus avoiding that patients accumulated more drugs than necessary. Patients would have to bring their medication plans and their health cards to pick the medicines at pharmacies. Medicines would be dispensed at any pharmacy regardless of the location of the prescriber.

The CatSalut defined two core requirements for EPI. First, all the data – i.e., prescriptions, dispensations, invoices, patients, drugs, health providers, doctors, pharmacies, pharmacists – should be integrated and accessible online by the diverse stakeholders – CatSalut, doctors, and pharmacists. Second, the processes of prescribing and dispensing should run in real time. Accordingly, the CHS would have information about the acts of prescribing and dispensing in real-time and would be able to influence both acts for instance by forcing the prescription of generics.

To fulfil these requirements and in line with the reference model defined by the Spanish Ministry of Science and Technology in 2002, the CatSalut proposed a model (see Fig. 5.3) consisting of a central system owned and managed by the CatSalut (called SIRE) that contained an integrated database with all the data. On

---

[4] A medication plan has a bar code that is read in the pharmacy (top right in Fig. 5.2) and includes (columns from left to right in Fig. 5.2): the drug, the dose and frequency, duration of treatment, doctor and health centre, temporal window with the validity of the plan, and comments and observations.

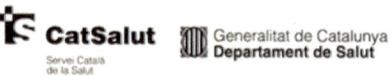

Data darrera modificació: 08.04.2011
Pàgina 1 de 2

Pla de medicació

Nom i cognoms del/de la pacient

TASA1030101002

Informació
per a la farmàcia

Tractaments de llarga durada

Medicament o producte sanitari i núm. de prescripció	Dosi i freqüència	Durada del tractament	Prescriptor/a i centre	Vigència	Comentaris
METFORMINA 850MG 50 COMPRIMI RECUB PELIC EFG P1E000152759	1 Unitat cada 8 hores	Segons evolució clínica	X. Vinyals (Col: 117018036) Medicina familiar i comunitària EAP Mataró Cirera Molins	del 02.01.11 al 02.01.12	Preneu-lo amb aliments.
HIDROSALURETIL 50MG 20 COMPRIMIDOS P1E000729153	0,5 Unitat cada 24 hores	Segons evolució clínica	D. Castelvií (Col: 117027063) Cardiologia Hospital de Mataró	del 02.02.11 al 02.02.12	En dejú, abans d'esmorzar.

Fig. 5.2 Example of the medication plan (printed on paper) that doctors give patients

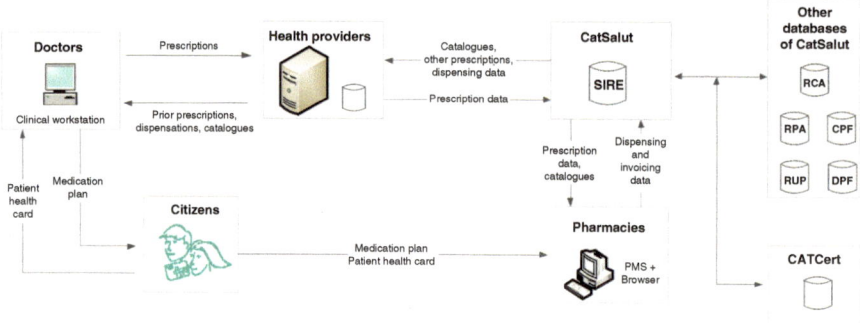

Fig. 5.3 Initial EPI model proposed by the CatSalut

the one side, the health providers would have to interconnect their systems with the CatSalut system (SIRE). On the other side, pharmacists would connect directly to SIRE – through a browser – for the dispensing and invoicing processes.

5.3.2 Phase 2: Mobilizing the Pharmacists' Installed Base (Mid-2004–Mid-2006)

Although CatSalut's model was framed as an efficient and effective way to conform to the two core requirements, the CCP argued that it was bypassed in the dispensing and invoicing and that was a threat to the existing pharmacy model. Such a direct

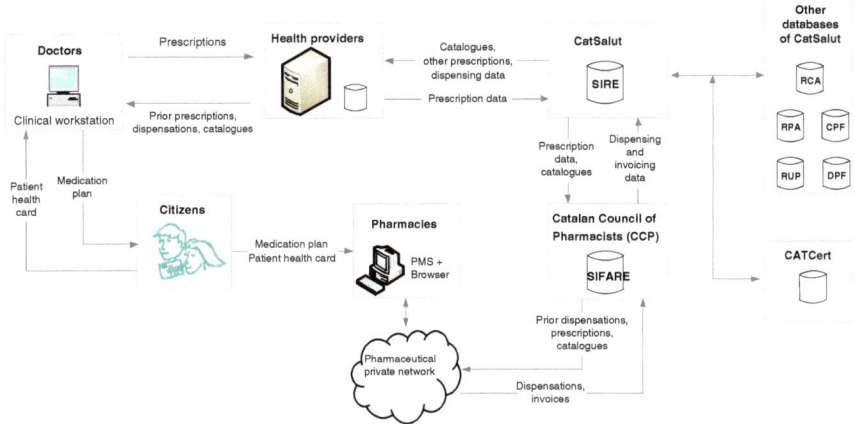

Fig. 5.4 Alternative EPI model proposed by the CCP

relationship between the CatSalut and pharmacists was against the terms of the existing pharmaceutical agreement. It weakened the position of pharmacists in front of the CatSalut who could more easily change the conditions that regulate pharmacies on an individual basis.

As a response, the CCP then proposed an alternative model on the pharmacists' side (see Fig. 5.4) consisting of a private network (VPN) that would interconnect all the pharmacies plus a central server (called SIFARE) that replicated the data of the CatSalut system that was needed for pharmacists – i.e., prescriptions, dispensations and data catalogues. Both the private network and SIFARE would be owned by the CCP. Community pharmacies would not have a direct access to SIRE (the CatSalut system) but instead to SIFARE (the CCP system) through the VPN, and the SIFARE would synchronize in real time with the SIRE for dispensing and invoicing. A vice-president of the CCP related the pharmacy model with the VPN in the following terms: "We are a network [the pharmacy model in Catalonia] that needs a network [the VPN]… Politicians argue for a capillary pharmacy model; that is, that pharmacies are spread throughout the country. We must transfer this network of pharmacies to the electronic world. It cannot happen that what is there physically does not exist electronically." Moreover, this new conceptual model guaranteed that all pharmacies would have the same conditions for dispensing and invoicing, and offered the opportunity for the professional development of pharmacists as they could implement new digital services on SIFARE and the VPN.

Initially, the CatSalut did not see the CCP's model (Fig. 5.4) favorably. The CCP was afraid that it could penalize the fulfilment of the two central requirements of data integration and real-time processes. Yet, the CatSalut saw that the CCP was a legitimized actor whose involvement in the project was critical for its success. Without the CCP, it would be very difficult to mobilize pharmacists. So, after some negotiations the CatSalut bowed to the interests of the CCP and the pharmacists, and accepted the CCP's model on May 2005. A manager of the CatSalut and leader of the EPI project retrospectively justified the final model in the following terms: "Why do pharmacies invoice us through the CCP? Well, I think it is something that is good for both of us. It is not the same to have 3,000 interlocutors as to have just one as with the CCP. Of course it has its good and bad aspects for both sides. However, for the CCP this means empowering the collective and serving in a role as representative of a collective. I imagine that the members of the CCP [pharmacists] are interested in somebody that brings them together and defends them in the negotiations. Moreover, this relationship structure is not new, it has some history."

The governance structure of the project also helped consolidate the CCP's model. It consisted of two main committees: a steering committee, and an executive committee later called follow-up committee, in which diverse members of the CatSalut, CCP, health providers and other stakeholders were present.[5] A manager of the CatSalut and leader of the EPI project depicted that committee structure as follows "This has been an integrative project from the first day... We started doing things all together [the sector]. Accordingly, we built this governance structure consisting of multiple committees that included all the agents."

In building the architecture for the model, the CatSalut opted for an architecture for SIRE based on web services. That is, the systems of health providers and those of the CCP would interact with SIRE through web services using SOAP and XML. The CatSalut developed two sets of web services (see Fig. 5.5): one set for prescribing that would be used by health providers, and another one for dispensing and invoicing that would be used by the CCP.

A main design decision of the CCP was that SIFARE should be as transparent as possible for pharmacists such that they would not be forced to use an additional information system for dispensing and invoicing. This meant that pharmacists should be able to integrate their existing pharmacy management systems (PMS) with SIFARE in a way that minimized the changes to their practices. To achieve so, the CCP boosted in 2005 a recognition program for PMS vendors that it had launched in 2004 aiming to guarantee that PMS vendors fulfilled the needs and requirements of community pharmacists set by the CCP and CHS. The initial scope of the recognition program had been that of patient's health card reading and data transmission for invoicing. In 2005 the CCP extended the recognition program to include e-prescription. The CCP developed a set of web services for SIFARE and an application program interface (API) exposed in a DLL for the convenience of PMS vendors. Those vendors who passed the recognition program got the API from the CCP to interconnect their PMS solutions with SIFARE. That is, getting that recognition became a necessary condition for PMS vendors to remain in the market. From the about 35 PMS solutions that existed in 2004, only 9 got the recognition. Of the nine recognized PMS, five PMS got the recognition in 2005, one in 2007 and three in 2008. Five of those nine recognized PMS were developed, commercialized and

---

[5] In 2014 this organizing structure was still running. The steering committee meets every quarter, and the follow-up committee meets monthly. Likewise, working groups are created when new domains of study are required (e.g. prescribing and dispensing by active ingredient, prescribing and dispensing of narcotics, professional filters, certification and authentication of professionals).

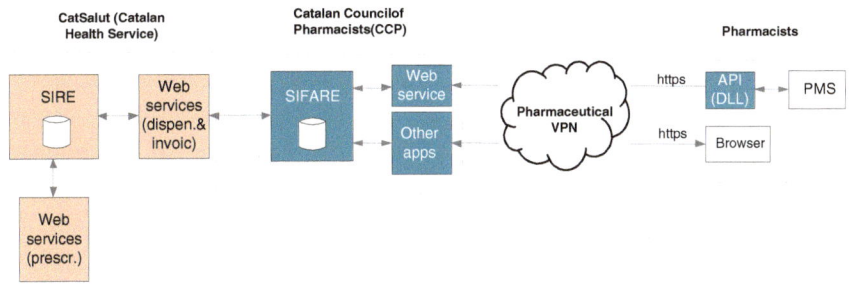

Fig. 5.5 EPI architectural components on the pharmacists' side.

supported by pharmaceutical wholesalers, and the other four by software vendors. The rest of PMS solutions were progressively discontinued.

Overall, the EPI architecture (Fig. 5.5) was modular in production. It decomposed the EPI into loosely coupled components: SIRE, SIFARE, and PMS that were interconnected through web services, and it influenced the role of actors in the project. For instance, the CPP would be in charge of (1) building the virtual private network (VPN) for pharmacies, (2) developing the SIFARE and (3) assuring that pharmacists integrated their PMS with SIFARE.

The security model, a central component of the EPI architecture, was defined by the Catalan Certification Agency[6] and included the following kind of requirements (eSignAct 2003): electronic certificate for professionals for their authentication (SAML authentication), digital signature of all the professional tasks, verification of signature, data encryption to ensure integrity and confidentiality, and obligatory use of patient health card and security code to access patient data. For the communication between SIRE and SIFARE they established a secure channel (SSL-Two-Way) ensuring the origin and destination of information and confirming that they are who they say they are. The CCP would act as a Registration Authority ensuring that any digital certificate is bound to the pharmacist to whom it is assigned in a way that assures non-repudiation.

Regarding the communications, pharmacies would be connected through a virtual private network (VPN). After a tender for the VPN in 2006, the CCP signed an agreement with a telecom provider. That agreement homogenized the service and price conditions for all the pharmacies, regardless of their location or size. Each pharmacy would have an asymmetric digital subscriber line (ADSL) and a backup integrated services digital network (ISDN) line to connect to the central server of the CCP – SIFARE. CCP would coordinate the rollout of the VPN with that of the EPI. From 2012 some pharmacies started setting up 3G back-up connections.

---

[6] The Catalan Certification Agency is a governmental agency that was set up in 2002 in order to implement and rollout the digital signature in all the Catalan governmental institutions and provide services to those organizations ensuring that the electronic transactions fulfill the legal guarantees.

5.3.3   Phase 3: Pilot and Rollout of EPI (Mid-2006–2010)

In 2005, the CatSalut had worked on a detailed list of functional requirements, and made a public tender for the development and implementation of SIRE. The goal was to launch a pilot by early 2006. With the first version of the SIRE web services for dispensing and invoicing, the CCP developed a first version of the SIFARE web services and the first API for PMS vendors. With that API, PMS vendors had to adapt their solutions for e-prescription, and install and configure the new version of the PMS in pharmacies.

   In 2006 the CatSalut and the CCP signed an appendix to the pharmaceutical agreement which established the clauses for the development of the pilot for the EPI, and made explicit the role of the CCP. This appendix helped stabilize the EPI by clarifying the roles of actors. On April 2006 a first pilot was inaugurated. However, due to repeated technical problems and errors, the CatSalut stopped the pilot and started a new version of SIRE that addressed those problems. On May 2007 the Catalan Parliament passed an act that regulated e-prescription (ePresDecree 2007; ePresOrder 2008). By the end of 2007, the CatSalut resumed the pilot involving five basic heath areas in two of the seven health regions of Catalonia (Girona and Terres de l'Ebre). The general practitioners, pharmacies and patients of those heath regions were gradually added into the pilot; the general practitioners decided which patients should be prescribed electronically. On May 2008 the pilot was satisfactorily completed. The pilot had involved 63 doctors, 39 pharmacies and 15,000 patients, and more than 300,000 prescriptions had been dispensed (Gilabert-Perramon et al. 2010). Then the rollout of the EPI in primary care started. It was organized into five phases, each involving one or more health regions (see Table 5.1).

   The fifth phase of the rollout involved the health region of Barcelona where there were about 2,200 of the more than 3,000 pharmacies in Catalonia. This last phase was also a very critical one as it could destabilize the whole project. First, since it took place in Barcelona, news about any failure would spread fast and that would have a greater political impact for sponsors. Second, it involved a considerable increase in the number of transactions, health providers, pharmacies, and patients. Accordingly, it required upgrading the technological infrastructure. On the side of pharmacists, the CCP re-scaled the hardware of SIFARE four times from 2006 to 2012 in order to accommodate the growth in the number of transactions derived from the scaling of EPI (see Table 5.3).

Table 5.1 Roll out of the EPI at primary care

Phase	Health regions involved	To start on
1	Girona, Terres de l'Ebre	May 2008
2	Camp de Tarragona	October 2008
3	Lleida, Alt Pirineu – Aran	October 2008
4	Catalunya Central	April 2009
5	Barcelona	May 2009

An important concern for the CCP was the cost of the technical infrastructure for the CCP and pharmacists. To overcome that concern, the CCP actively sought funding for SIFARE and VPN as well as the investments that pharmacists had to carry out (e.g. the connectivity services to the VPN, upgrading of PMS, the digital signatures, swipe card and swipe card readers). On the one hand, the main idea for funding the technological infrastructure of the CCP was that the reduction of cost related to the processing paper-based dispensations for invoicing (e.g. scanning and checking of dispensations) would be dedicated to pay the new technological infrastructure. Likewise, in 2008 the CCP got a subsidy from the Center of Innovation and Development of the Catalan Government. On the other hand, regarding the funding of pharmacists' investments, by early 2008 the CCP signed an agreement with a Spanish bank. According to that agreement, the bank would partially assume the connectivity costs of pharmacists and provide them with digital certificates and swipe card readers for free.[7] Later in 2010 the CCP received some financial aid from the Department of Health of Catalonia for the connectivity of pharmacies. Moreover, a condition for those PMS vendors passing the recognition program was that they would assume the costs of adapting their systems to interconnect with SIFARE and the costs of upgrading the PMS for their customers (the pharmacies).

Additionally, in order to support pharmacists during the rollout, the CCP created in 2008: (1) an e-newsletter to inform them; and (2) an IT Operations Center to support pharmacies in resolving technical problems, performing a baseline audit to check whether pharmacies were ready for e-prescription, informing them about the calendar for the rollout in their area, and support pharmacies in their daily practices with EPI. Later the CCP extended the scope of service of the IT Operations Center to include the monitoring of the infrastructure in order to detect failures before pharmacists realized them. The aim was to anticipate problems, keep pharmacists informed, as well as force and help the telecom provider to resolve incidents.

The rollout was completed during the third quarter of 2010. At that time all the more than 3,000 Catalan pharmacies were using the EPI. On August 2010 the prescriptions dispensed electronically accounted for 50% of all the prescriptions being billed[8] (see Table 5.2 for an evolution of electronic prescriptions being dispensed). In 2011 the CatSalut estimated that the e-prescription had saved around 5,100,000 patient appointments with primary care centers for collecting recipes. During 2011 the EPI was rollout at the specialized care and was completed by mid-2014. The rollout was extended to the geriatric residences and home care in 2012, and to mental care in 2013.

---

[7] Those conditions applied to pharmacies having a certain volume of business with the bank. In 2012 the funding agreement with the bank was still in place and the number of pharmacies benefiting from it had remained constant (around 1,300).

[8] In 2010 electronic prescription was only running at primary care, not at hospital and specialized care. The CatSalut encouraged the use of EPI among health providers by means of incentives defined in the multi-annual contracts that CatSalut signs with health providers.

Table 5.2 Electronic prescriptions being dispensed

Year	% (Electronic prescriptions/prescriptions billed[a])	Daily volume
2011	73,6	385.000
2012	85,3	430.000
2013	91,2	460.000
2014	95,4	522.100

Source: CatSalut
[a]Prescriptions billed includes the sum of electronic and paper-based prescriptions of all the primary care levels

5.3.4 Phase 4: Adaptation and Innovation on the Side of Pharmacists (2011–2013)

The functional evolution of the EPI has come from on the one hand, adaptations that are triggered by the CatSalut and the Catalan Spanish Governments, and on the other hand, new services that the CCP launches independently of the CatSalut.

In the first case, from 2006 to 2013 the CatSalut released 29 versions of SIRE web services with new functionalities (e.g. the inclusion of prescribing filters, the prescription by active ingredient, messaging among professionals, overdosing, and consult generic alerts). These functionalities reflect the approval of new laws, new requirements from the CatSalut and health professionals, and the new EPI rollouts at specialized and mental care, and geriatric residences. When the CatSalut creates a new SIRE web service for the dispensing and invoicing processes, the CCP immediately creates a new SIFARE web service and updates the API for PMS vendors. For instance, in 2012 the Catalan Government approved the "euro per prescription" tax that forced patients to pay an extra-euro for each drug dispensed at pharmacies (EuroPerPresAct 2012). To support this new tax the CatSalut developed three new web services. Then the CCP created three new services and the API 3 so that PMS vendors could adapt their applications to support such a tax. On average it takes between 6 and 8 months from the moment the API is delivered to PMS vendors until they update their PMS and install them in all the pharmacies. Similarly, in 2011 and 2012 the Spanish government passed two co-payment acts (copaymentReform 2011, 2012) which entailed that pensioners would have to partially pay medicines based on their income and with a monthly cap. The calculation of the final amount and the payment took place in the pharmacy when the patient picked the drug. This act entailed making changes to SIRE and SIFARE web services and to PMS.

However, it did not always happen that the release of a new version of an existing SIRE web service was followed by a new release of the corresponding SIFARE web service, and in turn, a change in the API for PMS vendors. That happened for instance, when a new feature included in a new SIRE web service was not mandatory (not required by law). Then the CCP might consider that the new feature did not add enough value to pharmacies, or that pharmacies were not ready, or that the CCP itself or the PMS vendors were not ready to implement that new version. Accordingly,

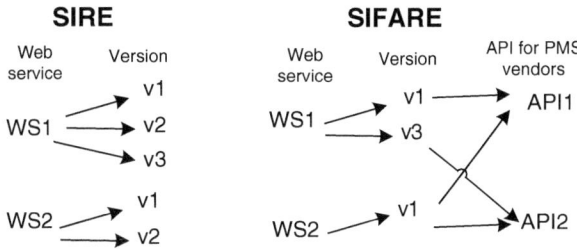

Fig. 5.6 Interdependencies between SIRE and SIFARE web services and API

the modular architecture of the EPI (Fig. 5.5) created a sequential interdependency between the CatSalut, the CCP, the PMS vendors and pharmacies in the development and release of new services (Fig. 5.6 illustrates this idea). This enabled the CCP to set the pace of evolution of the EPI by accommodating the changes triggered by the CatSalut to the needs and capacities of PMS vendors and pharmacists and its development resources.

The CCP has developed five versions of the API (which includes more than 30 web services): a first version in 2006 coinciding with the EPI pilot; a second one in 2009 before the massive roll-out in Barcelona; a third version in 2012 coinciding with two regulatory changes – the "euro per prescription" (EuroPerPresAct 2012) and co-payment act (copaymentReform 2011, 2012)–; a fourth version in 2012 to support the inclusion of paper-based prescriptions (e.g. generated at specialized care or other public mutual insurance companies) into EPI in order to dispense them electronically; and a fifth version in 2013 to support new professional services for pharmacists that are part of the SIFADATA initiative (which aimed to leverage on technology to digitalize pharmacists' processes and do analytics of the data at SIFARE).

On the other hand, the evolution of the EPI also came from new functionalities and services that the CCP developed on its own initiative –i.e., independently of the CatSalut. The rationale for those services was consistent with the vision of the CCP about the model of EPI. In particular, the CCP saw the EPI as an opportunity to re-professionalize the practice of pharmacists. For instance, from 2008 the CCP has been developing web apps to support pharmacists' work (e.g. tools to support the invoicing, management of alerts, management of users, and management of digital signature). Another example of a professional services tied to SIFARE was the SIFADATA initiative that the CCP launched by on 2012. This initiative involved redesigning other (than dispensing and invoicing) processes that pharmacists carry out daily and leveraging on the SIFARE and the VPN to digitalize them; this included for instance, the management of recipe and narcotics books, or the pricing of magistral formulae. In the case of the management of recipe and narcotics books, although most of the PMS stored those documents, pharmacists still had to periodically print those documents and carry them to the Department of Health. As part of the SIFADATA initiative the process was redesigned in a way that data would not only be locally stored at the PMS but also at SIFARE. Then pharmacists would electronically sign and submit the data stored at SIFARE to the Department of Health without any need to print them. With the development of this new kind of services, the CCP helped pharmacists by channeling their work practices through the PMS. At the same time the CCP boosted the use of the SIFARE and the VPN, and strengthened its role as service provider of pharmacists.

An assumption underlying this initiative was that the entry door for pharmacists to all those services must be the PMS. This requires the cooperation and involvement of PMS vendors who are expected to adapt their solution to the new services. In order to achieve so, the CCP leveraged the governance structure with PMS vendors. From the early stages of the project, the CCP created an advisory committee for technology and communications which brings together every quarter the CCP and the recognized PMS vendors to discuss about the status of the EPI and agree on its evolution – e.g. agree on the new requirements and services, on the pace of implementation of those services. What happened until 2012 was that, most of the adaptations that required developing new web services were triggered by the CatSalut, so eventually the PMS vendors had not choice implement them. However, with the development of professional services that are independent from the CatSalut, the PMS vendors cannot be obliged to implement them. Hence, PMS vendors became central actors in the strategy of the CCP regarding the new professional services. The CCP saw that for the launch of those professional services, the consensus with and involvement of the PMS vendors was much more critical. So the CCP felt the need to adapt the governing strategy with PMS vendors. To do so, in 2013 the CCP reoriented the focus of the recognition program more towards technical aspects and professional services.

Regarding those services that exploit the VPN, in 2011 the CCP set up a company called TicFarma seeking to transform all the pharmacies into a corporation which offered telecommunication services to the same pharmacies and pharmacists. With TicFarma, the CCP leveraged its ownership of the VPN to increase its bargaining power in front of telecom providers. TicFarma was a tool to: (1) reduce the connectivity costs for pharmacists, and (2) launch new telecommunication services for pharmacists. Moreover, the CCP used TicFarma's profits to pay the cost of the technological infrastructure consisting of the SIFARE and the VPN. Through TicFarma the CCP reinforced its role as a service provider for pharmacists.

5.4   Analysis and Discussion

Prior section has depicted the evolution of the Catalan e-prescription infrastructure (EPI) from the perspective of pharmacists. In particular, this chapter has narrated the transition from a paper-based asynchronous prescription model to a digital synchronous one. Our narrative has focused on how the Catalan Council of Pharmacists' (CCP) shaped that transition by appreciating the installed base and the potentialities of the EPI. Table 5.3 summarizes the evolution of the EPI according to several dimensions (timeline of events, regulations, and governance and architectural components).

Table 5.3 Evolution of EPI from the perspective of pharmacists

	Phase 1: genesis of EPI in Catalonia (2000–mid-2004)	Phase 2: mobilizing the pharmacists' installed base (mid-2004–mid-2006)	Phase 3: pilot and rollout of EPI (mid-2006–2010)	Phase 4: adaptation and innovation on the side of pharmacists (2011–2013)
Events	Spanish e-prescription project starts	Negotiations over the model for EPI between CatSalut and CCP	Pilot of EPI starts	CCP sets up TICFarma
	Pilot private e-prescription project in Catalonia	Tender for the VPN	1 PMS gets the recognition	Rollout at specialized care and geriatric centers starts
	Use of health card in dispensing	The development of EPI starts	Rollout of EPI stars (primary care)	CCP starts the SIFADATA initiative
	FirmaProfesional is set up	5 PMS get the recognition	3 PMS get recognition	New services at pharmacies (e.g. informing patients about treatments)
	Conceptual model of Spanish e-prescription is released	Agreement with a telecom provider for the VPN	Agreement with a bank to support pharmacies	Farmaguia mobile app
	Computerization of Catalan pharmacies	CCP becomes a Registration Authority	Rollout of EPI starts in Barcelona	
	Catalan EPI project starts		Rollout at primary care is completed	
			CCP launches web apps to support pharmacists' work	

(continued)

Table 5.3 (continued)

	Phase 1: genesis of EPI in Catalonia (2000–mid-2004)	Phase 2: mobilizing the pharmacists' installed base (mid-2004–mid-2006)	Phase 3: pilot and rollout of EPI (mid-2006–2010)	Phase 4: adaptation and innovation on the side of pharmacists (2011–2013)
Regulations and other social structures	Pharmaceutical agreement since 1995	Spanish Law on rational use of medicines	Catalan decree that regulated e-prescription	Co-payment acts
	Spanish laws for the cohesion and quality of the health system and about digital signature	CCP sets up a recognition program for PMS (data transmission and health card reading)	Order developing the decree	"Euro per prescription" tax
	Decree that regulates the use of health card	Setting up the Steering and Executive Committees for e-prescription	IT operations center to coordinate rollout and support pharma-cists	IT operations center extends its role
		CCP extends recognition program to include e-prescription.		Appendix to pharmaceutical agreement that reflects co-payment acts
		Appendix to pharmaceutical agreement		Changes to the recognition program (to support SIFADATA initiative)
		Advisory committee with PMS vendors		
Architectural components	Decentralized architecture with pharmacies using PMSs that were not connected to any central node and stored data locally	The centralized/hierarchical architecture is replaced by a new one involving two central nodes (Fig. 5.4) and modular (Fig. 5.5)	2 servers (up to 4 Million monthly dispensations)	Update of the VPN according to TICFarma requirements
	PMS progressively adapted to read health cards (data stored locally) and to use digital signature (data stored locally and asynchronous communication with central node)	The security model for EPI	SIFARE API 2 (before massive rollout in Barcelona)	SIFARE API 3 and 4 (to support co-payment reforms)
	Initial centralized/hierarchical architecture (only SIRE, Fig. 5.3)	SIFARE architecture (data stored at central nodes and locally at PMS)	6 servers (to support up to 6 Million monthly dispensations)	7 servers (to support up to 12 Million monthly dispensations)
		SIFARE API 1 (for the pilot)		SIFARE API 5 and new servers (to support new services from SIFADATA initiative)
		1 server (to support up to 100 Ks of monthly dispensations)		

On the one hand, our study shows how in building EPI, the exploitation and expansion of the installed base of pharmacists helped maintain the existing pharmacy model. Some of the technical components of EPI (e.g., SIFARE, the VPN, the security model) were built on and reinforced the installed base involving the pharmaceutical agreement and the pharmacy management systems (PMS). This also demonstrates that in building the EPI, the CCP thought in terms of what might happen – e.g. what might happen if the initial model for EPI proposed by the CatSalut (Fig. 5.3) was finally built. The CCP's concern was that the initial architecture proposed by the CatSalut could fragment the existing collective pharmaceutical agreement into individual agreements between CatSalut and pharmacists. So the CCP's counter-proposal for the EPI architecture protected the existing pharmaceutical agreement by avoiding any direct relationship between CatSalut and pharmacists.

Yet our narrative shows that the decision of the CCP to go for a new architectural model (Fig. 5.4) cannot be viewed simply as a radical shift at one point in time involving only individuals deliberate planning –i.e., choices and goals, matching means and ends–, but as a series of cumulative capabilities and events occurring from year 2000 that conferred legitimacy to the CCP –e.g., the pilot of e-prescription in the private health in 2001, the computerization of all pharmacies in 2003, the early version of the recognition program in 2004 to support the reading of individual health cards at pharmacies, and the implementation of health card recognition technologies.

On the other hand, this chapter also shows how the CCP also thought of EPI in terms of potentialities. For instance, on the side of pharmacists, the new recognition program and SIFARE API gave continuity to pharmacists' practices (pharmacists could keep using their PMS) while at the same time shifted the relationship between PMS vendors and pharmacists because the pace of updates and innovations of PMS would now be set by the pharmacists themselves (through the CCP). Moreover, the core components of EPI (SIFARE, VPN and recognition program) have enabled the CCP to act as a service provider and to foster innovation on new services for pharmacists (e.g. the SIFADATA initiative, TICFarma) and also for citizens (e.g. health information services offered through a portal www.farmaceuticonline.com, an app called farmaguia for locating pharmacists and informing about opening hours).

Finally, this chapter has presented a trajectory of an electronic prescription infrastructure. We argue that the longitudinal nature of our study (which covers the period 2000–2013), and our focus on the continuous causal interactions among multiple socio-technical components of the infrastructure has enabled us to give prominence to the role of the installed base in the evolution of the e-prescription infrastructure.

Acknowledgements This research was funded by the program "Internacionalització de la Recerca dels grups de recerca de la URL, un programa impulsat per la Universitat Ramon Llull amb la col·laboració de l'Obra Social 'la Caixa'".

References

CohesionAct. Ley 16/2003, de 28 de mayo, de cohesión y calidad del Sistema Nacional de Salud, en materia de prestación farmacéutica, BOE n.o 128 of May 29th 2003, Spanish Government, p. 20567–88; 2003.

copaymentReform. Real Decreto-ley 9/2011, de 19 de agosto, de medidas para la mejora de la calidad y cohesión del sistema nacional de salud, de contribución a la consolidación fiscal, y de elevación del importe máximo de los avales del Estado para 2011, BOE n°200 of August 20th 2011, Spanish Government; 2011.

copaymentReform. Real Decreto-ley 16/2012, de 20 de abril, de medidas urgentes para garantizar la sostenibilidad del Sistema Nacional de Salud y mejorar la calidad y seguridad de sus prestaciones, BOE n°98 of April 24th 2012, Spanish Government; 2012.

Cordobés A. Receta electrónica (I). Proyecto Pista y repercusiones sobre la oficina de farmacia. Offarm. 2002a;21(8):142–50.

Cordobés A. La receta electrónica (II). Proyectos de las comunidades autonomas. Offarm. 2002b;21(10):148–56.

ePresDecree. DECRET 159/2007, de 24 de juliol, pel qual es regula la recepta electrònica i la tramitació telemàtica de la prestació farmacèutica a càrrec del Servei Català de la Salut, DOGC n° 4934 of July 26th 2007, Catalan Government; 2007.

ePresOrder. 'ORDRE SLT/72/2008, de 12 de febrer, per la qual es desplega el Decret 159/2007', DOGC n°5081, Catalan Government; 2008.

eSignAct. Ley 59/2003, de 19 de diciembre, de firma electronica, BOE n.o 304 of December 20th 2003, Spanish Government; 2003. p. 45329–43.

EuroPerPresAct. Llei 5/2012, de 20 de març, de mesures fiscals, financeres i administratives i de creació de l'impost sobre les estades en establiments turístics, article 41, Capítol 21, CatSalut; 2012.

Gilabert A, Cubí R. La receta electronica en Cataluña (Rec@t):¿prescribimos o recetamos? Aten Primaria. 2009;41(6):298–9.

Gilabert-Perramon A, Prat A. La utilización de la tarjeta sanitaria individual (TSI) en las oficinas de farmacia. Informática y Salud. 2001;33:1713–4.

Gilabert-Perramon A, Lopez-Calahorra P, Escoda-Geli N, Salvadó-Trias C. Receta electronica en Cataluña (Rec@t): una herramienta de Salud. Med Clin. 2010;134(1):49–55.

Puig-Junoy J, Rodriguez-Feijoó S, Lopez-Valcarcel BG. Paying for formerly free medicines in Spain after 1 year of co-payment: changes in the number of dispensed prescriptions. Appl Health Econ Health Policy. 2014;12(3):279–87.

Yin RK. Case study research: design and methods. Thousand Oaks: Sage; 2003.

Open Access This chapter is distributed under the terms of the Creative Commons Attribution-NonCommercial 2.5 International License (http://creativecommons.org/licenses/by-nc/2.5/), which permits any noncommercial use, duplication, adaptation, distribution and reproduction in any medium or format, as long as you give appropriate credit to the original author(s) and the source, provide a link to the Creative Commons license and indicate if changes were made.

The images or other third party material in this chapter are included in the chapter's Creative Commons license, unless indicated otherwise in a credit line to the material. If material is not included in the chapter's Creative Commons license and your intended use is not permitted by statutory regulation or exceeds the permitted use, you will need to obtain permission directly from the copyright holder.

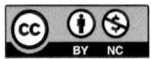

The ePrescription Initiative and Information Infrastructure in Norway

6

Ole Hanseth and Bendik Bygstad

6.1 Introduction

Several ePrescription initiatives were taken in Norway, the first in the early nineties. All failed, but, finally, an ePresecription II was built and widely adopted in the health care sector from 2011 onwards. There is a broad consensus that this solution and the initiative[1] behind it has been a great success. However, this success came after a long and painful "birth." The successful solution was developed with a strong focus on the involvement of GPs in the prescribing process even though the scope was intended to cover the whole chain. Later the solution was modified and extended in a number of ways: hospitals, support of multi-dose dispensing, becoming used as a crucial service for the national summary care record solution, and, hopefully, support for the rest of the primary care sector (i.e. midwives, public health nurses, home nurses, nursing homes as well as dentists).

The installed base, and the approaches for coping[2] with it, played a major role in the initiative, and was a key source of the challenges the initiative was

---

[1] The activities related to the ePrescription information infrastructure presented in this chapter, have been organized in different ways throughout its history. It started as a project. A couple of years later it was reorganized into a programme, and when the adoption process was getting momentum, the organizing of the activities changed into a more complex structure. For this reason, we use the term "initiative" to cover all these organizational forms which are described in more detail later in the chapter.

[2] The ePrescription initiative has never used the concept of "installed base" or related ones – at least we have never seen any traces of such concepts. Accordingly, the initiative did not have any deliberate strategy for dealing with the installed base either. We use the term "approach for coping with the installed base" for describing what would have been the initiative's operational strategy if it had been explicitly formulated.

O. Hanseth (✉) • B. Bygstad
Department of Informatics, University of Oslo, Postboks 1080, Blindern, 0316 Oslo, Norway
e-mail: oleha@ifi.uio.no; bendikby@ifi.uio.no

© The Author(s) 2017   73
M. Aanestad et al. (eds.), *Information Infrastructures within European Health Care*, Health Informatics, DOI 10.1007/978-3-319-51020-0_6

struggling with up to 2011. During 2011 they changed their approach to coping with the installed base. This change was an unintended result of an ad-hoc solution, a "quick fix," to a problem that had become urgent – the delayed development of a new EPR system by the vendor of such solutions having the largest market share. This change in the approach to coping with the installed base turned out to be a major contribution to the success of the solution – first the development of a solution that could be adopted by larger user groups and later the development of required of functionalities supporting multi dose dispensing and a major revision of all the involved.

All initiatives, also the latest one, has been based on the EDI paradigm with a strong focus on information sharing through message exchange between applications where the messages are specified and approved as standards and then implemented in the solutions. This approach is based on a classical specification driven approach to software development that implicit assumes that the new solution will be of a stand-alone kind developed from scratch. This contributed to make the initiative's approach to coping with the installed base schizophrenic: one the one hand the solution was designed as just extensions of existing applications like EPR systems and pharmacy applications (in addition to a central server and a secure network), on the other hand, it did not take seriously into account any challenges related to integrating the additional functionality to the existing installed base. This is true both for the existing applications and the platforms (PC hardware, operating system, network technologies, etc.) the applications were running on.

Methods

Our research approach was a case study conducted in the Norwegian health sector during a period of 7 years, from 2008 to 2015. Data collection included interviews with central stakeholders in the Ministry of Health, the Directorate of Health (who managed the project), and project developers and vendors, some of them several times during the study. In addition, we had access to the written materials of the project. This included the Government Budget documents, the project management documents, the system specifications and IT architecture documents.

Data analysis was conducted in the following steps. First a temporal analysis was done, focusing on the development over time. The identification of key events was done through interviews with central stakeholders and by a systematic analysis of the annual budgets of the Ministry of Health. Then a comprehensive analysis was conducted on the interplay of actors in the long project, such as government authorities, vendors, and users. Finally, we assessed and validated our findings by on-going presentations and discussions with key actors.

6.2   The Norwegian Health Care Sector

The Norwegian health care sector is primarily publicly funded. Until 2003 (most of) the hospitals were owned and managed by the 19 counties. By January 1st 2003 a reform was implemented. This implied that the government was taking over the ownership of the hospitals and organized them in 5, later four, regional corporations called Regional Health Authorities.

The primary care sector is managed at the municipal level. There are in total 428 municipalities in Norway – of these Oslo is the largest with app. 659,000 citizens and Utsira the smallest with only 203 citizens. GPs are either employed by municipalities or operating a private medical practice. These two groups are roughly of the same size.

Until March 1st 2001 the pharmacy sector was strictly regulated. Only pharmacists were allowed to own and run pharmacies and each pharmacist was allowed to own only one pharmacy. During 2001 the sector was liberalized and within a fairly short period more or less all pharmacies were taken over by large pharmacy groups, five in total, like for instance Boots.

6.3   Case Narrative

6.3.1   Establishment and Diffusion of a Solution for GPs

The ePrescription initiative starting 2004 was the most ambitious, well-funded, and professionally managed one among the efforts aiming at developing IIs for information exchange across institutional borders in the healthcare sector in Norway. Table 6.1 provides an overview of the timeline for the initiative.

In 2004, the Ministry of Health initiated a pilot study on electronic prescriptions. The background was a report in 2001 from the Office of the Auditor General that raised concerns on the accountability of prescription refunds from the Welfare Administration Agency. The following actors were included in the pilot study: the Norwegian Pharmacist's Union, National Insurance Administration (NIA), Norwegian Medical Association (representing physicians) and Norwegian Medicines Agency (NMA). The Directorate of Health managed the project.

The ePrescription project was established with direct funding of 40 million Euros from the Norwegian Parliament during 2005–2010. By the end of 2010 around 70 million Euros was spent on the project. During 2006 detailed requirements specifications and an architectural document was written, specifying an ambitious, fully integrated solution. Figure 6.1 illustrates the architecture of the II as it is presented in official project documents. The boxes represent the central data base server in the middle and applications (eight different EPR systems from six vendors used by hospitals and GPs, one pharmacy system used by all pharmacies, the MyPrescription module gives patients access to their prescriptions, and various applications run in three different government institutions). The blue arrows represent 31 different

Table 6.1 Timeline for the Norwegian e-prescription initiative

Timeline	
2001	Report from the Office of the Auditor General sent to the Parliament
2004	E-prescription project started
2006	Detailed design specification and architecture document released
2006	Invited EPR system vendors into the project
May 2008	First pilot. "Disaster"
2009	ePrescription exchange tested and accepted
June 2010	Pilot in Os municipality
Sept 2010	Pilot in Larvik
Autumn 2010	GPM developed
Spring 2011	GPM tested in lab
2011	Large scale deployment started
March 2012	Solution is deployed to about 280 GP offices and 134 pharmacies in 67 (of 428) municipalities distributed over 4 (of 19) counties. More than 1 mill prescriptions were sent
August 2012	Started extending the solution for Multi-Dose Dispensing (MDD)
Autumn 2012	GPM adapted to Dips and tested in hospital
2012	Started the development of version 2.5 of all standardized messages
June 2013	GMP adopted by all hospitals in the western health region
May 2014	First MDD pilot
Nov 2014	60 GP offices participating in MDD pilot

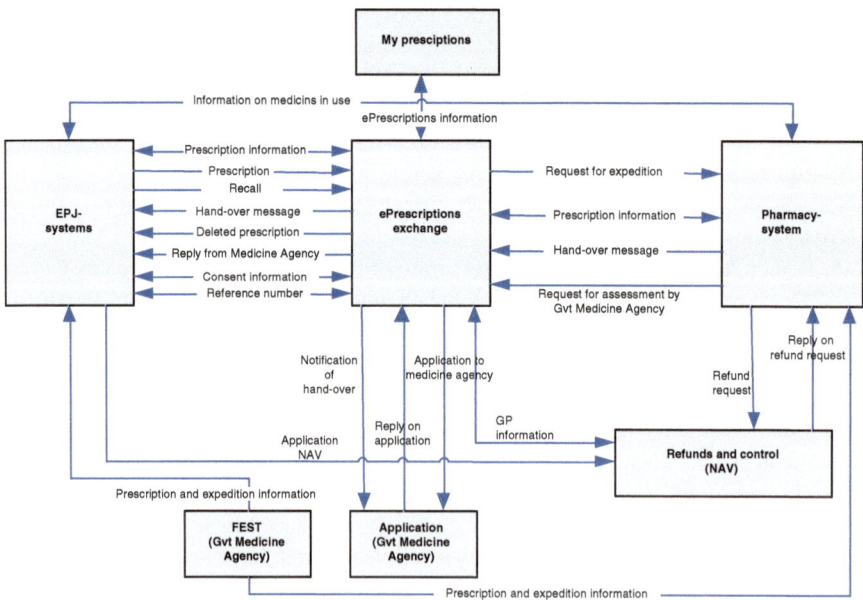

Fig. 6.1 The ePrescription solution: main components

(standardized) messages carrying information between the applications. It illustrates well the basic assumption of the EDI paradigm and ACA: information exchange is taken care of by enhancing existing applications.

The requirements specification of The Directorate of Health emphasized that the vendors and public agencies involved were responsible for their modules. The programme was organized in five projects. The six main EPR vendors were invited into one of the projects in 2006. Of the three suppliers of EPR systems for hospitals two were too busy to participate. In addition the suppliers of the hospital EPRs demanded a more specific requirement specification before they were willing to start development activities. Eventually, only the biggest vendor within the GP market, Profdoc,[3] agreed to develop a pilot version of electronic prescription. At this time Profdoc had two different EPR systems in the market and they had started to develop a new version that should replace both. They decided to develop an ePrescription module only for the new version. The ePrescription programme management accepted this. Later the two other vendors of patient record systems for GPs, Infodoc and Hove, also joined the initiative.

In May 2008 the first pilot implementation was inaugurated by the Minister of Health. It was carried out in a small town in the eastern part of Norway, and included the GPs and the local pharmacy. It turned out to be a disaster, and after 4 months a crisis was declared. Said the municipal health manager to the local newspaper; "the system is so slow, and has so many errors and deficiencies, that we will stop the whole pilot". The local authorities also raised concerns about patient safety. The main reason for the problems was not the ePrescription solution per se, but that the new version of Profdoc's new EPR system was full of errors and was very unstable. Somewhat unreasonably, the ePrescription project got the blame in an angry press.

The ePrescription Exchange was tested and accepted during 2009, while waiting for the vendors to complete and test their new versions. A new pilot was planned in March 2010, and contracts for large-scale operations were signed. The pilot testing started in Os municipality in Western Norway in June 2010, including two GP offices and one pharmacy. A second pilot started in Larvik in September 2010 including two pharmacies and a handful of GP offices. All GP offices in the pilots were using EPR systems from the same vendor, Infodoc (having app. 25% of the GP market for EPR systems). Infodoc's solution was the only one being ready for pilots at that time.

Infodoc integrated their patient record solution with the ePrescription II by developing a brand new version of their existing medication module. This new module included the functionality of the old plus those specified as part of the ePrescription programme. It was based on the same logic and user interface as the old one.

At the time the Os pilot was about to start it was uncertain when new EPR system from Profdoc would be ready. Actually, the new owners of Profdoc (CompuGroup Medical) was so unhappy about the progress (or rather lack of) of the development of the new product that they informed that management of the

---

[3] Profdoc was later taken over by the international company CompuGroup Medical and change name to CGM Norway. For reasons of consistency we use the name Profdoc only in this chapter.

ePrescription initiative that they were considering abandoning the whole project. Profdoc had at that time about 70% of the GP market for patient record solutions. Accordingly, having a solution for Profdoc users was absolutely necessary for the ePrescription initiative to succeed. So the programme management decided to develop a separate prescribing module with the functionality needed by GPs that could be used in combination with the two Profdoc solutions in use. This module, which later was given the name GPM, was running in parallel with, and only loosely integrated with, the EPR systems. That means that the users were filling in prescriptions using this module and all information exchange with other components of the ePrescription II was taken care of by this module and not the ERP systems. (This is explained in more detail below.)

The module was developed during the second half of 2010. The development costs were modest; around five MNOK. Users in lab settings tested the module during the first half of 2011, and real use testing and deployment started in the second half of 2011. Overall the tests were found to have a positive outcome. There were, however, challenges related to the fact that the GPM module was developed to run on later versions of available PC (Wintel) platforms while Profdoc's existing EPR systems were to a large extent running on old, some very old, ones.

All pharmacies in Norway were using the FarmaPro solution developed by NAF-Data;[4] NAF-Data started the development of a new version (v 5.0) of their solution in 2005 and planned, just like Profdoc, to implement the ePrescription module for pharmacies only as a part of the new solution. This solution should have been ready for deployment by 2008, but was delayed. In June 2011 it was still uncertain when the solution would be ready for full-scale deployment. At a meeting with the Minister of Health, the Minister made it clear that this uncertainty was beyond what she could accept. For this reason, and based on the positive experience with the GPM module, the management of the initiative decided to adapt this to the needs for users at pharmacies. This decision was, however, reversed. The initiative' management decided instead to put more pressure on NAF-Data so that they speeded up their development work. And so they did.

The evaluation of pilots concluded that they were successful - in particular user satisfaction was found to be high (PWC 2011). But some new challenges emerged. For instance, the evaluation also concluded that more or less all GPs needed to upgrade their ICT infrastructure – PCs, network bandwidth, and even printers – to be able to run the solution (ibid.). This again raised issues about who was to pay for this.

During 2011 Hove completed the extension of their medication module with the required functionality and its diffusion started. The same happened with the generic GPM module that was combined with Profdoc's two existing EPR systems. During 2012 Profdoc's new EPR, later called CGM Journal, was ready for deployment together with an integrated ePrescription/medication module. From early 2011 the ePrescription solution has been deployed at GP offices and pharmacies at a steady speed. By early march 2012 the solution is deployed to about 280 GP offices and

[4] NAF Data is owned by the Pharmacists' association in Norway.

134 pharmacies in 67 (of 428) municipalities distributed over 4 (of 19) counties. More than 1 mill prescriptions were sent. According to the plan the solution would be deployed to GPs and pharmacies in all municipalities by the end of 2013. By February 2013 1.200 GP offices were up and running using the GPM module while around 200 GPs using the new CGM journal solution. During the spring 2014 500–600 CGM customers had converted to the new CGM journal while Hove and Infodoc were taking over about 200 CGM customers during 2014.

The development of the GMP module for GPs, and the adaptation of this to hospitals, represented a change in the project's approach for how to cope with the installed base, and it was an ad-hoc modification of the architecture to speed up the development. This architectural change did indeed speed up the development activities by decoupling the solution from the ERP systems and their vendors' other development activities. These modules are seen as temporary solutions that will be used only until the "final" solutions are available. Whether they will be in use only temporarily or permanently remains to be seen.

6.3.2   The Hospital Sector

The primary healthcare system (the GP level, administrated by municipalities) issues 70% of the prescriptions; the rest is issued by hospitals. These are organized in four health regions, as separate state companies. In the autumn 2009 it became clear that the IT managers in the health regions had made very little preparations for integrating hospital EPRs (which are different from the GPs) with the ePrescription solution. Moreover, they raised comprehensive objections to the architecture of the solution. During some heated meetings in the winter 2009–2010 some kind of compromise was reached: the health regions would follow their own framework for integrating various old and new systems, while making an effort to implement a short-term solution for ePrescription. The South-East Health Region decided to postpone the integration of ePrescription until their preferred permanent solution was ready. This meant integrating the ePrescription solution with their regional chart and medication solution which has been under development for quite a few years and which was not expected to be ready until 2014–2016 (Nasjonal IKT 2009). The western region, however, was keener on adopting the ePrescription solution. Being informed about the existence and positive evaluation of the GPM module, the head of ICT in the western region asked the Health Directorate if they could get access to the module's software and adapt it to fit their needs, which the programme management gladly accepted. The western region started, then, in the second half of 2012 a project adapting the GPM module to the needs of users in outpatient clinics and hospital pharmacies and to run in combination with the Dips EPR system. Adapting the module was quite straightforward and pilot testing was successful. The main challenges involved were related to the security solution, modification of the GPM module and integration with Dips, and changes to the underlying communication platform. The security solution requires all physicians to sign the prescriptions they produce with an id card. For this reason they had to buy and install hardware that could read the cards and procedures for distribution of such id cards. The GPM module had to be modified a bit and extended with some additional functionality to satisfy the needs of prescription procedures in hospitals. This was primarily related to the prescribing of magistral[5] drugs. The GPM module was integrated with Dips in the following way: Dips has a menu where programs that can be started from Dips are listed. The GPM module was added to this menu. In addition, Dips transferred the patient id to GPM. Further, Dips added an API to its system that the GPM module could use to get access to information about the patient that may be important when deciding which drugs to prescribe. The prescription is not stored in Dips, but can be retrieved from the Prescription Exchange when needed. However, relevant information from the prescription can by copied from the prescription and pasted into a document that is added to the patient record. In addition, they also had to do some modifications in their communication platform used for the exchange of other kinds of messages (like lab orders and reports and admission and discharge letters). Finally, the version of the PharmaPro solutions used by hospital pharmacies had to be modified.

Deployment of the solution at the largest hospital in the region, Haukeland Hospital in Bergen, started at the beginning of January 2013 and fully implemented at all hospitals in the region by June 2014. Overall, ePrescription has been a great success in the western region. The costs related to the adaptation and integration of the generic module were modest, the deployment process smooth, and the users are very happy with the solution.

The western region's decision to implement ePrescription based on the generic module was taken against the recommendation of the Dips company. Dips started during spring 2012 a more ambitious project where ePrescription functionality will be an integrated part of their new module for handling of medication within hospitals which will be an integrated part of their EPR system. They argued that it would be better for the region to wait until this tightly integrated module was ready. The western region said they would continuously consider if they should switch to this alternative solution. So far, i.e. by late September 2015, they are very happy with the existing solution, but they plan to have a discussion about whether they should switch "soon."

Dips' integrated module was tested out in a pilot at UNN that started in 2014. The further adoption of this solution in the northern region has been very slow. However, it was successful implemented in one of the largest hospitals (called AHUS) in the South-Eastern Region during the first half of 2015. This solution will be adopted by the other hospitals in this region during 2015 and early 2016.

The hospitals in the Middle Region of Norway were using a patient record system developed by Siemens. The management of the region has announced that this solution will be replaced with a different one within the next few years. For this reason the regional management and Siemens have agreed to implement a simplest

---

[5] Magistral drugs are drugs which are produced at the pharmacy as specified by the physician on the prescription.

possible solution (i.e. minimal integration between the EPR system and the module) based on the GPM module. This solution was implemented in a pilot at three hospitals early in September 2015 and was planned to be scaled to the rest of the region later during 2015.

6.3.3   Adding Multi-dose Dispensing

Multi-dose drug dispensing (MDDD) is a service by which patients receive their medication packaged in bags with one unit for each dose occasion. The packaging is taken care of by machines. This service is intended for patients (mostly elderly) suffering from chronic illnesses for which they need to take several drugs throughout the day on (more or less) permanent basis. (There are about 70.000 such patients in Norway.) The traditional way of dealing with this is by means of a card (called ordinations card) filled in and signed by the patient's GP. A signed card is usually valid for 1 year. The card is taken care of by the patient herself or institutions responsible for the patients' home care or a nursing home. It is used as a prescription when the patient is buying drugs in a pharmacy. In addition, most patients are using a cassette containing the pills to be taken during 1 week. This cassette has one column for each day (seven in total) and one row for each time of the day a patient may take drugs (i.e. morning, noon, afternoon, evening). Such a cassette is then filled once a week either by the patient herself or a family member, but mostly by a home nurse or a nurse working in a nursing home. These processes are considered to contain two weaknesses which multi-dose (i.e. machine packaging) and e-prescribing solutions as expected to solve (at least partially). The first is that drugs may be mixed, for instance when the various pills are distributed across the cassette. Secondly, a patient may visit and receive prescriptions from more than one GP and she may be hospitalized for some reason and then being sent home with a number of drugs prescribed for a period. This may case various medication errors. The first of these problems are supposed to be solved by the multi-dose packaging machine and the second by the so-called drugs-in-use functionality in the ePrescription solution. The drugs-in-use functionality means that all ("active") prescriptions of one patient are compiled into one list. In addition, the GP of a patient taking drugs on permanent basis is given the responsibility of being the "editor" of the patient's drug-in-use list. That means that if a patient is admitted from hospital with some new prescriptions, the prescriptions are sent to the central database, the drug-in-use list is updated and sent to the GP. The GP then has to take action if necessary. Normally a multi-dose package contains drugs for 2 weeks. That means that in the electronic solution, a patient's drug-in-use list is sent to the Information System controlling the packaging machine every second week.

In Norway all pharmacies belong to one of the five chains (Boots, Apotek1 Vitus, Ditt apotek or Apotekergruppen). Each of these has one multi-dose machine serving all their pharmacies. The pharmacies started offering multi-dose packaged drugs about 10 years ago (2005).

Implementing support for multi-dose in the ePrescription solution started in August 2012. Specifications were worked out by a project group including the multi-dose project group in the Health Directorate and representatives for GPs and pharmacists. The first version of the specifications was approved by the Change Council (see below) 1 year later. These included modifications in the PrescriptionExchange (PE) module to generate and store the drug-in-use object and functionality for exchange of the new drug-in-use message between the PrescriptionExchange and the EPRs, FarmaPro, and the systems controlling the multi-dose packaging.

The EPR vendors were all hesitant in getting involved in this project, so the implementation started by adding the required functionality to the GPM module in addition to the Prescription Exchange and PharmaPro. The project managed to bring one of the chains of pharmacies, Apotek1, involved early on. A rather small team of actors, those responsible for GPM, PE, FarmaPro and Apotek1's system, then, succeeded in developing first a prototype and then through a few iterations a well working solution.

Apotek1 has a proprietary solution controlling the packaging machine, so coordination with Apotek1 about the required changes to their system has been rather smooth. Boots was enrolled into the project after the first version of the solution had stabilized. However, they have a system delivered by Visma, which is also delivered to other customers. Compared to Apotek1 this case involved a larger number of actors that had to reach agreement about how to implement the required functionality and the coordination of the implementation has been more demanding. Currently the Boots solution is in test. It was assumed to be approved before Christmas 2015.

Piloting multi-dose (based on version 2.4 of the standardized ePrescription messages) started in Jevnaker municipality in Eastern Norway in May 2014. They started with a small and controlled pilot with a limited number of actors and then gradually scaling up by including municipalities with a larger number of GPs and pharmacies from the autumn 2014. From September to November 2014 about 60 GPs in the municipalities Sandnes, Klepp, Time and Gjesdal were included in the pilot.

Among the EPR vendors Hove was the first to start implementing multi-dose functionality in their System X EPR system. Currently (September 2015) their solution are in "integration test." Infodoc plans to be ready for a pilot during 2016 while it is still unclear when CGM will adapt their solution (CGM Journal) using the integrated module for prescribing. When the other suppliers of multi-dose dispensing (Vitus, Ditt apotek and Apotekergruppen) will integrate their solutions with ePrescription is still unclear. So at the moment (September 2015) only municipalities using Apotek1 as multi-dose dispenser and GPs using Profdoc's old EPRs combined with the generic GPM module can participate in the pilots.

The pilots have been evaluated by two master students as their master thesis project (Ertesvåg and Tselischeva 2014). They found that overall the users very satisfied with the solution, however, desirable improvements of the solution were identified.

6.3.4   Other Developments

In addition to the changes to the ePrescription II mentioned above, a number of smaller changes have been made after the large scale rollout started. This includes a more or less continuous process of making the solution more robust. A number of smaller changes have also been made because of changes in regulations of the prescribing of drugs. This includes changes in the regulation of patient reimbursement for drugs and procedures for how to apply for individual patients to get reimbursed for specific drugs.

One important change is the definition of few new messages and functions that integrate ePrescription with the more recent national Summary Care Record II. These two IIs are integrated in the sense that all data from the PE are also copied to a similar service of the Summary Care Record (SCR) II. So every night all updates of the PE during the last 24 h are copied to the SCR data base. The reason for this copying is that the two IIs are under different jurisdictions. The ePrescription II are only allowed to store prescriptions as long as they are valid (or "active") while the SCR II stores this information for 3 years.

Some work has also started to adapt the II to new user group. Most important among these are employees of the elderly care sector like home nurses and nurses working in nursing homes. Unfortunately, the regulations established for the ePrescription deny nurses access to the II. However, they are allowed to access the SCR II which also includes the same information about prescriptions. Public health nurses in municipal service and midwives have some rights to prescribe some drugs (for instance contraceptives) and they are planned to be given access to ePrescription. Further, work is going on to provide ePrescription to dentists. Giving these user groups access to ePrescription requires the vendors of the applications they using to be modified for this purpose. Most vendors seem to plan to integrate their solutions to the II by means of the GP module. Visma has already started adapting their Profil solution and will start running a pilot later in 2015.

During 2012 activities started aiming at a major revision of the II with a focus on specifying new version of the standardized messages. The overall scope of the activities was approved in February 2013. This activity is defined as the specification of version 2.5 of the messages. This new version will include modifications representing a huge range of smaller and bigger modification of the functionality of the II based on practical use of the II, corrections of errors discovered, and modifications triggered by regulatory changes. The new version of the message standards are first implemented in the PE and GP modules. PE was scheduled for being able to send and receive version 2.5 messages by October 10 2105. It is not clear when other modules will be modified.

6.3.5   Operations and Governance

When the full-scale rollout started an operational model and governance structure was established. First of all, the only way of getting access to the II was through connection to the National Heath Network. The PE service was operated by the data center Evry. In the Health Directorate a permanent organization was established for coordinating the maintenance and further development of the II. They also established a governance structure. The main elements of this structure are the Change Council and the Change Forum. The latter were constituted by representatives of the "operational resources" from all actors, i.e. representatives of vendors etc. The Change Council includes representatives from user groups and health care authorities.

6.4   Concluding Discussion: Installed Base Strategy

The ePresecription II was built and widely adopted in the health care sector. There is a broad consensus that the solution and the initiative behind it has been a great success.[6] However, this success came after a long and painful "birth." The first running pilot was operational about 6 years after the initiative started and having spent about 500 million Norwegian kroner (about 55 million Euros) of funding from the Norwegian government. In addition, the vendors involved allocated substantial resources to the initiative not covered by the grant from the government.

The solution being piloted and subsequently adopted was developed with a strong focus on the ordinary prescribing practices of GPs and similar dispensing practices of pharmacies, i.e. the production of a prescription for an individual patient during the patient's visit and the dispensing of the prescribed drug when the patient visits the pharmacy. Later, the solution was successfully extended with required functionality to support a broader range of practices related to prescribing, dispensing and consumption of drugs, i.e. prescribing in hospitals, support of multi-dose dispensing, becoming a platform for the national summary care record solution, and, hopefully, support for the rest of the primary care sector (i.e. midwives, public health nurses, home nurses, physicians working in nursing homes, and dentists).

We see the approach to coping with the installed base followed by the initiative as a key source of the challenges it was struggling with up until the successful pilots started in 2010 as well the later successful diffusion and extensions of the overall solution (or II). Initially the ePrescription initiative was based on the dominant EDI paradigm with a strong focus on information sharing through message exchange between applications. According to this approach the messages are specified and approved as standards and then implemented in the solutions. This EDI paradigm is based on a classical specification driven approach to software development that implicit assumes that the new solution will be of a stand-alone kind developed from scratch. This contributed to make the initiative's approach to coping with the installed base a bit schizophrenic: One the one hand the initial design was drawing extensively upon the existing installed base as the overall solution, or II, was

---

[6] By the end of 2014 about 75 % of all prescriptions were transferred between prescribing physicians and pharmacies by using ePrescription II.

designed as just extensions of existing applications like EPR systems and pharmacy applications (in addition to a central server and a secure network). On the other hand, the design did not take seriously into account any challenges related to integrating the additional functionality to the existing installed base. This is true both for the existing applications as well as the platforms (PC hardware, operating system, network technologies, etc.) the applications were running on. This strategy turned out to be problematic for a number of reasons:

- The number of independent actors (vendors, authorities, health care institutions, professional associations representing various user groups) involved;
- The complexity of and amount of work needed to modify all applications according to the specifications;
- A huge number of users are running ole software running on old computing platforms (PC hardware, operating system, networking technology, printer, etc.) which they might have to upgrade (i.e. replace);
- The level of details the actors had to reach agreement about;
- The degree of coordination of all activities; etc.

The struggles the initiative was fighting until 2010 clearly illustrates this. Up to that point, Profdoc was the only vendor seriously working on the development of a module supporting GPs' practices. However, due to the complexity of this module they decided to develop the module only as a part of their new product. And when the development of that product was delayed, the whole ePrescription initiative was stalled. Other vendors and the hospital sector were too busy with other, and for them more urgent, tasks to be seriously involved in the ePrescription initiative. The ePrescription strategy presumed that all stakeholders involved or affected (vendors, GPs, municipalities, government agencies, etc.) had the capacity and willingness to do exactly what they were assumed to – and in a coordinated manner. These assumptions were proven not to be valid.

A key factor leading to the end of failure stories and the "birth" of the successful solution was a change in approach for how to relate to and deal with the installed base. The GPM module represented this change in "installed base approach". The generic prescription module, GPM, embeds a different strategy for relating to the installed base. It draws equally much on the installed base as a resource, but it is much more loosely coupled to this, and accordingly demands much less modification of the installed base, and accordingly resources to be spent by vendors as well as on coordination among independent actors. Furthermore, this module could be developed by the Health Directorate without the involvement of Profdoc or any other vendor.

The GPM module turned out to have a positive impact on the establishment and evolution of the ePrescription II far beyond Profdoc users. The module was, next, used by the ICT unit of the hospitals in the western region, meaning they could adopt and use ePrescription without waiting for Dips to develop an integrated module. Then the middle region did the same. In this case Siemens did not want to develop a module on their own because they were informed that their product would be replaced with another within a few years. Finally, the module is planned to be used by vendors of patient record systems for home nurses, public health nurses and nursing homes. The generic GPM module has also play a crucial role in the prototyping and piloting of support for multi-dose dispensing and version 2.5 of the messages. The module gave the project group in the Health Directorate opportunities for developing support for multi-dose dispensing through an experimental and evolutionary approach together with users without involving vendors and without being dependent on their engagement from the very beginning. The GPM module then also allows the users to adopt this service before the vendors make changes in the EPR solutions. And the vendors may want to do so until the specifications of a solution that works well have stabilized.

The development of the GPM module was anything but a strategic decision. It was a "quick fix" to an extremely urgent problem. And as such, it did definitively not represent a deliberate change in the initiative's strategy for how to cope with the installed base. But over time, however, the role that this module could play contributed to a change in the overall development approach. This change happened as those involved discovered the possibilities the module opened up for speeding up the adoption of the II among users of various vendors' patient record systems. This change of overall approach is most visible in the development (prototyping, piloting) and diffusion of the support for multi-dose dispensing.

The change in architecture and development approach was taking place in parallel, and dependent upon, changes in the organizing and governance structures of the initiative. When the adoption and diffusion of the II were getting momentum, more formal governance structures were established as described above. This happened at the same time as more and more of the development activities were transferred from vendors to the project group in the Health Directorate. We see the combination of these changes (i.e. changes in architecture (flexibility in integration between EPR systems and the prescribing module); development approach (from specification driven to a prototyping/evolutionary approach); and organizing and governance structures) as the key to the (final) success of the Norwegian ePrescription initiative.

References

Magne Ertesvåg og Elena Gennadjevna Tselishcheva. Elektronisk «Legemidler i bruk» – et blikk inn i fremtiden. Evaluering av pilotprosjektet «Legemidler i bruk» i «Reseptformidleren», inkludert elektronisk multidose i e-resept.

Nasjonal IKT. 2009. http://www.nasjonalikt.no/filestore/Dokumenter/Saksdokumenter/2009/MotereferatSGNIKT091204.pdf.

PWC. Evaiering av e-resept I poilot. 2011. https://docs.google.com/viewer?a=v&pid=sites&srcid=ZGVmYXVsdGRvWFpbnxuZmFlcGp8Z3g6NWQzZjgyMDI1ODk4YTTFjNg.

Open Access   This chapter is distributed under the terms of the Creative Commons Attribution-NonCommercial 2.5 International License (http://creativecommons.org/licenses/by-nc/2.5/), which permits any noncommercial use, duplication, adaptation, distribution and reproduction in any medium or format, as long as you give appropriate credit to the original author(s) and the source, provide a link to the Creative Commons license and indicate if changes were made.

The images or other third party material in this chapter are included in the chapter's Creative Commons license, unless indicated otherwise in a credit line to the material. If material is not included in the chapter's Creative Commons license and your intended use is not permitted by statutory regulation or exceeds the permitted use, you will need to obtain permission directly from the copyright holder.

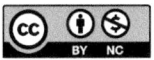

Cultivating the Installed Base: The Introduction of e-Prescription in Greece

7

Polyxeni Vassilakopoulou and Nicolas Marmaras

7.1 Introduction

E-prescription was introduced in Greece during times of financial turbulence with the aim to enhance control over pharmaceutical expenditure and also, to improve doctor-pharmacy collaboration and patient safety and to support evidence-based policy development. In that sense, the introduction of e-prescription is not yet another technology project but rather, a socio-technical intervention with infrastructural nature. In this chapter we explore the national e-prescription service's surprisingly swift deployment. Specifically, we identify how a series of pragmatic tactical decisions allowed building upon a "good-enough" installed base by exploiting its latent potential without perpetuating all of its weaknesses. Furthermore, we show how hedging against obsolescence was practiced through continuously addressing exogenous shifts in the installed base. Finally, we point to the pivotal role of the technical architecture implemented for enabling installed base cultivation. A combination of novel technological affordances, standards and architectural patterns made possible the development of a technical solution which supports openness, evolvability and scalability.

In our study we position e-prescribing within the overall Greek health system and we describe how the new electronic service evolved to inscribe specific

P. Vassilakopoulou (✉)
University of Agder, Postboks 422, 4604 Kristiansand, Norway

University of Oslo, Oslo, Norway
e-mail: polyxenv@uia.no

N. Marmaras
National Technical University of Athens, Heroon Polytechniou 9,
15780 Zografou, Athens, Greece
e-mail: marmaras@central.ntua.gr

© The Author(s) 2017   89
M. Aanestad et al. (eds.), *Information Infrastructures within European Health Care*, Health Informatics, DOI 10.1007/978-3-319-51020-0_7

prescribing policies, to provide clinical decision support, and to facilitate the processes and roles of policy and financing stakeholders. Our case description spans the period from 2010 to 2015.

Data Collection

To (re)construct e-prescription's trajectory: extensive documents' review including legislation and guidelines, policy documents and strategic plans, press releases (from Social Security Funds, the Ministry of Health, and IDIKA), public consultation documents, presentation documents from various professional and academic events, posts in professional electronic forums, articles in specialised press and journals.

To develop an understanding of the e-prescription solution: on-site observations of e-prescription use in pharmacies. The observations were repeated in 2 month intervals. Additionally, we studied the user manuals for pharmacists and doctors.

To elicit practitioners' perspectives: seven semi-structured interviews.

The remaining of the chapter is structured as follows: in Sect. 7.2 we present an overview of the Greek healthcare system and the situation with respect to information systems, in Sect. 7.3 we present the rationale for the introduction of e-prescription in Greece, we provide an overview of the e-prescription service and we describe its evolution over time, then, in Sect. 7.4 we discuss the relationship to the installed base. Finally, in Sect. 7.5 we provide some concluding remarks.

7.2   Healthcare in Greece

7.2.1   Overview of the Greek Healthcare System

Healthcare delivery in Greece is based on both public and private providers (mainly in primary care and diagnostic tests). The Greek national health system (ESY) was established after a major healthcare reform in 1983 with the aim to guarantee universal healthcare coverage for all (universal healthcare rights are stipulated by the Greek Constitution). Public health provision is coordinated by seven Health Regions that are supervised by the Ministry of Health. Secondary healthcare is provided by public and private hospitals and clinics. Primary healthcare is provided through rural health centers and provincial surgeries in rural areas, the outpatient departments of regional and district hospitals in urban areas and contracted doctors with private practices (OECD 2013a). Unlike what is common in many other European countries, Greek residents do not have to register with General Practitioners (GPs) and GPs do not have a gate-keeping role. Individuals can access the entire spectrum of specialists for consultations and can be directly referred by them for reimbursable tests and examinations. Because of the structure of healthcare provision, and the lack of a GP referral system, free choice of provider is a key characteristic of the system. The ownership of pharmacies is limited to pharmacists. Pharmacies are licensed by the government on the basis of criteria for population coverage and distance from the nearest existing pharmacy.

Key health indexes for the Greek population are good. In the 2000 report by the World Health Organization on health systems' performance, the Greek healthcare system was ranked 14th worldwide in terms of overall performance and 11th on level of health (World Health Organization 2000). During recent years, healthcare cost containment has been the main Government's concern. This concern is induced both by the rise in healthcare services demand (due to the aging population, the increase of patients living with chronic conditions and citizens' pressures for increasing the supply of quality healthcare services) but also, by the need to address the ongoing public debt crisis.

As in nearly all European countries, the public sector is the main source of healthcare financing. Financing is provided mainly by social security funds (although out-of-pocket-payments and direct health financing from the national budget of the central government are also significant). Most of the funds are public entities (legal persons governed by public law), and while they are autonomous, they operate under the control of central government. The funds cover both pensions and healthcare for particular socio-professional groups (i.e. there are different funds for farmers, public servants, etc.) on the basis of personal contributions but the state also contributes to their financing. The number of funds was brought down from 130 to 13 in 2008 (OECD 2013a) and there is further consolidation underway. For healthcare, the aim is to merge all healthcare coverage schemes (that relate to different funds) to a single one. On March 2011, the healthcare schemes for farmers, freelance non-professional workers and public servants were subsumed by the scheme for non-public sector salaried employees (IKA). All together came under the umbrella of a new organisation named "National Organisation for Health Services Provision" (EOPYY, incorporated with Law 3918/2011) which started operating in 2012. EOPYY is still being expanded to cover the beneficiaries of all other social insurance funds and is gradually becoming a single public buyer of healthcare goods and services. Figure 7.1 provides an overview of the main actors involved in healthcare regulation, provision and financing.

Aggregate public spending for health is moderate compared to EU and OECD averages (OECD 2013b). Although the overall expenditure is moderate, the statistics indicate room for improvement especially within pharmaceuticals where the annual expenditure both per capita and as a share of the Gross Domestic Product is high (about 40% more than the EU average) (OECD 2013b). This high expenditure has been a key concern for the Government also because health goods are predominantly financed by public funds (74% of expenditure is publicly financed in Greece while only 54% in Europe as an average (OECD 2013b)).

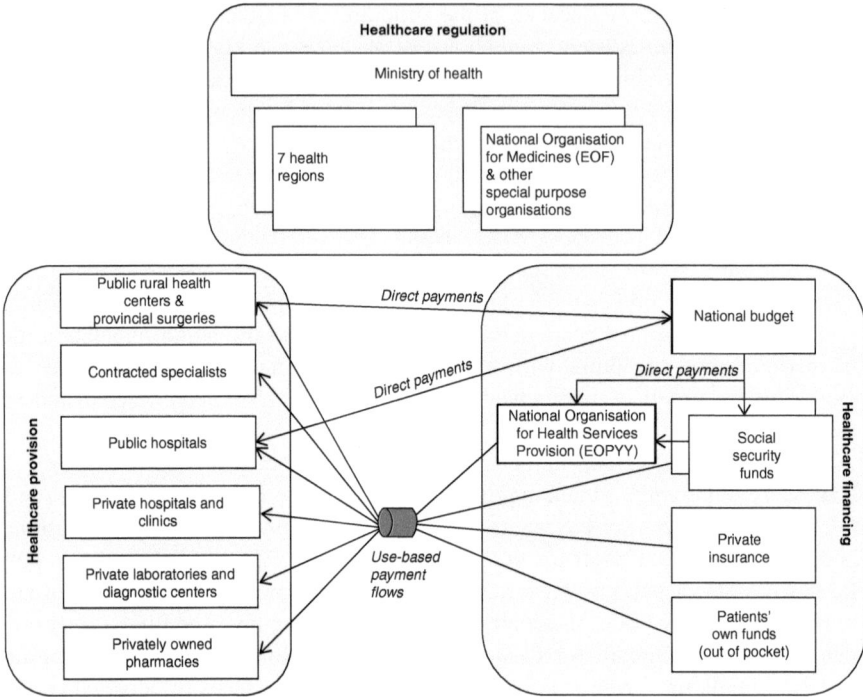

Fig. 7.1 Greek healthcare: regulation, financing and service provision (as of 2015)

7.2.2 Information Systems in Greek Healthcare

Initial efforts for the introduction of information systems within Greek healthcare date back to the 1980s (Fragidis and Chatzoglou 2011). Nevertheless, although a series of national plans were drafted and pursued (e.g. most recently, the national 2002–2006 Action Plan "ICT in healthcare" and the national eHealth roadmap 2006–2015), the progress achieved has not always been significant.

Notwithstanding the delays, there has been a clear positive trend in information systems' use over the years. Practically all pharmacies use information systems. Within primary care, as of 2013, 99% of GP practices had computers in the consultation room as opposed to only 66% back in 2007, 99% of practices were connected to the internet or a dedicated GP network and 24% had their own website (European Commission DG Communications Networks Content and Technology 2013). The electronic storage of medical patient data is relatively common among GPs although it is not universally exercised: around 70% of GPs store electronically the medical history of their patients and more than 60% register electronically their clinical notes, symptoms and ordered tests (idem). Health information exchange is much less developed among GPs (idem): only around 22% receive laboratory reports electronically and around 20% exchange medical patient data with other healthcare providers and professionals (excluding prescriptions), electronic interactions with patients are also limited (27% of GPs).

As of 2013, practically all hospitals (99%) used computer systems; billing management (90%) and discharge letters (76%) were the most common hospital applications (European Commission Joint Research Centre Institute for Prospective Technological Studies (JRC-IPTS) 2014). Hospital-wide electronic health record systems shared by all clinics were used in around half of the hospitals (52%) another 13% used multiple local systems, while 35% had no health record system in place (idem). Only 24% of hospitals exchanged health information (excluding prescriptions) with entities outside the hospital (e.g. other hospitals, external specialists, GPs) (idem).

Medical data exchange has been impeded by the lack of a single personal identifier for all Greek residents up till recently (the obligatory social security number – AMKA was only introduced in October 2009 (Greek Ministry for Labour 2012)), the delays in establishing a secure network (the secure network "Syzefxis" that connects all public entities including healthcare was only initiated in 2004, became operational in 2006 and it is still under development although it has now achieved significant coverage) and the multitude of solutions with different logics and limited standardization (Emmanouilidou and Burke 2012; Bogdanos et al. 2008).

7.3   The Introduction of E-Prescription

7.3.1   Rationale for E-Prescription and Key Milestones

Greece introduced e-prescription to enhance control over pharmaceutical expenditure, to improve doctor-pharmacy collaboration and patient safety and to capture data required for evidence-based policy development. The aspired benefits were clearly set-out in the law that provides the legal basis for e-prescription (Law 3892/2010). The year when the e-prescription law passed (year 2010) the Greek economy was facing a severe public debt crisis which captured global attention. In return for loans from the International Monetary Fund and European Institutions, the Greek government agreed to accelerate reforms including structural reforms of the healthcare sector and the introduction of new electronic tools. The strong financial motivation behind the e-prescription initiative is demonstrated by its inclusion in May's 3rd 2010 "Memorandum of Economic and Financial Policies" between Greece and the International Monetary Fund and subsequently in the "Hellenic National Reform Programme 2011–2014" issued on April 2011.

The introduction of e-prescription was swift: development started in 2010, a pilot was run in October of the same year and the official launch was on January 24th 2011 (Table 7.1). By the fall of 2011 around 40% of prescriptions were covered, and by fall 2013 almost full coverage was reached (Papanikolaou 2013). E-prescription was one of the initiatives that contributed to the reduction of the total pharmaceuticals' expenditure by approximately 33% between the years 2009

Table 7.1 Greek e-prescription: key facts

Function	Users	Temporal evolution	
Guide prescribing behaviour, support registration and circulation of prescription and dispensing information	General practitioners and specialists in primary care, private and public hospitals	Initiated in 2010	
		Launched in January 2011 (pilot October 2010)	
	Pharmacists		
	Reimbursing authorities	Almost full coverage (98%) by 2013	
	Public health policy makers		

	Fall 2010 (pilot)	Fall 2011	Fall 2012	Fall 2013
Pharmacists	~8,500	~8,500	~10,800	~10,800 (98% of total)
Doctors	~4,100	~10,100	~37,500	~41,000 (90% of total)
Prescriptions (monthly)	~8000	~2,500,000	~4,500,000	~6,000,000 (98% of total)

and 2011 (Greek e-Government Centre for Social Security 2011). In the next sections we present the trajectory followed starting with a brief presentation of the situation before the introduction of the new electronic service.

7.3.2 Information Handling Before the Introduction of E-Prescription

Before the introduction of e-prescription prescribing was supported by "prescription booklets" issued by Greek social security funds. These booklets were kept by the patients and used during their interactions with doctors and pharmacists. The booklets were personalised: they contained a photo, identity information such as name, birth date, address, registration id (for the fund's internal registry), national tax id and a unique identification number per booklet. Each booklet contained fifty double-sided prescription pages and their carbon copies (a white coloured original and a yellow coloured copy). Each prescription page had on the one side fields to be used by the prescribing doctor (including doctors' information, diagnosis, drugs description and quantity) and by the dispensing pharmacist (including pharmacist information, drugs' cost and patient's cost share) and on the other side a template for attaching identifying adhesive labels from the packaging of the drugs dispensed. These labels are mandatory for all drugs circulating in Greece. Drugs carry a serial number that identifies each pack uniquely. Serial numbers are used for preventing reimbursement fraud and monitoring consumption and expenditure. The booklet format was defined in 1998 (presidential decree 82A/1998) and revised in 2008 to include the national insurance number (AMKA) and a barcode. Figure 7.2 presents the standard prescription template that was in use before the introduction of e-prescription.

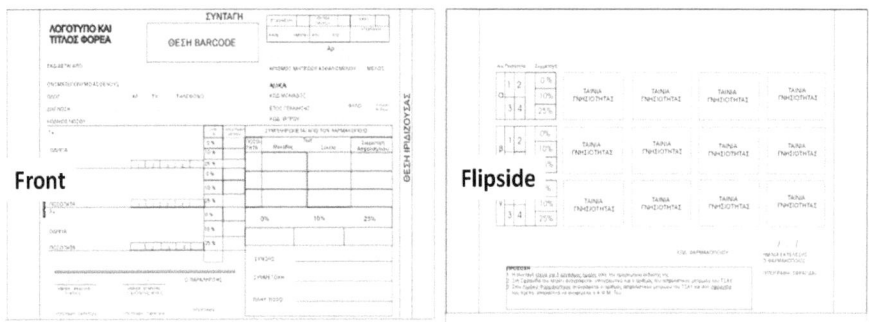

Fig. 7.2 Paper prescription template

Patients carried with them their prescription booklets when visiting a doctor. Doctors would use a page for prescribing drugs, sign and stamp the page and hand the booklet back to patients. Afterwards, patients could visit any pharmacy, hand the booklet to the pharmacist who would then complete the remaining fields on the front of the prescription page, sign and stamp, tear off the page (the yellow copy remained in the booklet), fetch the prescribed drugs from storage, detach the identification labels from the drug packages and attach them to the page, handover the drugs to the patient and collect payment (patient's share of cost). Periodically, pharmacists would send to social security funds lists with filled prescriptions attaching the white prescription pages in order to be reimbursed. The booklet's yellow pages served as records for the medication history of each patient.

For social security funds, processing prescriptions' data required resources and a dedicated infrastructure. For instance, IKA (the largest social security fund) conceptualised a project in 2005 for the electronic processing of the white prescription pages received. A request for proposals was published in 2007 and a contract was signed in 2009 for the development of a scanning and processing system and its initial operation for 2 years (with a total cost of approximately 6 million Euro). The system was in place in April 2010 and made possible the scanning, checking and clearing of 2.5 million prescriptions per month (IKA 2009; Hararis 2011). The systems that social security funds have developed for scanning, checking and clearing prescriptions are part of the overall prescriptions' installed base and had to be eventually linked to the e-prescription solution (see also Sect. 7.3.4).

7.3.3 Information Handling After the Introduction of E-Prescription

A graphical representation of the Greek e-prescription service is provided in Fig. 7.3. Web-based access is provided to prescribing doctors and pharmacists. Access is controlled at the user level (registered users go through a username and

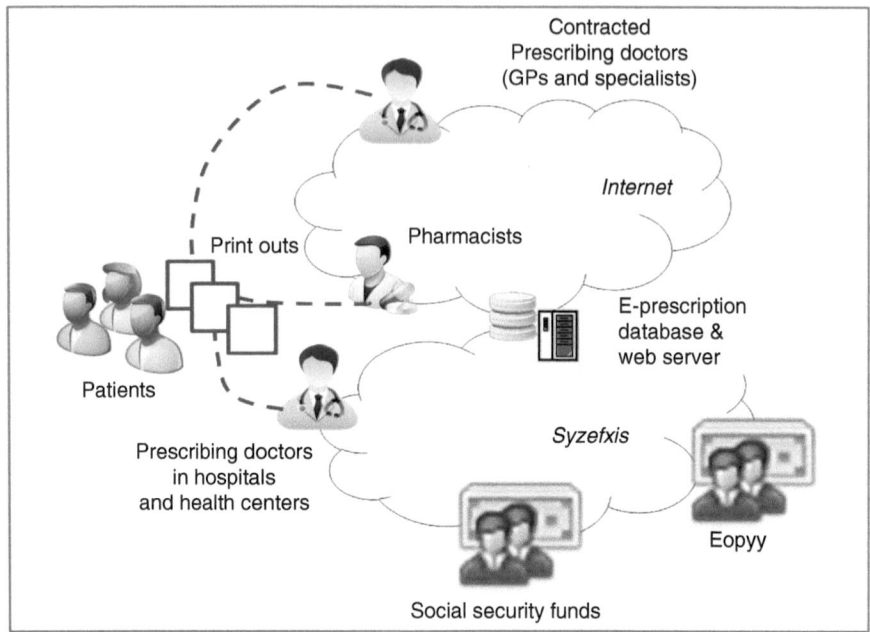

Fig. 7.3 E-prescription in Greece

password identification process) and a central repository of all prescriptions is maintained nationally. Hospitals access the service over the closed secure network Syzefxis, all other healthcare users use their private internet connections. Prescribing doctors register key information (including the patient's name and social security number, the diagnosis encoded according to ICD-10, and the medications prescribed) and then, print a summary page which is handed to the patient. Patients can visit any pharmacy in order to obtain prescribed medications. Pharmacists take the printed prescription summary page and scan the barcode to retrieve the prescription from the national central repository (alternatively they can type). Before delivering medications, pharmacists scan the medication packages' barcodes which are then matched to prescription details. In case of mismatch an error message appears on the screen and processing cannot be completed.

As with the previous fully paper-based process, pharmacists detach package labels and attach them to the prescription printout before handing over medications to patients and collecting payment (patient's share of cost). The bottom part of the printout contains designated positions for placing the labels (Fig. 7.4). Periodically, pharmacists send to reimbursement authorities lists with the prescriptions they filled attaching the printouts that include the identification labels of the medications dispensed. Doctors can use e-prescription for retrieving the full prescriptions' history per patient (pharmacists do not have access to this functionality). Patients do not have direct access to e-prescription data.

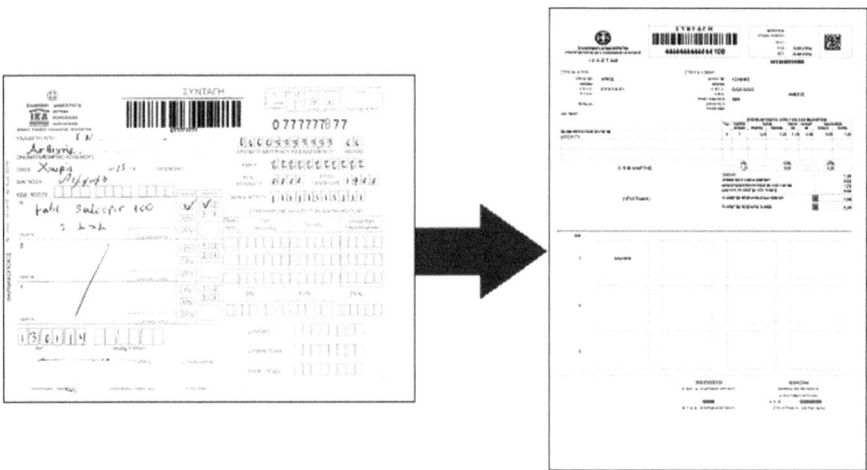

Fig. 7.4 Prescriptions in Greece: from booklet pages to printouts

The e-prescription solution is hosted and maintained by the Greek e-Government Centre for Social Security (IDIKA) which has developed it in-house. IDIKA is supervised and controlled by the Greek Ministry of Labour, Social Security and Welfare; it is mainly financed by the social security funds and is responsible for the implementation of information and communication technology within the social security sector. E-prescribing was initially piloted in October 2010 for patients covered by one specific social security fund (the fund for self-employed workers – OAEE). For the piloting of the service almost all pharmacists were enrolled along with doctors contracted by the specific fund (see also Table 7.1). In January 2011, the service was officially launched and three more social security funds were added: the fund for non-public sector salaried employees (IKA) which is the largest in the country, the fund for farmers (OGA) and the fund for public servants (OPAD). In 2012 a number of additional funds were included: in April, the fund for seafarers (NAT), in May, the fund for bank employees (TAITEKO), in November, the fund for employees in the mass media (ETAP MME) and in December, the fund for lawyers, engineers, doctors, dentists, veterinarians and pharmacists (ETAA). Each addition necessitated information exchange with additional fund-specific registries. The establishment of the new "National Organisation for Health Services Provision" (EOPYY) which started operating in 2012 and gradually assimilated the healthcare insurance schemes of multiple funds (as described in Sect. 7.2.1) helped in the establishment of common rules but the different funds retained their separate registries.

The software development for e-prescription was initially contracted to external providers and the first versions launched were not developed in-house. Two low-budget contracts were signed with two relatively small software houses (the total value including contract extensions for accommodating additional social security funds was approximately 200,000 euro (ΑΓΓΕΛΟΠΟΥΛΟΥ 2012)). At the beginning of 2012 IDIKA started the in-house development of a new e-prescription solution which was successfully launched in May 2012 (Sfyroeras 2012b). The new in-house development aimed to remedy a series of issues: slow response times and concerns about scalability, reliability and usability. It also provided the opportunity for expansions and service improvements in a flexible incremental way. The in-house development was an interim solution which became necessary as the procurement of the fully-fledged solution through a public tendering process (which was initiated in 2010) was delayed due to administrative procedures (Pangalos and Asimakopoulos 2015).

7.3.4   System Evolution

The in-house version of e-prescription was launched in May 2012 and included enhanced functionality. For instance, it supported the automatic retrieval of basic patient information, it provided doctors the option to use multiple affiliations (i.e. doctors working both for a private practice and a private clinic), it simplified the repeat prescriptions' process and offered improved search functionalities. This was the start of a continuous effort for incremental improvements and extensions.

Connections and Extensions
The initial versions of e-prescription were only accessible via web browsers. There was no connectivity to the EPRs already in use by doctors or to pharmacy information systems (PISs). A major improvement was the publishing of Application Programming Interfaces (APIs) that allowed connectivity with doctors' and pharmacists' systems. In the spring of 2012 IDIKA initiated discussions with system providers for the APIs that were under development. The APIs were initially tested in 400 pharmacies during August 2012 (Πετρόχειλος 2012). They were subsequently used by multiple system providers connecting the majority of pharmacies (by the end of 2012). In 2015 the APIs for doctors' EPRs were launched (Tagaris 2015). The web service APIs developed adhere to REST architectural constraints (RESTful APIs) and to the Clinical Document Architecture (CDA) markup standard to specify the encoding, structure and semantics of exchanged documents. The introduction of the APIs and their exploitation by third party system providers not facilitated everyday work for pharmacists and doctors that could now conclude their tasks without having to use multiple applications. Figure 7.5 provides an overview of the key architectural components for e-prescription (adapted from Asimakopoulos (2012)). The figure depicts also the link with the scanning and processing systems (for prescription printouts and attached medication labels) of the social security funds (Scan SFF). This was an additional extension implemented during the same period. The e-prescription team collaborated also with the European project epSOS for cross-border interoperability of summaries of electronic health records and

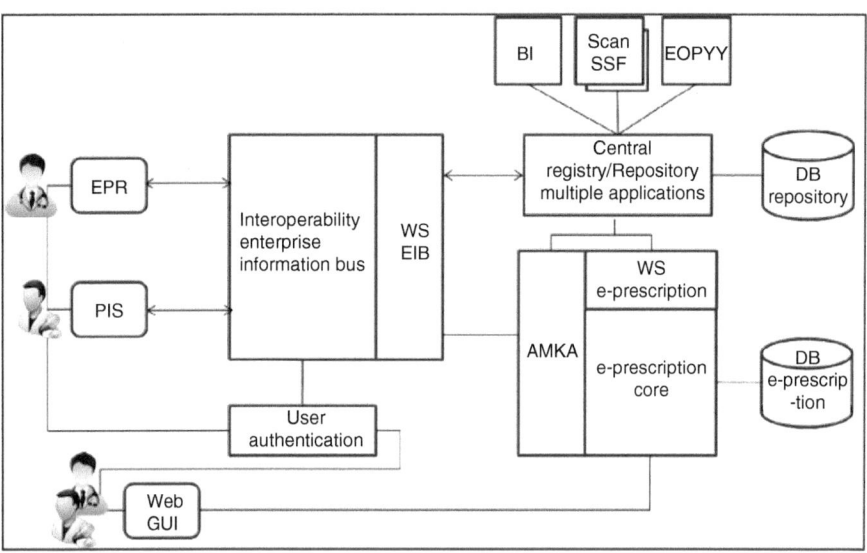

Fig. 7.5 Key architectural components of the Greek e-prescription

e-Prescriptions. Hence, the system can process epSOS friendly prescriptions for cross-border healthcare.

The publishing of APIs and the subsequent adaptation of the local EPRs and PISs, made possible for doctors and pharmacists to prescribe and dispense medications without having to shift between the web interface and their local systems. Still, doctors that needed not only to prescribe medications but also to order diagnostic tests (e.g. diagnostic imaging and blood tests) had to access an additional system (named e-diagnosis) via a web interface. The electronically supported process for test ordering is similar to the process for electronic drug prescribing: doctors register key information (including the patient's name and social security number, the diagnosis encoded according to ICD-10, and the tests ordered) and then print a summary page which is handed to the patient. Patients can visit public or private contracted laboratories and diagnostic centers for performing the tests. The e-diagnosis system for test ordering was initially launched in October 2010 (for patients covered by the social security fund for public servants – OPAD) and was developed and maintained by a private software company. In May 2011, it was decided to simplify use by applying a common user authentication scheme for both e-prescription and e-diagnosis but the two systems were kept separate. After the successful launch of the in-house version of e-prescription, IDIKA decided to extend its functionality by including test ordering. In January 2013, a new extended version of e-prescription was launched that made possible for doctors to prescribe drugs and order tests from within the same environment.

As medications are reimbursed mainly by social security funds, information about patients' affiliation with a specific fund is needed for prescribing medications (to apply specific reimbursement rules). When e-prescription was first introduced the funds were maintaining multiple electronic registries for their members and several of those registries were incomplete (for example, most registries did not include information about children that are fund beneficiaries when one of their parents is a fund member) (Sfyroeras 2012c). Before the introduction of e-prescription, doctors and pharmacists would find information about a patient's affiliation by simply looking at the prescriptions' booklet. The booklets also contained information on the status of patients as insured members (status relates to the payment of dues to the fund – benefits can only be claimed if dues are paid). For the digital process both affiliation and status information needed to be electronically available. IDIKA was already responsible for the national registry for social security (AMKA-EMAEΣ) that contains national social security numbers (AMKA) and basic information per individual (name, date of birth, parents' names). The AMKA registry did not contain information about the status of individuals' relationship with particular funds. In an initiative parallel to e-prescription, a new system named ATLAS that includes a new national registry for all healthcare beneficiaries was developed and launched by IDIKA in 2014. ATLAS links multiple registries and supports the flow and storage of information on insurance status and social insurance contributions. ATLAS is not dedicated to healthcare, it is also meant to support the calculation of pensions. This new system was linked to e-prescription in the summer of 2014.

Inscriptions of Administrative Rules and Clinical Knowledge

Overall, several rules related to reimbursement are inscribed to e-prescription. To start with, the electronic service was designed to replicate the simple constraints of the paper-based system that was previously in place. Up to three different medications can be included in one prescription (see also Fig. 7.4); in case that more are needed, separate additional prescriptions have to be issued. Furthermore, specific rules for medication quantities are also in place – rules differ for chronic patients, specific types of medications etc. Since June 2012, substance-based prescribing (instead of naming pharmaceutical products) was electronically imposed. The classification of active ingredients of medications is based on the ATC international classification system. This new rule (substance-based prescribing) was subsequently relaxed so e-prescribing was readjusted. Recently, (September 2015) the rule was reintroduced in the system after yet another change in the reimbursement regulations. The rules for patients' cost-sharing are also inscribed in the electronic solution (and are being updated each time they change). The general rule is that patients contribute 25% of medications' cost but there are many special patient and/or therapy-specific categories for which the contribution is 10% or even 0% (e.g. chronic patients, pregnant women, patients with transplanted organs, etc.). Additionally, there are rules for the maximum amounts that patients may pay. Specific constraints on what can be prescribed by doctors according to their specialty are also implemented. Additionally, there are specific rules for prescribing doctors that limit the number of prescriptions that can be issued and define upper bounds (caps) for the total permitted cost per prescription (since 2013 different methods for calculating caps were applied based on simple data analytics e.g. by taking into account the prescribing history of individual doctors or specific specialties and geographic areas).

The rules inscribed to e-prescription are not only related to costs and reimbursements. Therapeutic prescribing protocols for a series of conditions (i.e. diagnosis-based prescribing guidelines) have also been electronically implemented. Practically, this means that e-prescribing gradually extended to become a decision support tool for doctors. The protocols include medication of "first choice", secondary medications, alternative therapies and rare cases. The medication options are described on the basis of active substance. These protocols are developed by specially appointed committees for condition categories defined by the National Organisation for Medicines (EOF) and are approved by the Central Health Council (KESY). A total of 160 protocols were developed and approved on October 2011. The first protocols were launched within e-prescription in October 2013 (for osteoporosis) and since then, their number has been continuously increasing. Up to September 2015 15 different protocols were implemented (e.g. for dyslipidaemia, diabetes, arterial hypertension and rheumatological conditions) while there are several more under development with the aim to be launched before the end of 2015 (for dementia, Parkinson disease, epilepsy, chronic obstructive pulmonary disease, chronic bronchitis, asthma).

Working Around Complications in National Plans

The national eHealth roadmap 2006–2015 included a plan for the introduction of smart cards in healthcare. The smart cards would be used both for identification and authorisation purposes (for patients and healthcare providers) and also for storing data (administrative identification, clinical emergency data, prescriptions and insurance status) (Angelidis et al. 2010). Small-scale experimentations with smart cards for healthcare have been taking place in Greece since the 1990s (Karounou and Vassilakopoulos 1995). However, the plan for national level deployment of smart cards for health has not been materialised till today. The exploration of the whole spectrum of issues that impede the national deployment of smart cards for health in Greece is outside the scope of this chapter but we can briefly mention issues related to the cost and complexity of extending the existing physical infrastructure to include card readers, the need for large-scale organisational and regulatory adaptations and discussions/disputes around data security and data ownership. Nevertheless, as smart health cards are part of the national plan the introduction of e-prescription was linked to the use of the cards and that was clearly stated when the consultation process for the development of the new electronic prescription services was initiated back in 2010 (the use of PKI-based smart cards was part of the requirements).

IDIKA was also involved in small-scale experimentations with smart cards. Specifically, a pilot was launched in 2012, in the prefecture of Corinthia were 2500 individuals insured by the social security fund for municipal employees (TYDKY) were provided with personalized smart cards. The pilot was discussed in public by IDIKA management: the stated aim was to explore and prepare for national scale implementation; it was also announced that IDIKA was planning to provide 60.000 smart cards to healthcare providers (covering all prescribing doctors and pharmacies) to enhance e-prescribing security (Πετρόχειλος 2012). The use of smart cards for e-prescription was never scaled-up but the pilot showed the preparedness of the system to accommodate the national strategy for smart cards in healthcare.

The government's intention for nationwide deployment of smart cards in healthcare has been recently reconfirmed and the current plan is to use the cards both for healthcare and social benefits (Greek Ministry of the Interior and Administrative Reform 2015). Still, the necessary arrangements for nationwide deployment are not in place while the e-prescription service is deployed nationally. Given the current situation, the much awaited security enhancement of e-prescription is being currently implemented with the introduction of USB tokens for healthcare providers (launched in June 2015). While till recently access healthcare providers were accessing e-prescription using their user name and password, with the introduction of the tokens authentication is performed by the combination of the password and the USB token (two-way authentication).

The new authentication component is an outcome of the large-scale e-prescription project that was awarded to a consortium of companies. As already mentioned the in-house developed system is a makeshift solution that was put in place for the interim period required to implement the system acquired through a public procurement process. This process was initiated with a public consultation on the design and implementation of the e-prescribing system (February–March 2010). This was followed by another public consultation which was specific to the implementation stages for e-prescription (April 2010). Subsequently, the tendering documents were made available for public consultation in April 2011. After that, a two-step tendering process was initiated. An open call for the project (budget Euro 24,6 million – duration 36 months) was published in September 2011, four consortia were pre-selected (March 2012) and subsequently three of them submitted proposals (August 2012). The proposals were evaluated through a lengthy process that culminated in the contract award (June 2014). The value of the contract was significantly lower than the original budget (approx. 40% lower) and the duration was set to 18 months. The new e-prescription solution was still under development at the time of writing.

The overall system evolution described in this section is graphically represented in Fig. 7.6. The figure depicts key milestones for the system-in-use and also for the public procurement process (for the fully-fledged solution) which has been running in parallel.

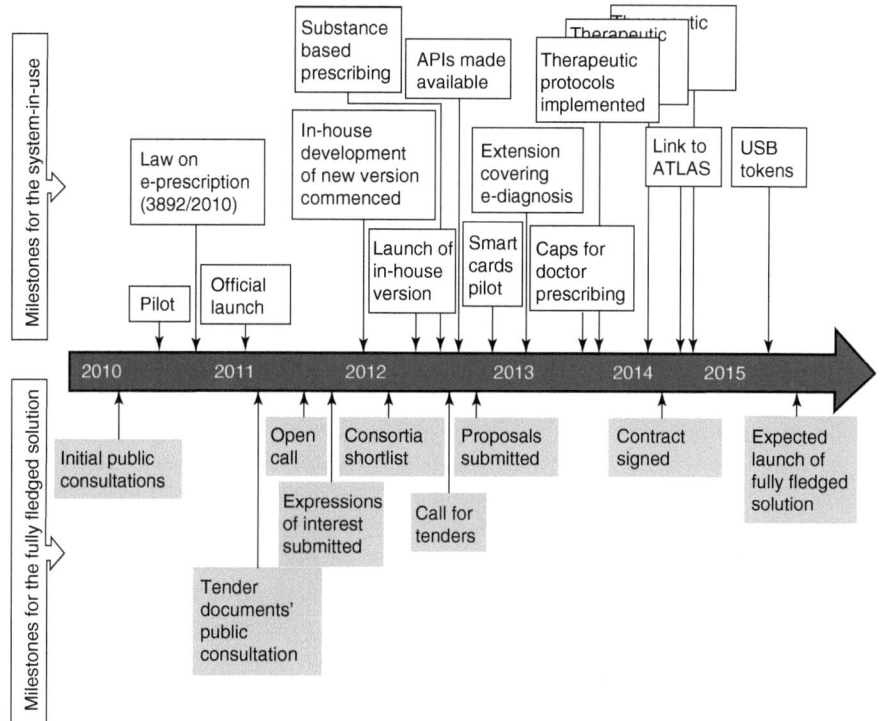

Fig. 7.6 Key milestones for the Greek e-prescription case

7.4   Discussion: Relationship to the Installed Base

7.4.1   Building Upon an Installed Base That Is "Good Enough" Without Perpetuating All Weaknesses

Gaps in the backbone of the country's information infrastructure caused difficulties to previous eHealth initiatives. Efforts to harmonize Greek healthcare with European "best practices" have repeatedly failed to deliver expected results and some of them were abandoned altogether (Economou 2010). Heath data exchange was impeded by the lack of a single personal identifier for all Greek residents (each social security fund used its own registry with its own identifiers) and the lack of a secure network to connect healthcare facilities. A number of recent initiatives with infrastructural nature filled some of these gaps and created a more favourable environment for the initiation of e-prescription. A new secure network (Syzefxis) supports connections among public institutions and provides gateways to the internet. A single national social security number (AMKA) was introduced in October 2009. Furthermore, computer-based information systems were present in practically all hospitals, primary healthcare units and pharmacies although as recently as 10 years ago this was not the case (see also Sect. 7.2.2). Additionally, standards for information codification like the International Classification of Diseases (ICD), the Anatomical Therapeutic Chemical (ATC) classification and HL7 Clinical Document Architecture (CDA) were already mature and readily available. E-prescription was built upon these enabling components and would have been challenged without them. Moreover, software architectural styles that allow client-server separation of concerns and simplify modular implementation (such as REST) were established. So, the development of the software capitalised on relevant technical knowledge and experience.

The installed base included also a complicated arrangement of multiple social security funds and national actors including the Ministry for Health, the Ministry for Labour Social Security and Welfare, the National Organisation for Medicines, Doctors and Pharmacists Associations. All these actors were involved by setting rules and providing datasets required for digitising the prescribing process. The Chief Executive Officer of IDIKA stated in an interview in 2012 that the main challenges faced were not related to the technical development but rather to the coordination of all involved actors (Sfyroeras 2012a). He also stated that the lack of interoperability among systems and the absence of a national registry for the beneficiaries of healthcare were assessed as showstoppers by some participants during the early stages of the initiative. Moreover, he pointed to other key components that were missing when the development of e-prescription started: lack of a full list of medications available in Greece (not just a list of approved medications), lack of a common identifier for medications, lack of a unified doctors' registry (multiple registries in place).

Although a number of key components were missing, the new system was not merely built upon the installed base perpetuating all of its weaknesses. Instead, several initiatives were taken to fill some of the gaps. For example, it would have been possible to circumnavigate problems with the national medications' list by allowing users to enter free-text medication descriptions. This would facilitate the circulation of messages between doctors and pharmacists but would be an inefficient solution for monitoring prescribing practices. The lack of standardised medications' lists is a problem in many other countries including USA were free-texting of e-prescription medications is common (Dhavle and Rupp 2014). However, in the Greek case, it was decided not to follow such an approach, instead, comprehensive lists were created and maintained, new registries were put in place, and new connections were implemented.

Overall, a pragmatic approach was adopted: some gaps were filled while others were worked around. For instance, for almost 5 years access control to e-prescription was rudimentary. Authentication was performed by means of user name and password. The implementation of mechanisms for two-factor authentication required the deployment of a physical infrastructure (smart cards or usb tokens) which was costly and logistically demanding. Hence, it was initially postponed and was eventually implemented in 2015.

7.4.2   Handling Continuous Exogenous Shifts in the Installed Base

The situation within the installed base kept changing during the 5-years trajectory not only as a result of initiatives triggered by the need to put e-prescription in place but also because multiple initiatives related to wider reforms within healthcare took place. The institutional environment changed with the establishment of the National Organisation for Health Services Provision (EOPYY) which started operating in 2012 and is gradually becoming a single public buyer of healthcare goods and services. Additionally, a number of social security funds were merged. Furthermore, the distribution of roles and responsibilities among existing actors changed. For example, since October 2012 the price lists for medications are issued by the National Organisation of Medicines and not by the General Secretariat for Trade. The e-prescription service had to adapt to all these changes. Moreover, new potentially useful infrastructural components were created after the initial launching of e-prescription. For instance, therapeutic prescribing protocols were made available in 2011 and were subsequently progressively included in e-prescription.

Although several of the installed base changes were planned and known in advance, e-prescription would not be developed by taking them for granted as it is not uncommon to experience delays or even radical twists in national plans (a good example is the situation with smart cards for health where there is practically no significant advancement till today). Consequently, all decisions had to be based on the situation at hand while maintaining openness to accommodate changes. Part of the overall uncertain situation was the public procurement process for a fully-fledged system which was under way but without any certainty about the timing of the delivery. Hence, there was a need to adapt swiftly and cost-effectively since it was already known that the system in use would be replaced at some point. What was pivotal for this continuous effort to develop and maintain e-prescription through adaptations was the clear ownership and dedication by a single institution (IDIKA). This institution took the seemingly paradoxical decision to develop in-house at the beginning of 2012 a new version (even though the fully-fledged solution was already planned), replacing the one that was in place and was already reaching its limits (see also Sect. 7.3.3).

7.4.3   Installed Base Cultivation vs. Specifications-Driven Development

The tactics described in the two previous sections can be summarised as pragmatic exploitation and expansion of a "good enough" installed base, and continuous adaptation to exogenous shifts within this base. This can be characterised as a "cultivation" approach. In that approach, the installed base is not considered as a given and stable foundation for further developments that can be fully planned. Instead, the dynamics of this base are acknowledged and hence, interventions are attempted in an active interplay with it (Ciborra 1992; Ciborra and Hanseth 1998). Such an approach towards the installed base necessitates a requisite technical design that supports openness, evolvability and scalability. These were key characteristics of the new version of the system that was developed and launched in 2012. Specifically, the architectural configuration of the new system (Fig. 7.5) allowed loose coupling among components, offered the possibility for continuous new releases and supported component modifiability to meet changing needs.

A cultivation approach to the installed base entails incremental and evolutionary development which is drastically different to the conventional specifications-driven approach that was followed in the past for national systems. For instance, the tax authorities' system was launched after 7 years of systematic design and implementation efforts (Prasopoulou 2012), while the system for social security reached countrywide implementation after almost two decades of planning and multiple discontinuities in the design and development process (Avgerou and McGrath 2007). For the procurement of the fully-fledged system the specification-driven approach was also adopted and it would be interesting to know how e-prescription would turn out without the prior experience of cultivation for over 5 years.

7.5   Concluding Remarks

E-prescription played a key role for the establishment of new rules and norms disrupting existing practices within healthcare. The introduction of the new electronic service was legitimised by referring to the expected economic impact (Greek e-Government Centre for Social Security 2011; Sfyroeras 2012a; Vassilakopoulou and Marmaras 2015) and to obligations towards the International Monetary Fund and European Institutions. The need for cost containment was undisputed as expenditure on pharmaceuticals had reached very high levels: per capita pharmaceutical expenses in $ purchasing power parities (PPP) rose from 461 in 2004 to 840 in 2009 (OECD 2015b). The government managed to reduce the annual bill for pharmaceuticals by €1.8 billion between 2009 and 2013 (OECD 2015a). This significant cost cutting cannot be attributed to e-prescription alone. It was the outcome of several concurrent measures some of which were related to e-prescription e.g. favouring the use of generic medicines via substance-based prescribing and introducing caps per prescribing doctor. Additional measures not related to e-prescription include a new reference pricing model that takes into account the three EU countries with lowest prices, and the renegotiation and reduction of pharmacy and wholesaler margins on reimbursed drugs (OECD 2013a; Siskou et al. 2014; Deloitte Centre for Health Solutions 2013). The sense of crisis certainly facilitated change nevertheless, this by itself is not sufficient. The overall outcome was made possible by a combination of institutional leverage, novel technological affordances, and pragmatic tactical decisions.

Open Access This chapter is distributed under the terms of the Creative Commons Attribution-NonCommercial 2.5 International License (http://creativecommons.org/licenses/by-nc/2.5/), which permits any noncommercial use, duplication, adaptation, distribution and reproduction in any medium or format, as long as you give appropriate credit to the original author(s) and the source, provide a link to the Creative Commons license and indicate if changes were made. The images or other third party material in this book are included in the work's Creative Commons license, unless indicated otherwise in the credit line; if such material is not included in the work's Creative Commons license and the respective action is not permitted by statutory regulation, users will need to obtain permission from the license holder to duplicate, adapt or reproduce the material.

References

Angelidis P, Giest S, Dumortier J, Artmann JH. Country brief: Greece. European Commission, DG Information Society and Media, ICT for Health Unit; 2010.

Asimakopoulos A. 2012. Διαλειτουργικότητα τρίτων εφαρμογών με το Σύστημα Ηλεκτρονικής Συνταγογράφησης. Interoperability Day 2012. Athens.

Avgerou C, McGrath K. Power, rationality, and the art of living through socio-technical change. MIS Q. 2007;31:295–315.

Bogdanos C, Lagouros M, Ekonomou L. 2008. Healthcare information systems in Greece: system and human integration. Commun Inform Technol:196–200.

Ciborra C. From thinking to tinkering: the grassroots of strategic information systems. Inf Soc. 1992;8:297–309.

Ciborra C, Hanseth O. 1998. Toward a contingency view of infrastructure and knowledge: an exploratory study. Proceedings of the international conference on Information systems. Assoc Inf Syst:263–72.

Deloitte Centre For Health Solutions. Impact of Austerity on European pharmaceutical policy and pricing. staying competitive in a challenging environment. Deloitte LLP, London; 2013.

Dhavle A, Rupp M. 2014. Towards creating the perfect electronic prescription. J Am Med Inform Assoc:22;e7–12.

Economou C. Greece: health system review. Health Syst Transit. 2010;12:1–180.

Emmanouilidou M, Burke M. A thematic review and a policy-analysis agenda of Electronic Health Records in the Greek National Health System. Health Policy;2012;109(1):31–37.

European Commission DG Communications Networks Content & Technology. Benchmarking deployment of ehealth among general practitioners – final report – country profile: Greece. Luxembourg: Publications Office of the European Union; 2013.

European Commission Joint Research Centre Institute For Prospective Technological Studies (JRC-IPTS). European hospital survey: benchmarking deployment of ehealth services. Luxembourg: Publications Office of the European Union; 2014.

Fragidis LL, Chatzoglou PD. 2011. The use of electronic health record in greece: current status. Computer and Information Technology (CIT), 2011 IEEE 11th International Conference, IEEE, p. 475–80.

Greek E-Government Centre for Social Security 2011. Press release 10 Nov 2011.

Greek Ministry for Labour, S. S. A. W. 2012. Τι είναι ο AMKA (what is the social security number).

GREEK Ministry of the Interior and Administrative Reform. 2015. Press release: key points of the speech by Deputy Minister J. Katrougalos in the 5th eGovernment Forum (ΣΗΜΕΙΑ ΟΜΙΛΙΑΣ Γ. ΚΑΤΡΟΥΓΚΑΛΟΥ ΣΤΟ 5ο e-GOVERNMENT FORUM). Athens, 3 June 2015.

Hararis G.. IKA/EOPYY prescriptions processing system. Results after 20 months of productive operation. Annual Greek ICT Forum. Athens; 2011.

IKA. 2009. Press release on the system for automated prescriptions' management – Δελτίο Τύπου για το Σύστημα Αυτοματοποιημένης Διαχείρισης Συνταγών του Ιδρύματος. *23rd September 2009* [Online]. Available: http://www.ika.gr/gr/infopages/press/20090923.cfm. Accessed 12 Sept 2015.

Karounou V, Vassilakopoulos G. 1995. Plans and experiments with health cards in Greece. Studies in Health Technology and Informatics, 26: Health Cards '95, 229–32.
OECD. Greece: reform of social welfare programmes. Paris: OECD Publishing; 2013a.
OECD. Health at a glance 2013: OECD indicators. Paris: OECD Publishing; 2013b.
OECD. 2015a. Country note: how does health spending in Greece compare?
OECD. OECD health statistics 2015 – frequently requested data. In: OECD editor. July 2015, Last updated: 7 July 2015 ed; 2015b.
Pangalos G, Asimakopoulos D. 2015. The new Greek national e-prescription system: A powerful ehealth tool for improving services to citizens and administrative control. NHIBE 2015: New Horizons in Industry Business and Education. Skiathos.
Papanikolaou C. The Greek EU Presidency's plans in 2014: ehealth forum & beyond. 3rd EU-US eHealth marketplace and conference. Boston; 2013.
Prasopoulou E. Addressing contextual influences during ICT innovation for public sector reform: the case of TAXIS. In: Papadopoulos T, Kanellis P, editors. Public sector reform using information technologies: transforming policy into practice. Hershey: IGI Global; 2012.
Sfyroeras V. 2012a. Interview with the CEO of IDIKA. Pharma and Health Business; p. 26–9.
Sfyroeras V. 2012b. Ηλεκτρονική Συνταγογράφηση: Προβλήματα και Προοπτικές. Σεμινάριο Ερμούπολης για την Κοινωνία της Πληροφορίας, Syros.
Sfyroeras V. 2012c. Το σύστημα της ηλεκτρονικής συνταγογράφησης. PHARMACY MANAGEMENT ΚΑΙ ΕΠΙΚΟΙΝΩΝΙΑ. p. 68–9.
Siskou O, Kaitelidou D, Litsa P, Georgiadou G, Alexopoulou H, Paterakis P, Argyri S, Liaropoulos L. Investigating the economic impacts of new public pharmaceutical policies in Greece: focusing on price reductions and cost-sharing rates. Value Health Reg Issues. 2014;4:107–14.
Tagaris A. 2015. Ο ρόλος της ΗΔΙΚΑ στην Εθνική στρατηγική για την η-υγεία (The role of IDIKA in the National strategy for e-health). 11ο πανελλήνιο συνέδριο για τη διοίκηση, τα οικονομικά και τις πολιτικές της υγείας (11 th panhellenic conferemce for health management, economics and policiew). Athens.
Vassilakopoulou P, Marmaras N. Investigating technology-induced transitions in healthcare: work practice adaptations within their overall context. Health Policy Technol. 2015;4:277–85.
World Health Organization. The world health report 2000. Health systems: improving performance. Geneva: Office of Publications, World Health Organization; 2000.
Αγγελοπούλου Α. 2012. Βλάσης Σφυρόερας: Γρήγορη και φιλική η νέα πλατφόρμα συνταγογράφησης. Ιατρικός Τύπος, 29 May 2012.
Πετρόχειλος Χ. 2012. Σημαντική η πρόοδος στην ηλεκτρονική συνταγογράφηση παρά την έλλειψη πόρων και προσωπικού. Ιατρικός Τύπος, 2 Nov 2012.

Open Access This chapter is distributed under the terms of the Creative Commons Attribution-NonCommercial 2.5 International License (http://creativecommons.org/licenses/by-nc/2.5/), which permits any noncommercial use, duplication, adaptation, distribution and reproduction in any medium or format, as long as you give appropriate credit to the original author(s) and the source, provide a link to the Creative Commons license and indicate if changes were made.

The images or other third party material in this chapter are included in the chapter's Creative Commons license, unless indicated otherwise in a credit line to the material. If material is not included in the chapter's Creative Commons license and your intended use is not permitted by statutory regulation or exceeds the permitted use, you will need to obtain permission directly from the copyright holder.

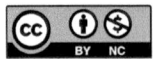

England's Electronic Prescription Service

Infrastructure in an Institutional Setting

8

Ralph Hibberd, Tony Cornford, Valentina Lichtner,
Will Venters, and Nick Barber

8.1   Introduction

Primary care computing in the UK has been presented as a national success story for health informatics development and use (Benson 2002a, b). Despite each UK nation having its own devolved National Health Service and developing its own systems, primary care health professionals in England, Northern Ireland, Wales and Scotland all use electronic patient records, on-screen prescribing decision support, and electronic prescription printing. Recently this has been augmented by the adoption of electronic transmission of prescriptions (ETP), with each devolved nation's NHS developing their own version to meet local needs. The subject of this chapter is the solution adopted by England's National Health Service (NHS), which takes the institutional form of the Electronic Prescription Service (EPS).

England's EPS was designed to support the processing and management of increasing primary care prescription volumes, which have shown a consistent growth of around 5% a year for the last two decades. Currently, England's 56 million citizens receive over 1,000 million prescription items from NHS primary care services. Whilst the potential for electronic prescription transmission has been long recognised, the development and deployment of EPS as a national system has taken over 13 years (2003–2015). As of early 2016, deployment is

R. Hibberd (✉) • T. Cornford • W. Venters
Department of Management, London School of Economics and Political Science,
Houghton Street, London WC2A 2AE, UK
e-mail: R.E.Hibberd@lse.ac.uk

V. Lichtner
School of Healthcare, University of Leeds, Woodhouse Lane, Leeds LS2 9JT, UK

N. Barber
Department of Practice and Policy, UCL School of Pharmacy,
29 Brunswick Square, London WC1N 1AX, UK

© The Author(s) 2017
M. Aanestad et al. (eds.), *Information Infrastructures within European Health Care*, Health Informatics, DOI 10.1007/978-3-319-51020-0_8

ongoing, although the service looks to be gaining widespread acceptance as it has now been installed in 98% of the 11,844 community pharmacies, and 78% of the 7,803 GP practices in England (Health and Social Care Information Centre 2016).

In this chapter, we examine the making of EPS and the forces that shaped its present form and status. EPS has been assembled as an operational service from decades of technical development and pilot implementation efforts brought together within a specific project under the NHS National Programme for Information Technology (NPfIT) – the decade long centrally mandated initiative running from 2002 to 2013. It also drew heavily from (and at times changed) the established work practice in primary care. Our analysis adopts three interlinked temporal perspectives to trace the influence of existing systems, old and new infrastructures and wider interests in the way EPS has been assembled. These are expressed as; (1) a causal past represented by history and the installed base, (2) a concurrent present of established practices and change programmes seeking to influence them, (3) desired futures as reflected in policy goals and visions. Thus EPS is assembled from its past, its present and its future(s). This process is traced out using three interwoven perspectives; the realization and negotiation of *constraints* found in the wider NHS context that limit change, as *inertia* arising from limited resources and weak incentive structures, and in a purposive *fidelity* to existing institutional culture, seen here most directly in the history, practices and ethos of the NHS (Fig. 8.1).

This chapter draws data from a commissioned evaluation of EPS (see Box on Methods and Data), reported in Cornford et al. (2014), although the analysis here is new. In particular we focus on how the EPS entering wide scale use today (2016) draws on extant technologies and installed bases of infrastructures, and how this relates to and reflects the practices and interests of multiple stakeholders. EPS draws from, and contributes to, the long history of UK health informatics (Fig. 8.2). This is a history characterised by incremental development and pilot deployments, recurring local and national initiatives, and successive policies looking for service transformation through technology. The history begins with the computerisation of hospital admissions and hospital pathology laboratories in the 1960s (Brennan 2005), and continues into the present with a promise of an Integrated Digital Care Record (NHS England 2013). This history is punctuated by occasional failures, for example with the Care Records Service (CRS) component of the National Programme for Information Technology (Matheison 2011). Still, the NHS continues to pursue, with undimmed enthusiasm, the new frontiers of health informatics. Thus current informatics policy is focused on supporting a transformed service that embodies integrated patient-centred care, accountability in care provision, and the capture and curation of aggregated data for NHS management, research and the promotion of better health and healthcare (NHS England 2013).

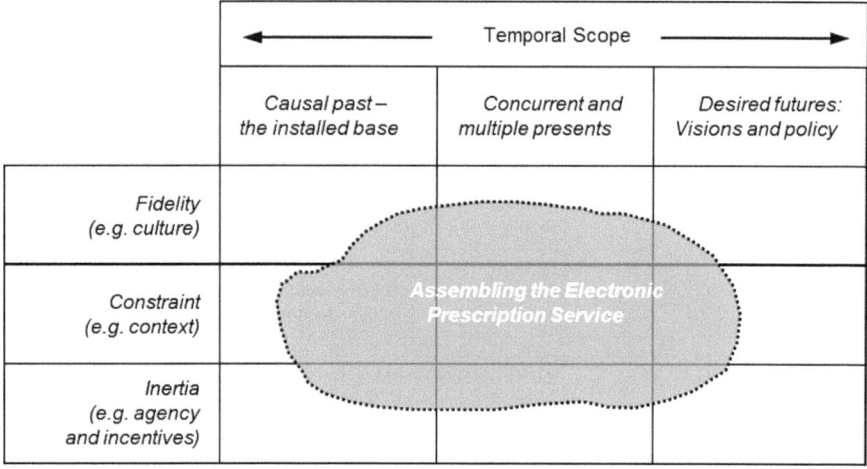

Fig. 8.1 The analytical model used

Methods and Data

This chapter draws from work conducted as part of the Evaluation of the Electronic Prescription Service in Primary Care, a project which ran from 2008 to 2013 and was funded by the Connecting for Health Evaluation Programme (Cornford et al. 2014; Hibberd et al. 2012; Petrakaki et al. 2012; Lichtner et al. 2012). In writing this chapter we identified from the project data key exemplars of where the installed base, which can be thought of as a multi-layered set of socio-technical systems, based on Cornford et al. (1994), constrained or influenced the development of the service.

The evaluation encompassed both a historical analysis and an examination of the contemporary development of the service through interviews with key stakeholders from the agencies and software companies developing the systems, end-users in the form of patients, GPs and community pharmacists, as well as observations of practice. This data provided an understanding of the intent of the system, its operation in various settings, and examples of operational surprises which often revealed unforeseen influences of the installed base.

The EPS has undergone further development since the evaluation research ended. To reflect this we also examined contemporary public literature from the EPS delivery agency, the Health and Social Care Information Centre, and from practitioner organisations, such as the Pharmaceutical Services Negotiating Committee, an organisation that has been an influential stakeholder in the development of the EPS.

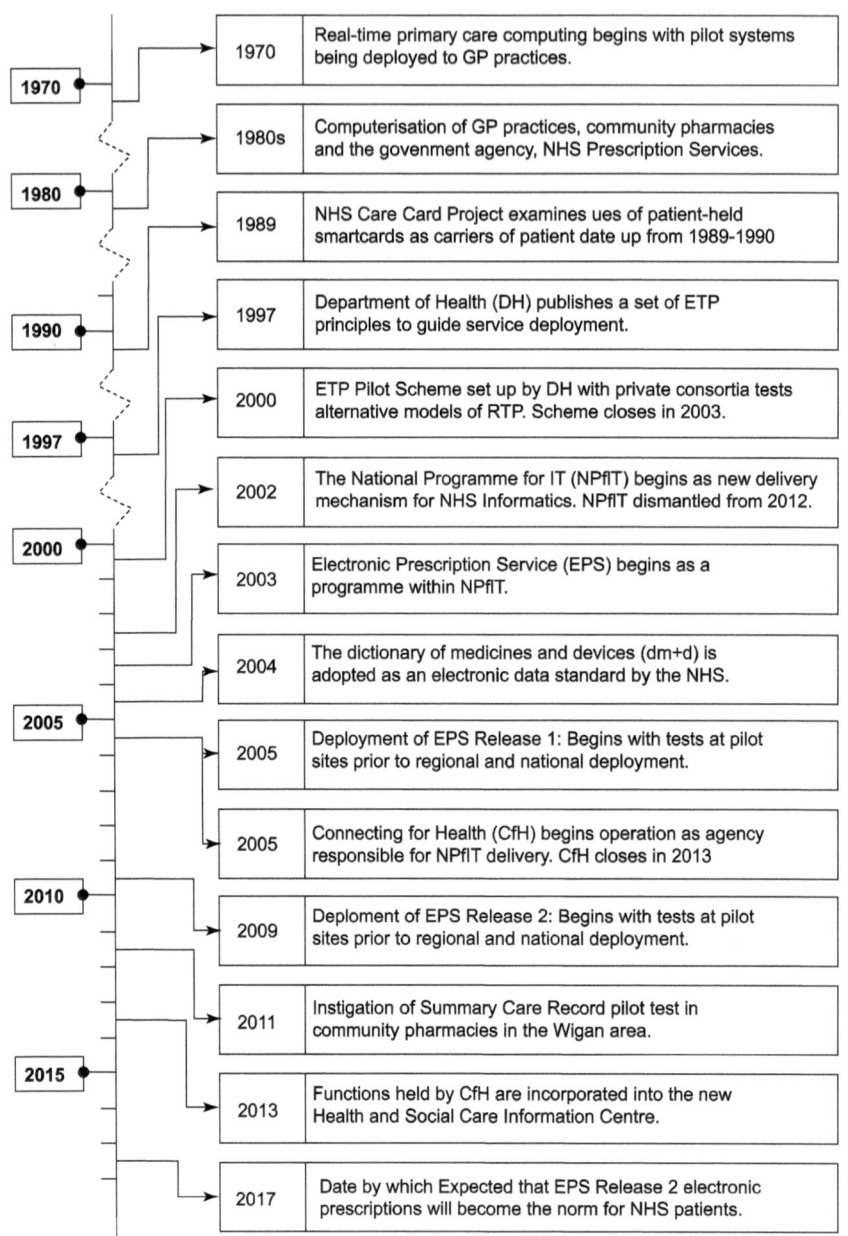

Fig. 8.2 Timeline of electronic prescription development in England

8.2   Primary Care and Health Informatics in England

The NHS commissions and delivers healthcare at a population level, supporting the development of health informatics to help achieve its broader remit for care. Funding for the service is through both general taxation and the charging of capped co-payments for some services, including primary care prescriptions. It commissions care from both public and private healthcare facilities. The NHS has also developed an unenviable reputation for reorganization of its core management structures (Talbot-Smith and Pollock 2006). Current policy, following the Health and Social Care Act of 2012, places emphasis on devolution of decision-making, service commissioning and budgeting. This landscape might appear incompatible with national informatics programmes such as EPS, and indeed EPS did emerge from a different economic and political era, being conceived in 2003 as part of the National Programme for Information Technology (NPfIT) that sought to direct informatics initiatives from the centre (Takian and Cornford 2012).

From its foundation in 1948 primary care in the NHS has been delivered mostly by private sector providers (Talbot-Smith and Pollock 2006). A rough division can be drawn between those who diagnose, prescribe and refer on to secondary care, typically general practitioners (GPs) and those licensed to provide therapeutic aids and drugs to patients, typically community pharmacies in high street shops. Both constituencies represent private businesses providing services to NHS patients though local and national commissioning contracts.

The devolved structure of primary care presents a challenge to new informatics based initiatives, insofar as any new service requires that primary care providers adopt compatible systems that are themselves supplied through competitive private sector markets, and to assent to sharing of data with both other primary care service providers and NHS secondary use services (Cornford et al. 2014). Thus NHS primary care providers and their informatics contractors, can and do at times hesitate and resist when asked to deploy new services and systems. Provision and use of health informatics services also reflects, in most cases, espoused health policy visions and strategies and come with some associated incentives. Thus, in the case of EPS there is a policy vision of community pharmacy as a resource that can support prescribers and patients by undertaking a greater role in the management of drug therapies for patients with chronic illness.

8.2.1   Prescribing, Dispensing and Reimbursing Primary Care Drugs

The typical pattern of prescription management in primary care is for the general practitioner to issue a prescription and for a community pharmacist to dispense against this, as appropriate. This division was first enshrined in the 1911 National Insurance Act which removed from prescribers the right to provide therapeutic drugs as part of a single care package (Anderson 2006). This had the effect of supporting an emerging pharmacy profession that gained greater and greater importance over the next 80 years as an ever-expanding catalogue of pre-packaged ready to use, experimentally proven drugs displaced the remedies traditionally compounded by pharmacists (Wade 1993).

More recently, during the period from 1979 to 2013, the average number of prescription items dispensed in primary care per capita each year has increased from 6 to 19 (Government Statistical Service 1991; Comptroller and Auditor General 1992; Health and Social Care Information Centre 2015), with those over 60 years of age receiving on average over forty prescription items per year. Increasing life expectancies and the associated increases in co-morbidities suggest that the prescribing and dispensing activities of primary care will become more central to care, more complex and could also have greater potential for harm (Banarjee et al. 2011). In response, community pharmacy has been promoted as needing to have a greater role in management of therapeutic drugs (Zermansky 1996), which is reflected in policy around service digitalization and repeat dispensing (Cornford et al. 2014).

8.2.2 Computers in English Primary Care

Development of EPS has been able to exploit a substantial installed base of NHS primary care informatics which has emerged from over three decades of initiatives in community pharmacies, GP practices and by the agency responsible for reimbursing primary care contractors for therapeutic drugs dispensed, NHS Prescription Services (Hayes 2008). But despite computerisation efforts in all three of these constituencies since the 1980s, it was not until the EPS programme in 2002 that a concerted effort was made to digitize the exchange of prescription data. Prior to this data flowed between the three main constituencies using hand-written, and more recently, computer-printed, paper prescription forms, officially known as the FP10.

Of these constituencies, GP practices have the longest history of computerisation, stemming back to batch processing experiments in the 1960s and real-time computing with a shared primary and acute care electronic patient record in the 1970s (Hayes 2008). The advent of the personal computer in the 1980s, schemes to support the adoption of primary care computing such as the Micros for GPs scheme (Project Evaluation Group 1985), and a reorganization that placed emphasis on documenting care provision as well as experiments in GP fundholding, led to the development of GP practice computing in earnest with many vendors entering the market (Brennan 2005; Hayes 2008). The numbers of vendors of GP practice systems subsequently declined through the 1990s, following the imposition of mandatory accreditation, but adoption of computerisation increased, reaching 96% of GP practices by 1996 (Hayes 2008).

Adoption of these systems by GP practices was initially driven by the value that the systems held for these businesses in the face of contractual change. In community pharmacy, computerisation was also driven by business concerns. In the 1980s pharmacy wholesalers recognized the opportunity for computers to support pharmacists in managing stock, and themselves in supporting ordering. These early systems, initially promoted and supplied by wholesalers, were subsequently developed as a platform that could integrate new clinical functionality. Thus as new professional requirements, such as maintaining patient medication records (PMRs) and creation of printed labels for dispensed items, came into force, these software systems were adapted (Shepherd 2008).

Given that it was the business opportunities provided by computers that drove the adoption of informatics by primary care providers, it would have been surprising if NHS Prescription Services (NHS PS) had failed also to adopt new informatics in support of its role of remuneration for prescription drugs dispensed. Although some prescriptions do attract a fixed patient co-payment (currently £8.20 ≈ €10.00 per prescribed item), the majority of funding for primary care dispensing is from the NHS, and is managed by NHS PS. Pharmacies make claims for the costs of dispensing therapeutic drugs to NHS PS using the prescriptions they have dispensed. Thus a prescription represents an invoice to be checked and paid as well as an authorisation to supply therapeutic drugs. It also provides a means to capture data on prescribing practices, and to collate data that can show how prescribers and GP practices are prescribing in comparison to their local and national peers (NHS Prescription Services 2011b, 2012).

NHS PS started computerisation in the 1970s as it became apparent there were no longer sufficient numbers of recruits to support the paper intensive process (Shepherd 2008). A later automation initiative, the Capacity Improvement Programme (CIP) launched in 2007 during EPS development, was similarly a response to concerns over the year-on-year prescription volume increases (NHS Prescription Services 2008, 2011a). The CIP was however still focused on the paper based system, using sophisticated optical character recognition to render prescription forms into digital data for processing.

8.2.3 Early ETP Experiments and Pilots

Computerisation of the NHS in the 1980 and 1990s inspired two in-vivo ETP experiments prior to the development of EPS. The first of these was the NHS Care Card programme of the late 1980s, which used the then novel technology of microprocessor based smartcards held by patients to transfer health record and prescription data between suitably equipped health care providers (NHS Management Executive 1991). Although this experiment, run in parts of England and Wales, did successfully demonstrate the service's concept, concerns over the cost and durability of the smartcards, and also of the lack of a back-up network to transfer data in case of smartcard failure, led to the abandonment of this solution (Hayes 2008; NHS Management Executive 1991).

At the turn of this century, ETP was revisited with a second NHS experiment using the new technology of electronic data interchange (EDI) and web services. The ETP Pilot Programme of 2000 invited private sector consortia to set up regional pilot projects in order to support the development of a set of standards that could underpin an England-wide ETP service (NHS Prescription Pricing Authority 2000).

From the start it was proposed that the outcomes of the ETP Pilot Programme would be reflected in a new ETP service that would be deployed in English primary care by 2004, although this timetable was later revised to 2008 as it became apparent that the institutional texture of the primary care environment was more complex than imagined. Some suppliers in the pilot believed that this could also provide an opportunity for at scale deployment of their pilot service, but the ETP Pilot Programme closed in 2003, as originally envisaged (Mathieson 2003).

The conclusions drawn were that the solutions developed were unable to meet stated institutional requirements around ensuring continuity of existing business flows between GP practices and community pharmacies (Department of Health 2004; Sugden 2003). More importantly, the pilot systems were incompatible with the new NPfIT vision of service integration, national systems, and shared resources (Brennan 2005). However, the vision of ETP as an EDI and network-based service remained and influenced the subsequent EPS.

8.3   Assembling the Electronic Prescription Service

EPS at its simplest just offers more reliable data transfer between the three main stakeholders using a digital version of the existing FP10 prescription form. Still, the influence of EPS inevitably leads to practice change across these institutional settings. Claims made for consequential change were often expressed as benefits to be realized and illustrate the service's expected influence on practice. Anticipated benefits included support for faster, more efficient prescription processing, reduced risk through elimination of transcription errors and the availability of electronic cancellation, reduced clinician prescription management workload, and increased patient convenience. Another suggested benefit, which was not pursued, was the expectation that the service could provide a proxy record of patient adherence to treatment through a record of dispensing events (Harvey et al. 2014). Concurrent changes in prescription management (discussed below) would later bring repeat dispensing prescriptions into the dialectic around EPS, and became more dominant as managers and policy makers became familiar with the possibilities this could offer (Cornford et al. 2014).

8.3.1   Transforming the Prescription

The benefits of EPS follow from one principal goal, replacing the paper form – known in the NHS as an FP10 – as the legal prescription by an electronic and digitally-signed equivalent. This form has traditionally been handed from prescriber to patient to dispenser and then passed onto NHS PS for reimbursement. Over the years, the FP10 has evolved to encompass a number of different functions for prescription management. The example shown below (Fig. 8.3) is for a repeat prescription. The left hand side represents the prescription which is dispensed against and will be used by the

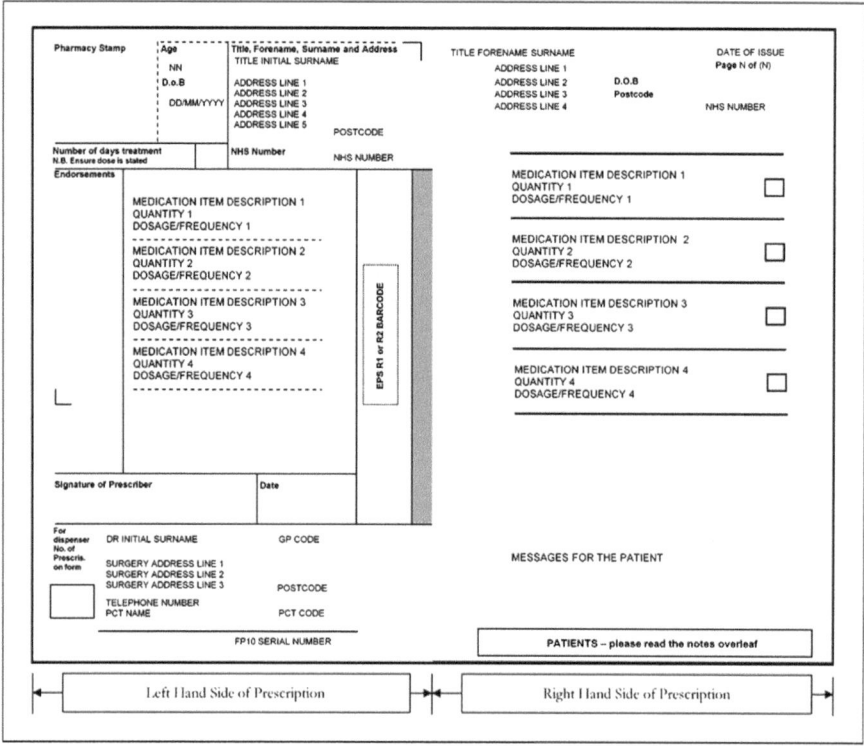

Fig. 8.3 English primary care FP10 prescription form (Gooch 2007a, b). Copyright © 2016, Re-used with the permission of the Health and Social Care Information Centre, also known as NHS Digital. All rights reserved.

dispenser to claim for what has been dispensed. The right hand side of the FP10 is a tear-off reorder form for use by the patient. Re-ordering is allowed for a set number of times until a review date has been reached, without the need for a GP consultation on each occasion. The right hand side also can be used by the GP practice for health promotion messages, or to advertise services, such as flu vaccination, which GP practices and community pharmacies might compete to provide. The back of the form (not shown) includes a signed declaration for those claiming free prescriptions.

Development of the EPS coincided with changes in how prescriptions can be managed. Prior to 2015 prescribers issued either acute or repeat prescriptions (Table 8.1). However, concerns over the capacity of GP practices to effectively monitor repeat prescriptions (Zermansky 1996) led to a new model of prescription management, the repeat dispensing prescription, where the activities of monitoring and control of prescriptions for chronic illness were handed to community pharmacy. This in turn triggered calls for change in the institutional relationship between prescribers and dispensers, principally around giving dispensers access to the concurrently developed national electronic Summary Care Record (SCR).

Table 8.1 Types of Prescription Used in English Primary Care (Cornford et al. 2014)

Type	Application	Management
Acute prescription	A one-off prescription for short term illness issued following a consultation between patient and general practitioner (GP)	The prescription is presented to the community pharmacist. Clinical checks are conducted by the pharmacist to ensure the prescription is appropriate for the patient. If the prescription is appropriate the relevant drugs are dispensed to the patient
Repeat prescription	Prescription is issued for the management of a long-term condition following a consultation between patient and GP. It is agreed by both parties that the prescription can be re-issued a set number of times until a review date without further consultations	Prescription is presented to the community pharmacist and checked and dispensed against as for acute prescriptions. The prescription is re-ordered from the GP practice using an order form printed with the prescription, and will be re-issued unless a review date has been reached or there are concerns over patient adherence
Repeat dispensing (introduced 2005)	Prescription is also used for long-term condition management. All issues of a prescription that the patient is expected to need until the review date are issued as a single batch. On paper these prescriptions are sent to a single pharmacy. With the use of electronic prescriptions each issue is a separate entity that can be dispensed against at any pharmacy	A batch of prescriptions is handed to the community pharmacist. Each issue is dispensed against when requested by the patient. Prescriptions are dispensed against in the same manner as an acute prescription with the addition of a check by the community pharmacist of patient's use of the medicine

8.3.2 Architecture

As a part of the NPfIT portfolio of projects EPS was explicitly designed alongside efforts to build services that met agreed national informatics standards. NPfIT was based on commitment to a common infrastructure through which constituent components such as EPS, SCR, the Care Records Service and others could connect and exchange data. At the core of this was a data-center and communications backbone, known as the Spine, providing common services and enabling the transfer of data between NHS computer systems. NPfIT also established a national secure network for the NHS – known as N3. The services used by EPS included the N3 network, extended to include links to high street pharmacies, and two principle Spine Services to manage the delivery of prescriptions: an Identity Agent service to establish the validity of prescribing and dispensing endpoints, and the NHS Smartcard to implement role based access control for prescribers and dispensers (Fig. 8.4). In addition a new underlying drug dictionary (dm+d) was developed – described below.

EPS functionality for prescribing and dispensing would however be delivered to health professionals by the vendors of community pharmacy and GP practice software, and to do so would make use of these core infrastructures and central data

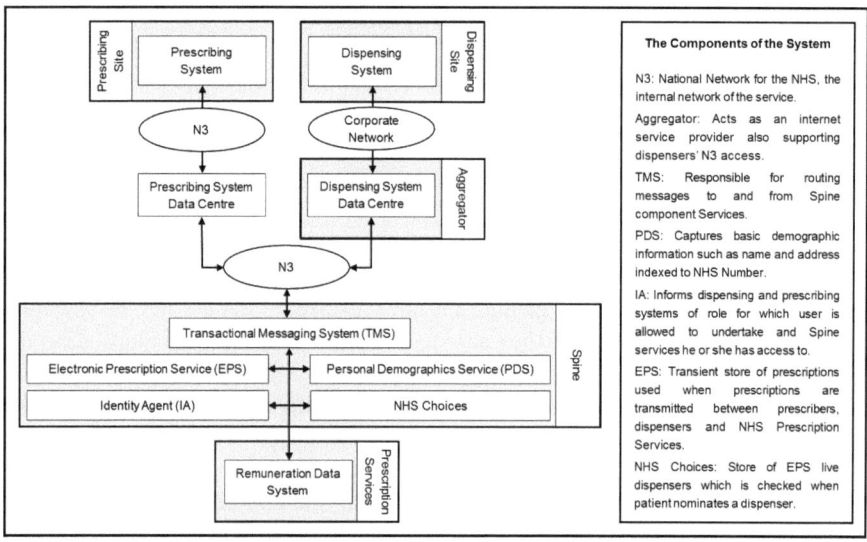

Fig. 8.4 Components of the electronic prescription service (Health and Social Care Information Centre n.d.). Copyright © 2016, Re-used with the permission of the Health and Social Care Information Centre, also known as NHS Digital. All rights reserved.

services. A set of output-based specifications were made available to software vendors that described how the EPS software for doctors and pharmacists should manage and process electronic prescriptions (Gooch 2007a, b). Compliance of software with these specifications was assessed through a multi-stage common assurance process (CAP) managed centrally (NHS Connecting for Health 2012). These specifications provided a partial definition of the operation of the service, but details as to the management of user interfaces and circumstances for the creation of paper versions of the electronic prescriptions was placed in system suppliers' hands.

Electronic Drug Dictionaries

Prior to EPS there was no single database of therapeutic drugs available for use within GP practice systems, system vendors choosing from a number of commercial suppliers, such as First Databank Europe, or opting to develop their own, as EMIS, a major software supplier, did. In parallel NHS Prescription Services compiled a monthly Drug Tariff based on manufacturer data, marketing authorisations, and latterly, dispensing volumes. One consequence of EPS was that a new and common underlying database to describe medicines as they were prescribed, dispensed and paid for was developed, the dictionary of medicines and devices (dm+d). This ontology can represent therapeutic drugs at multiple levels depending on how the data was to be used. To support access to existing decision support systems manufacturers might chose to map dm+d coding to their own dictionaries, which also allows the development of decision support across multiple international markets

8.3.3   Release Strategy and Deployment

EPS was structured and delivered to users as two sequential releases. The releases differed in their functionality and the demands made on dispensing and prescribing health professionals. This approach allowed for tests of the technical infrastructure to be conducted in the first release, including networking and the Spine services developed for NPfIT (Brennan 2005).

EPS Release 1 (EPS R1) focussed on augmenting the paper prescription with digital data (Fig. 8.5). A unique identifier for each prescription was created at the time of prescribing and printed on the prescription as a barcode. A digital copy of the prescription was then sent to the Spine. A pharmacy could scan this barcode and download a digital copy to be used to populate the patient medication record (PMR) in the pharmacy system and help in stock control and label creation. Although a dispenser could forward the digital version of the prescriptions to NHS Prescription Services, this functionality simply served as a test of prescription transmission with no immediate benefit for community pharmacy. In many ways EPS R1 was a partial parallel run of digital and paper systems side by side from which much was learned about the network and the software.

EPS release 2 (EPS R2) expanded the administrative and clinical functionality and enabled electronic and paper artefacts to trade legal status (Fig. 8.6). In EPS R2 the digital message has the legal status as a prescription, and is dispensed against and used to claim for remuneration. In addition, new clinical functionality in the form of repeat dispensing prescriptions and safety functions, such as electronic cancellation of prescriptions were added, with the expectation of more timely and effective delivery of prescription drugs to patients as well as efficiency benefits for GPs, pharmacists and NHS PS.

At the time that EPS R2 was ready to be deployed NHS primary care was composed of a number, of local health authorities, known as Primary Care Trusts (PCTs). In order to issue digitally signed electronic prescriptions, the PCT had to have Secretary of State Directions (e.g. permission). This was issued based on the readiness of the PCT to manage the local deployment process. Control over which prescribers could issue electronic prescriptions was at the discretion of the PCT. A GP practice would only be allowed to use EPS R2 when at least 80% of their existing prescription volumes could be sent to dispensing sites that had EPS available. This ensured both that there were local places to send prescriptions to, and helped avoid market distortion.

However, whilst a prescriber might be authorised to issue electronic prescriptions, not everything prescribed could be sent electronically, specifically certain schedules of controlled drugs –drugs that can be abused or employed for nefarious purposes (Department of Health 2014). Following a high profile case of murders committed using diverted controlled drugs, the department responsible for drugs policy, the Home Office, revised the Misuse of Drugs Act to restrict the

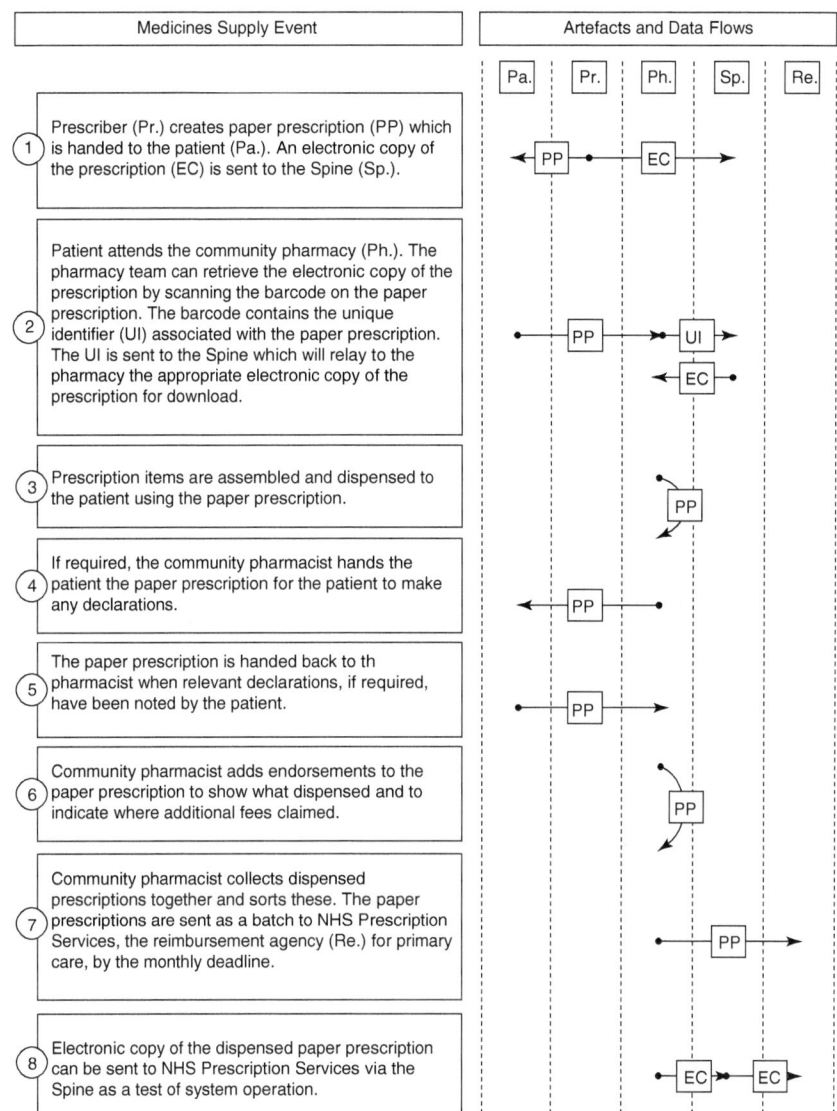

Fig. 8.5 Operation of the electronic prescription service release 1

opportunities for diversion. So, despite the potential that EPS had in restricting and auditing supply, it was not until July 2015, that the Misuse of Drugs Act and other regulations were amended to allow for full electronic prescribing of controlled drugs (Department of Health 2015).

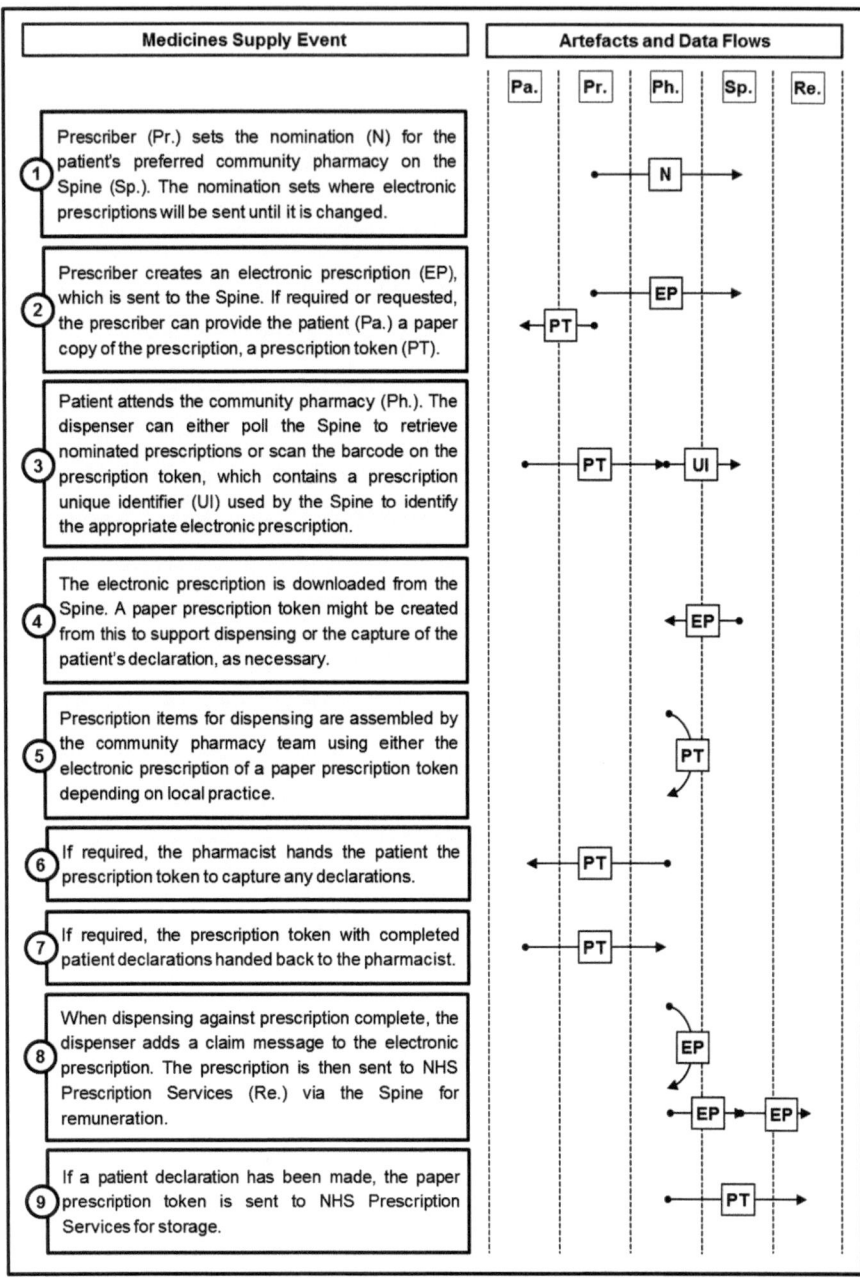

Fig. 8.6 Operation of the electronic prescription service release 2

8.4   Assembling EPS as Past, Present and Future

In this section we consider the nature of the work needed to assemble the EPS we see today. We do this using a model that identifies the work of assembly in terms of *constraints* imposed within the context of EPS development and deployment, *inertia* resulting from unaligned incentives and lack of resources, and finally concern to maintain *fidelity* to the mission of the broader NHS, its culture and practices (Fig. 8.1).

8.4.1   The Physical and Material in a Digital World

We start by considering EPS in its technical/architectural form employing a range of digital services to support communication of relationships about the physical world in terms of medicines, people and locations. General communication standards introduced across the NHS by NPfIT such as ebXML, HL7 and the clinical coding terminology SNOMED CT, provide underlying substrates for this communication. Other specific new services were developed, for example, electronic verification of users and sites by Spine Identity Agent which check both validity of role-profiles on individuals' Smartcard and the identity of endpoints through Organisational Data Services (ODS) codes. As noted above, the therapeutic drugs that can be prescribed using EPS are described in a new electronic dictionary of medicines and devices (dm+d) developed for EPS.

These protocols, databases and services each fulfill necessary roles and functions in the new EPS, but EPS must also show some fidelity to established structures, practices and professional roles within the NHS. A primary example is the FP10 prescription form. The FP10 endures within EPS in many ways and links it to the past and facilitates its viability in the present. The continuing presence of the FP10 within EPS is in part a means of overcoming inertia and institutional constraints in implementation and also a demonstration of fidelity with the past. Retaining elements of the FP10 in the assembly ensures a better 'fit' of the new EPS in the wider health care context, both conceptually and practically. The FP10 also endures in a printed form, although without legal status. For example, a printout may support the FP10's traditional role in collecting patients' signed declarations for prescription charge exemptions as well as meeting dispensers' needs for a portable representation of the prescription, a picking list, against which to assemble drugs when dispensing. Similarly, a prescriber may wish to give a patient a paper copy of their drugs to keep, even if the prescription itself is electronically transmitted. And we know that 'handing over the prescription' is a common way that doctors politely terminate a consultation.

In the new electronic world, just as with paper prescribing, an EPS prescription can be composed of multiple prescription messages, each message constrained to a maximum of four prescription items. This constraint, originally imposed by the physical size of the FP10 form, endures in EPS reflecting the need to replicate existing FP10 processes, for example in its role as a dispenser's picking list. This fidelity is reinforced by the inertia implied in the delivery model used for EPS, in which providers of existing prescribing and dispensing software were invited to integrate relevant functionality into their *existing* software systems. As a result many aspects of EPS software design, in particular interfaces, drew directly on existing processes for FP10 handling in GP practices, Community Pharmacies and NHS Prescription Services.

8.4.2   The Reinvention of Services

EPS is constrained and shaped by the complex and multiple institutional and technical relations in which it is embedded. The confluence of multiple institutional presents place constraints on how and what EPS can do or change, and can conspire to reduce the service functionality and availability. These constraints invite resolution over time through such things as regulatory change (e.g. controlled rugs), workarounds and re-purposing of infrastructures. Indeed, work-arounds are a common and an essential part of EPS's ability to respond to challenges and reshape itself over time.

This is also seen in the ways that the NHS Smartcard is repeatedly renegotiated as a part of EPS. The NHS Smartcard implements a Role Based Access Control (RBAC) model in which access to services are associated with specific privileges for individual's roles stored in the Spine's Identity Agent (NHS Connecting for Health 2011). A health professional's NHS Smartcard has to be in an attached reader for the session and a password entered at the start of a session. This is broadly suitable to work practices of prescribers in primary care and such use, for example by doctors preparing prescriptions, predates EPS.

This model was not, however, found appropriate for dispensers in community pharmacy and indeed was never designed to encompass 'non NHS' persons in private organisations – the status of a community pharmacist, either as a permanent or locum staff. The result is that new models of Smartcard use emerged in the form of work-arounds. First, for EPS R1, given access is only to an electronic copy of the patient's prescription, information that the community pharmacy already has, the solution found was simple. Each community pharmacy was issued with an NHS Smartcard that acted as a proxy for the site, and which represented shared rather than a personal roles and privileges. But this 'fix' could not work in EPS R2 where dispensers gained access to Spine services that support inspection and amendment of patient data, which requires an audit trail (NHS Connecting for Health 2010).

For EPS R2, community pharmacies moved to the model used by NHS clinicians. In this model the Spine Identity Agent records the identity of the clinician, the clinician's roles and the sites at which this role is enacted, each site being identified by an ODS code. Locum community pharmacists, moving often from site to site, posed a problem if their ODS mapping requires frequent updates. The solution found was to create a virtual organisation for dispensing staff, initially community pharmacists but later dispensing technicians too, which was given the ODS code FFFFF, the 5-F code (NHS Connecting for Health 2010). This workaround allowed an EPS R2 user access to limited patient data. However, it is now policy that pharmacists have access to the Summary Care Record (SCR) – a national summary of the individual health record including medicines prescribed, seen as an essential tool to support pharmacists in safe therapeutic drug supply. This created a need to reinvent the process once again to provide a more detailed audit trail. Now locum staff access the SCR by the 'emergency' access button *plus* manually inputting the ODS code for the site where they are working (Royal Pharmaceutical Society 2014).

8.4.3 Ruthless Standardization

> We will improve the leadership and direction given to IT, and combine it with national and local implementation that are based on ruthless standardisation. (Department of Health 2002)

NPfIT, the large national programme within which EPS was initiated, started out with a mantra of 'ruthless standardization'. It took time to dilute and finally wash this idea away. EPS as it has been delivered is very much a child of this policy and the retreat from it. Initially NPfIT proposed that all GP systems would be replaced with just one of two national 'solutions' incorporating EPS. In time there was revolt as GPs realised they would be coerced into giving up systems they knew and trusted. To placate them, in 2006 a new model of GP software procurement was established, GP Systems of Choice (GPSoC). This allowed GP practices theoretically to adopt any software that offered GPSoC functionality including EPS and the Summary Care Record (NHS Connecting for Health 2008).

The GPSoC model of approval based around output-based specifications (OBS) only defined how *electronic* messages would be handled. So controlled drugs initially fell outside of EPS and thus also fell outside of the OBS. Consequently, with no guidance available as to how to manage prescriptions which contained both EPS and non-EPS items, no common model was proposed for managing these situations. Some software suppliers choose to prevent any part of a prescription containing controlled drugs being transmitted electronically, others choose to create an electronic prescription for non-controlled drugs, and in parallel a paper prescription for the out-of-scope controlled drugs. Receiving drugs from GP practices with systems adopting the latter model caused confusion and inconvenience in their own work practices and for patients. This was only resolved when the law on controlled dugs changed.

A more active approach to addressing inertia and limited resources is seen in the structuring of development of pharmacy systems and the lengthy period of software testing required by the Common Assurance Process (NHS Connecting for Health 2008). This stepped assurance process for both dispensing and prescribing systems, moved from safety case analysis through to in-vitro testing with test messages in a sandpit environment through to in-vivo testing in a limited number of sites with a test set of messages, and later, real prescriptions. This detailed programme provided a mechanism through which to focus resources and supplier attention. Deliberate selection of early implementation sites on the basis of their readiness also allowed for the gradual expansion of the service and provided some quarantine for problems arising and unexpected events.

8.5   What Can the Electronic Prescription Service Teach Us?

Looking back over the history of EPS, what stands out is how much of EPS is formed by hybridisation of the digital and the physical/material. EPS was conceived to be new and powerful, embodying policy visions of transformation, but it had also to fit within existing processes and work practices, mimicking existing data flows, and co-opting core artefacts such as the FP10. Thus a flexible and evolving assembly of the digital and the physical was necessary for EPS to come into existence. Further, it is from the institutional environment as much as the installed base of infrastructures that the necessary conditions and resources for EPS are mobilised, assembled and sustained. Of course in this they also create (assemble) the conditions for complications, as we saw with regard to management of prescriptions for controlled drugs in the early implementation of EPS and the multiple reconfigurations of the NHS smartcard RBAC system.

EPS also illustrates how inertia, as represented in the limited capacities of dispensing and prescribing system suppliers to resource change, can be managed through institutional arrangements such as testing and controlled deployment. NPfIT and those managing the deployment used the power to establish specific arrangements to overcome inertia and channel limited resources within the supply network and in the context of use. Even a programme with unprecedented political commitment behind it, as NPfIT had at the outset, had to remain flexible. So our final message drawn form EPS is that the search for new opportunities within and beyond the installed base is driven by a creative search across institutional spaces as much if not more than across technological spaces. The installed base is in this way more diverse, and more pliable than we might at first think, and introduction of innovation rests on the opportunities and routes carved through.

References

Anderson S. From 'bespoke' to 'off-the-peg': community pharmacists and the retailing of medicines in Great Britain 1900–1970. In: Curth L, editor. From physick to pharmacology: five hundred years of British drug retailing. Aldershot: Ashgate; 2006.

Banarjee A, Mbalmu D, Ebrahim S, Khan A, Chan T. The prevalence of polypharmacy in elderly attenders to an emergency department – a problem with a need for an effective solution. Int J Emerg Med. 2011;4:22.

Benson T. Why general practitioners use computers and hospital doctors do not – Part 1: incentives. Br Med J. 2002a;325:1086–9.

Benson T. Why general practitioners use computers and hospital doctors do not – Part 2: scalability. Br Med J. 2002b;325:1090–3.

Brennan S. The NHS IT project: the biggest computer programme in the world... ever. Oxford: Radcliffe; 2005.

Comptroller and Auditor General. Community pharmacies in England. London: Her Majesty's Stationery Office; 1992.

Cornford T, Doukidis G, Forster D. Experience with a structure, process and outcome framework for evaluating an information system. Omega. 1994;22:491–504.

Cornford T, Hibberd R, Barber N. The evaluation of the electronic prescription service in primary care: final report on the findings from the evaluation in early implementer sites. London: University College London; 2014.

Department of Health. Delivering 21st century IT support for the NHS: national strategic programme. London: Department of Health; 2002.

Department of Health. Electronic prescription service: ETP principles. 2004. http://www.dh.gov. uk/en/Healthcare/Medicinespharmacyandindustry/Prescriptions/ElectronicPrescription Service/DH_4070920. Accessed 5 Mar 2012.

Department of Health. The proposals to include schedules 2 and 3 controlled drugs within the scope of the electronic prescription service: consultation document. London: Department of Health; 2014.

Department of Health. Proposals to enable the electronic prescribing of schedules 2 and 3 controlled drugs: response to consultation. Leeds: Department of Health; 2015.

Gooch R. Dispensing system compliance specification. Leeds: NHS Connecting for Health; 2007a.

Gooch R. Prescribing systems compliance specification. Leeds: NHS Connecting for Health; 2007b.

Government Statistical Service. Department of Health Statistical Bulletin: prescriptions dispensed by Pharmacy and Appliance Contractors – England 1979–1989. London: Department of Health, London; 1991.

Harvey J, Avery A, Hibberd R, Barber N. Meeting user needs in national healthcare systems: lessons from early adopter community pharmacists using the Electronic Prescription Service. BMC Medical Informatics and Decision Making. 2014;14:16.

Hayes G. The history of primary care computing in the UK. In: Hayes G, Barnett D, editors. UK health computing: recollections and reflections. Swindon: British Computer Society; 2008.

Health and Social Care Information Centre. Prescriptions dispensed in the community: England 2004–14. Leeds: Health and Social Care Information Centre; 2015.

Health and Social Care Information Centre. Statistics and progress: latest statistics (8th Apr 2016). 2016. http://systems.hscic.gov.uk/eps/stats. Accessed 8 Apr 2016.

Health and Social Care Information Centre (n.d.) Components of EPS. http://systems.hscic.gov. uk/eps/library/components. Accessed 14 Sept 2015.

Hibberd R, Barber N, Cornford T, Lichtner V. The evaluation of the electronic prescription service in primary care: interim report on the findings from the evaluation in early implementer sites. London: University College London; 2012.

Lichtner V, Venters W, Hibberd R, Cornford T, Barber N. The fungibility of time in claims of efficiency: the case of making transmission of prescriptions electronic in English general practice. Int J Med Inform. 2012;82:1152–70.

Mathieson S. Scrapping the National Programme for IT: a journey not a destination. The Guardian, 22 Sept [Online]. 2011. http://www.theguardian.com/healthcare-network/2011/sep/22/npfit-ends-cfh-andrew-lansley-bt-csc. Accessed 14 Sept 2015.

Mathieson S. All good things come to an end. The Guardian, 10 Jul [Online]. 2003. https://www. theguardian.com/technology/2003/jul/10/medicineandhealth.onlinesupplement. Accessed 8 Apr 2016.

NHS Connecting for Health. A guide to GP systems of choice. Leeds: NHS Connecting for Health; 2008.

NHS Connecting for Health. Migration of community pharmacy users from eps release 1 functionality to eps release 2 functionality including addendum for UIM users. Leeds: NHS Connecting for Health; 2010.

NHS Connecting for Health. Smartcards. 2011. http://www.connectingforhealth.nhs.uk/systemsandservices/eps/stuff/faq/smartcards/smartcards. Accessed 31 Dec 2013.

NHS Connecting for Health. Spine compliance. 2012. http://www.connectingforhealth.nhs.uk/ industry/compliance. Accessed 5 Mar 2012.

NHS England. Safer hospitals, safer wards: achieving an integrated digital care record. Leeds: NHS England; 2013.

NHS Management Executive. The care card: evaluation of the exmouth project. London: Her Majesty's Stationery Office; 1991.

NHS Prescription Pricing Authority. Electronic transmission of prescriptions. Impact: prescribing and dispensing newsletter, Dec 2000 [Online]. 2000. http://www.nhsbsa.nhs.uk/ PrescriptionServices/Documents/PPDImpact/imPACTdec2000.pdf. Accessed 8 Apr 2016.

NHS Prescription Services. Implementation of the Capacity Improvement Programme by the Prescription Pricing Division. 2008. http://www.nhsbsa.nhs.uk/1618.aspx. Accessed 4 Mar 2012.

NHS Prescription Services. CIP Q and A. http://www.nhsbsa.nhs.uk/PrescriptionServices/Documents/PrescriptionServices/CIP_Q_and_A_2009-11.pdf. 2011a. Accessed 4 Mar 2012.

NHS Prescription Services. Prescription Cost Analysis (PCA) data. 2011b. http://www.nhsbsa.nhs.uk/PrescriptionServices/3494.aspx. Accessed 21 Mar 2012.

NHS Prescription Services. ePACT. 2012. http://www.nhsbsa.nhs.uk/PrescriptionServices/815.aspx. Accessed 21 Mar 2012.

Petrakaki D, Barber N, Waring J. The possibilities of technology in shaping healthcare professionals: (Re/De-)professionalization of pharmacists in England. Soc Sci Med. 2012;75:429–37.

Project Evaluation Group. General practice computing – evaluation of the 'Micros for GPs' scheme: final report. London: Her Majesty's Stationery Office; 1985.

Royal Pharmaceutical Society. Summary care records: a quick reference guide. London: Royal Pharmaceutical Society; 2014.

Shepherd I. Computing in the pharmacy. In: Hayes G, Burnett D, editors. UK health computing: recollections and reflections. Swindon: British Computer Society; 2008.

Sugden R. Electronic transmission of prescriptions evaluation of pilots: summary report. London: Department of Health; 2003.

Takian A, Cornford T. NHS information: revolution or evolution? Health Policy Technol. 2012;1:193–8.

Talbot-Smith A, Pollock A. The new NHS: a guide. Abingdon: Routledge; 2006.

Wade O. British National Formulary: its birth, death, and rebirth. Br Med J. 1993;306:1051–2.

Zermansky A. Who controls repeats? Br J Gen Pract. 1996;46:643–7.

Open Access This chapter is distributed under the terms of the Creative Commons Attribution-NonCommercial 2.5 International License (http://creativecommons.org/licenses/by-nc/2.5/), which permits any noncommercial use, duplication, adaptation, distribution and reproduction in any medium or format, as long as you give appropriate credit to the original author(s) and the source, provide a link to the Creative Commons license and indicate if changes were made.

The images or other third party material in this chapter are included in the chapter's Creative Commons license, unless indicated otherwise in a credit line to the material. If material is not included in the chapter's Creative Commons license and your intended use is not permitted by statutory regulation or exceeds the permitted use, you will need to obtain permission directly from the copyright holder.

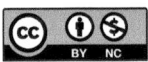

The Challenges of Implementing Packaged Hospital Electronic Prescribing and Medicine Administration Systems in UK Hospitals: Premature Purchase of Immature Solutions?

9

Hajar Mozaffar, Robin Williams, Kathrin M. Cresswell,
Neil Pollock, Zoe Morrison, and Aziz Sheikh

9.1   Introduction

This chapter explores the difficulties experienced in recent attempts to implement 'packaged' Hospital Electronic Prescribing and Medicine Administration (HEPMA) systems in NHS England. Though electronic prescribing was originally conceived as a pharmacy technology, it has become the occasion for integrating various other kinds of digital information (e.g. laboratory test results) at the point of care and for sharing this information across the care pathway. HEPMA in the United Kingdom (UK) has thus served as a stepping stone in developing hospital-wide infrastructures that directly support both diagnosis and care delivery. Considerable effort was needed to *integrate* HEPMA modules within the hospital information

H. Mozaffar • N. Pollock
Business School, The University of Edinburgh, 29 Buccleuch Place, Edinburgh, UK, EH8 9JS
e-mail: Hajar.mozaffar@ed.ac.uk; neil.pollock@ed.ac.uk

R. Williams (✉)
Institute for the Study of Science, Technology and Innovation, The University of Edinburgh, High School Yards, Edinburgh, UK, EH1 1LZ
e-mail: Robin.Williams@ed.ac.uk

K.M. Cresswell • A. Sheikh
Centre for Medical Informatics, The University of Edinburgh, Doorway Number 3, Teviot Place, Edinburgh, UK, EH8 9AG
e-mail: kathrin.beyer@ed.ac.uk; aziz.sheikh@ed.ac.uk

Z. Morrison
Business School, University of Aberdeen, Edward Wright Building, Dunbar Street, Aberdeen, UK, AB24 3QY
e-mail: Zoemorrison@abdn.ac.uk

© The Author(s) 2017   129
M. Aanestad et al. (eds.), *Information Infrastructures within European Health Care*, Health Informatics, DOI 10.1007/978-3-319-51020-0_9

infrastructures and to *interface* them with external systems – and other parts of the health system, notably primary care. The difficulties besetting attempts to implement HEPMA as Commercial Off The Shelf (COTS) packaged software have highlighted the gap between the generic workflow models embedded in standardised COTS solutions (many of which were developed overseas) and the diverse practices of particular UK hospitals. Similar problems arose with previous attempts to implement packaged enterprise systems (ES), but were ameliorated through a protracted social learning (Sørensen 1996) process involving vendors, suppliers and various intermediaries. Comparing HEPMA and ES highlights the current immaturity of the HEPMA market. This is characterised by: the relatively embryonic linkages between HEPMA vendors and their potential market of users; users' lack of understanding of the exigencies of exploiting packaged solutions; vendors' limited understanding of user requirements and poorly elaborated strategies to address diverse user needs in generic solutions.

Stakeholders managing health systems in many countries have invested substantial efforts to implement and deploy electronic or ePrescribing systems (Mozaffar et al. 2014; Cresswell et al. 2013) to support prescribing decisions in health organisations (Aarts and Koppel 2009; Bates et al. 1998). The National Health Service (NHS) in England has similarly invested considerable resources in these systems. It describe these systems as:

> *The utilisation of electronic systems to facilitate and enhance the communication of a prescription or medicine order, aiding the choice, administration and supply of a medicine through knowledge and decision support and providing a robust audit trail for the entire medicines use process. (NHS Connecting for Health, England)*

9.1.1 The UK Context for Hospital Electronic Infrastructures

Health care in the UK is primarily provided through the publicly-funded National Health Service (NHS). With over a million employees, the NHS is an exceptionally large and complex organisation (Hibberd et al. 2016). There are differences between the NHS in each of the devolved administrations (England, Scotland, Wales, Northern Ireland). This chapter focuses on developments within NHS England, which is by far the largest. Hospitals are run by regional health authorities, originally known as Primary Care Trusts, with primary care delivered by multiple independent General Practitioners. Despite a very long history of hospital computerisation stretching over 60 years, the development of hospital electronic infrastructures was seen to be held up, *inter-alia*, by the fragmentation of procurement between hospitals and trusts. Repeated attempts to improve integration culminated in a major national initiative: the National Programme for Information Technology (NPfIT) in which, as well as creating a central transaction processing 'Spine' (Hibberd et al. 2016), selected software applications were to be centrally procured and implemented in NHS hospitals (Sheikh et al. 2011; Robertson et al. 2011). This initiative however encountered numerous problems and, as a result, the Department of Health instituted a change of direction from a 'centrally driven strategy of replace all' to 'locally chosen and implemented systems' (Robertson et al. 2011; Sheikh et al. 2011).

NHS calls to improve the quality, safety and efficiency of healthcare, coupled with substantial financial support, have provoked widespread interest in the timely implementation of HEPMA systems in UK hospitals (Buntin et al. 2011; Black et al. 2011; McKibbon et al. 2011) and attracted a number of UK and overseas suppliers. Electronic prescribing is already well established in England's primary care (Avery et al. 2007; Fernando et al. 2004; Hibberd et al. 2016). Over the last decade, several attempts have been made to implement HEPMA systems in secondary care. In 2013 only 13% of hospitals had hospital-wide HEPMA systems (Ahmed et al. 2013). This is however expected to rise rapidly as a result of the £500 Million *Safer Hospitals Safer Wards* technology fund launched in 2013 and a policy target of complete implementation across the NHS by 2020 (Carter 2015). The move towards local selection of systems has resulted in hospitals being faced with a range of options, none of which are however currently perceived as fully meeting the needs of the English market (Mozaffar et al. 2014).

Whilst the first generation of HEPMA systems was developed within hospitals, today we see a marked shift away from home-grown solutions towards COTS 'packaged' software (Mozaffar et al. 2014). There are a number of reasons for this move. These include the very substantial costs associated with developing and maintaining bespoke systems (and the stalled progress and anticipated failure of a flagship project to jointly develop an integrated solution within/for English hospitals[1]), the perceived advantages of packaged solutions (in terms of functionality/price, dependability, maintenance) and problems with limited interoperability between providers (Schiff et al. 2003; Westbrook et al. 2012). However, standard COTS solutions, built around generic models of the user organisation, may be far removed from the workflows of particular adopter organisations, necessitating a considerable effort to configure and customise software or to adjust local working practices (Pollock and Williams 2008). Despite these investments, the HEPMA market in England is faced with a great deal of uncertainty and is undergoing rapid change and evolution (Aarts and Koppel 2009; Mozaffar et al. 2014). As well as intense policy pressures and incentives to adopt HEPMA, hospitals are confronted by the lack of maturity of current supplier offerings, their limited tailoring to the English context, the diversity of systems and lack of knowledge about the available options. These factors all contribute to the challenges that hospitals face in procuring, implementing and realizing the benefits of these systems (Wolfstadt et al. 2008; Bates et al. 2003; Cresswell et al. 2013; Mozaffar et al. 2014).

---

[1] Thus the Lorenzo patient system being collaboratively developed under NPfIT encountered such serious delays that its wide adoption is seen as increasingly unlikely. Tameside Hospital NHS Foundation Trust recently awarded the highest possible risk rating to its Lorenzo project, citing "potential risks to patient safety quality, information governance and performance trajectories" (HSJ 2014).

In this chapter we examine the problems that have arisen in the supply, procurement and implementation of packaged HEPMA solutions. We explore the reasons for this in terms of the state of development of the HEPMA market – encompassing the strategies and capacities of both vendors and adopters. Our analysis brings to bear insights from the Biography of Artefacts and Practices (BoAP) perspective (Pollock and Williams 2008) that emerged from our previous long-term programme of research into the evolution of the Enterprise System market. BoAP draws also upon recent related analytical advances in relation to the conceptualization of information infrastructures and to the formation and maturation of technological fields. As we outline below, this suggests that analysis of the development of information infrastructures (IIs) needs to engage with the exigencies surrounding technology supply and the increasing resort to commercially-supplied solutions. For example (Koch 1997), highlighted the choice between "bricks and clay" when building corporate IIs: between procuring integrated solutions or configuring together large numbers of small infrastructure components. The latter offers greater scope for adopter organisations to exercise choice in the selection of components and (because they tended to be technologically simpler) greater potential influence over their design. Integrated solutions offered less flexibility but transferred the integration challenge to the supplier. They could also operate as a platform onto which other offerings might be erected (Koch 2007). This in turn suggests that theories of the installed base need to go beyond a focus on the evolution of individual IIs and take on board the complex sets of relations linking multiple vendors and their adopter communities. We will explore this conceptual framework in our Discussion.

Methods

This chapter draws upon an extended national research programme investigating the implementation and adoption of HEPMA systems in English hospitals funded by the National Institute for Health Research (NIHR). In this chapter we re-examine these findings in relation to the goals of this book to understand the development of health infrastructures and examine the influence of the installed base.

We draw particularly upon a study of the current status of the English HEPMA market (Mozaffar et al. 2014, 2015; Cresswell et al. 2013; Crowe et al. 2010). We collected qualitative data from both suppliers and adopters of various HEPMA systems in England. Data collection, undertaken over the period October 2012 to October 2014, involved a combination of semi-structured interviews with staff of six English hospitals adopting HEPMA and of four system vendors, ethnographic observations (totalling 21 h) of user groups and hospital practices, a supplier round-table discussion, and collection of publically available documents. Interviews and data analysis were conducted in tandem – research foci and theme emerged inductively over a number of iterations. Table 9.1 summarises the data sources and collection methods.

Table 9.1 Data collection methods

Method	Data source	Focus of enquiry
Semi-structured interviews (ranging from 45 min to 2 h)	Four suppliers	(a) The current status and trajectory of growth of HEPMA systems in England;
	Six hospitals	(b) Strategies in design, development and adaptation (Anglicization) of the system;
		(c) The problems faced during implementation and their possible causes; and
		(d) The supplier-user relationship throughout the project lifecycle
Observations	Two user group meetings	(a) The technological contents of the discussion;
		(b) The supplier-user relationships; and
		(c) Decisions being taken.
Focus group	Supplier round-table discussion	(a) Challenges and opportunities for suppliers from the early stages of project initiation to implementation;
		(b) Suppliers' experiences of go-live and system stabilization; and
		(c) Suppliers' views on system optimization and enhancements

9.2 Understanding the Uneven Success of HEPMA

Overall there had been a relatively low uptake of these products by English hospitals and implementation has been slow (Mozaffar et al. 2014). This market was undergoing rapid cycles of change with many suppliers entering and offering a wide range of products in terms of functionality and architecture. Our analysis suggests a range of explanations for the current uneven growth and variable success of HEPMA systems in England, rooted in suppliers' strategies and adopters' current reactions to the technology and the market.

9.2.1 How HEPMA Systems Are Constituted: Extension of Non-clinical Systems

Our earlier study on the spectrum of available HEPMA systems in England identified a wide range of systems including 13 hospital-wide applications and a range of specialty systems in implementation or use across English hospitals (Mozaffar et al. 2014). Nine of these systems were developed outside England and were introduced into the English market over the past decade.

We studied four HEPMA systems. None were initially designed as HEPMA systems.

One of the products in our sample involved a pharmacy stock control system, which was extended with the addition of HEPMA functionality including what is sometimes described as computerized physician order entry (CPOE) and computerized decision support (CDS). This medication-focused system offered basic integration between the two modules but it was not a fully integrated hospital information system. This was a standalone application that covered inpatient needs, discharge prescribing, and pharmacy stock control. Interfacing strategies were used to connect this system with other systems used in hospitals. During this the course of this study, plans were made to extend this system by designing and developing the discharge prescribing system.

There were two multi-modular integrated 'systems', which arose through the expansion of insurance or billing systems for U.S. hospitals into integrated hospital-wide systems with the additional modules covering various areas such as inpatient and outpatient prescribing, electronic medical record, clinical imaging and labora-tory, linked into an integrated whole with one underlying database. The final system was initially designed as an electronic patient chart system and then expanded over time to include a scheduling system and HEPMA modules (initially only inpatient prescribing, though during the course of this study, plans were made to extend this system by designing and developing the discharge prescribing system). Thus, we saw that the promotion of HEPMA functionalities had pulled in product offerings and component technologies from different sources with different historical paths, which resulted in packages with rather different architectures and configurations.

Members of adopting organisations noted that the two U.S. 'integrated systems' emerged by adding multiple modules to what was originally a billing/insurance management system, formed around calculating the costs of drugs and saw this as an important factor in the problems in implementing and using these systems. They often described these as 'non-clinical systems', to draw attention to the fact that they arose as an extension of an already existing product with a different focus.

> *...over the years they have progressed from the original billing system or pharmacy stock control systems to now be basically sold as EPMA* [ePrescribing and medication adminis-tration] *systems .... It's just a billing system... the funding for the hospital was gained rais-ing bills from the patients they treated. So they needed a full audit trail to know what went on with the patient so they can charge the right amount of money. So again they were origi-nally billing systems but they started to tag on clinical functionality on them (Adopter Interview, P1)*

These users questioned the clinical merits of offerings that were not initially designed as clinical systems, but emerged by adding HEPMA functionality to non-clinical systems:

> *...in recent times there has been a lot more influx on the market. The EPMA systems are generally changing to focus on the clinical functionality... but whether you could say that the system is totally designed around the clinical users interface is a debatable question... if you want something to be a clinical tool then it should be clinical enabling and not some-thing like clinical disabling ... do we want to collect clinical information to make clinical judgment better or do we want it to manage the process that we are doing when we are trying to treat patients (Adopter Interview, P1)*

The non-clinical origins of these systems were seen as resulting in interface designs and workflows that were not centred around patient care pathways. A clinician, using the HEPMA system built around a stock control system, felt that system design might usefully take a different starting point:

> ...*our starting point is not just prescribing a drug, our starting point is actually saying you come in with this condition therefore your pathway is this. (Adopter Interview, P2)*

We observed a wide range of HEPMA systems shaped by the history through which they were constituted. In general the trend was to add HEPMA functionalities to already existing (non- ePrescribing) systems or to adapt existing systems to accommodate the newly required functions. These systems had inherited some of the characteristics of their source system and this affected their usability. Despite significant technical differences between the solutions, we encountered homologous problems. In particular, in the process of expanding the scope of systems, suppliers seemed to have underestimated the complexity of HEPMA as a clinical system and the particularity of user activities (a failing that closely mirrored criticisms of early ES offerings two decades earlier).

9.2.2 Adoption of Systems That Had Been Developed Outside England

Mozaffar et al. (2014) highlighted that more than half of the systems available in England originated in other countries. Respondents attempting to implement these systems in English hospitals frequently drew our attention to this point which they saw as representing a major problem, as:

> ...*their* [US] *way of working is very different to the U.K. based working (Adopter Interview, P2)*

The lack of alignment between 'foreign' supplier offerings and UK hospitals' internal processes and needs was seen as a major barrier to implementing these systems.

> ...[Product Name] *is a U.S. system and it works very well for a U.S. hospital, but some things in the U.K. are quite different specially around medicines practices and we are still working with* [Supplier Name] *to see if we can get some of their products changed to better reflect our workflow (Adopter Interview, P4)*

This became clearer when adopters expressed a desire to see England-specific solutions being developed around 'generic' English hospitals' needs.

> *In terms of medicine there are a number of issues we have with* [Product Name] *and most of these are issues that aren't just local to* [Place Name] *they're issues that we think are indicative across other U.K. sites... (Adopter Interview, P4)*
>
> *Well a lot of it is U.S.-based but they have to customize it to the U.K. market because we are different, so I mean that's why we have had a number of meetings with them and with the* [Product Name] *user group to explain, you know, we're different and they know this but we keep having to remind them. (Adopter Interview, P5)*

Overseas suppliers emphasized that they were aware of the differences between the two countries and highlighted that they had particular ways of catering for these needs, in particular by offering England-specific versions of the application.

> *An interface to a formulary vendor for medications is standard in the U.S. but we obviously had to go above and beyond knowing that there are different requirements, there's different information on drugs in the U.K., you know, how they're numbered and tracked is different, you know, DM&D* [Dictionary of Medicines and Devices – unique identifier given by NHS] *number does not exist in our U.S. software (Supplier Interview, P6)*

However, despite pressure from hospitals and end-users, participants in user group meetings complained that many suppliers had been slow to create England-specific solutions.

Some vendors appeared reluctant to invest the significant resources needed to implement these changes, particularly where they only had a small presence in the English market. Other suppliers (and particularly those with a stronger foothold in and expectation of a larger share of the market) were deploying strategies to create England-specific versions of the products. However the challenge seemed to be more substantial than they had anticipated. As they began to implement these systems in English hospitals, they were confronted by growing numbers of requests to adapt the systems to local practices and preferences, which forced them to take on board multiple cycles of modification to their products. However at the time of the study, with only a handful of hospitals having implemented their system, the majority of these systems were in the early stages of being 'anglicized'. Hence, what we observed were products in their infancy with respect to English-specific requirements which arose as a result of differences in national systems and policies (e.g. between private insurance-funded health care in the United States of America [USA] and the public-funded UK NHS) and particular hospital practices (e.g. differences in discharge processes). Some of these overseas suppliers had prior experience and knowledge of the English market. However they tended to develop their English version as an extension of their current non-English HEPMA system. We interviewed one supplier which had had live implementations in England of an older product for over a decade, but which was also offering its new HEPMA product to the English hospitals.

> *...at that point after several hospitals* [in the USA] *were up running live and stable with the software that's pretty much the version that we took as our initial like U.K. kind of starting point... And basically where we started there were certain items that we knew, we knew were going to be different, for example in the U.K. wait lists, 18 week waiting, CDS reporting those are like three kind of big areas that, you know, don't exist in the U.S. [American] software so we literally had to start with some of those areas and we just started from what we knew the requirements were in the* [Old Product Name] *environment and fit those to the, you know, the* [New Product Name] *product, you know, the new version.(Supplier Interview, P7)*

NHS England is seen as a target for many overseas suppliers from Europe and the English-speaking world, though it is only a secondary market for many U.S.A. producers. It is not uncommon for systems to be initially developed for local customers within a national market before being redeveloped for the international markets

(Pollock and Williams 2008). As a result, system architectures may be sub-optimal for the English market. Users who were attracted by the powerful functionalities offered by non-English systems found themselves caught in an unanticipated and slow process of joint system redevelopment with the supplier in a protracted implementation. Suppliers entering the English HEPMA market found themselves needing to address in a compressed timeframe: (1) the NHS policy context and generic English hospital's needs; and (2) the widely differing specific needs of individual adopting hospitals. This in turn called for some way of prioritizing user requirements and selectively developing solutions.

9.2.3   Suppliers' Configuration and Customization Strategies

Suppliers of packaged organisational technology solutions need to develop effective strategies for addressing the diversity of user demands for modifications and new functionality. Experienced suppliers had learnt the need for strategies to cater for increasing diversity as their user-base grew in size. This required them to develop a strategic vision for their software product and its longer-term development, to keep control over the overall architecture of their product as it moved forwards, in the face of the plurality of adopter demands. This allowed them to decide which change requests they would entertain, which changes they would be unable to support, and which changes could only be undertaken by end-users themselves (Pollock and Williams 2008).

In order to retain overall control over architecture in the face of diverse users, software packages are designed around a basic set of organisational functionalities - a 'generic kernel' (Pollock and Williams 2008). Libraries of 'templates' are built upon this kernel, catering for commonly encountered workflows and practices. Such software packages are 'user-configurable', meaning that they incorporate preprogrammed features, which can be selected to meet the needs of various environments through setting up parameters rather than rewriting program codes (Davenport 2000). However if the range of pre-defined configurations is limited and does not meet particular user needs, adopters may be forced to seek to alter the programme. Issues then arise about whether this will be incorporated into the package (with programming and testing imposing a significant effort and expense for the supplier) or whether it will be an *ad-hoc* customization (which the adopter may have to pay/take responsibility for). If too many local customizations are made by an adopter, reliability may suffer and upgrades may become difficult to implement (Fincham et al. 1995).

In the case of HEPMA systems in England, suppliers were pursuing various product development strategies but had made very uneven progress in developing their strategies. Some had rather rudimentary arrangements for incorporating user requirements into the system. Others had begun to develop a more organised approach to assessing change requests, generalizing needs and building system enhancements. Moreover, at this stage, most HEPMA solutions in England seemed to be 'too limited' in terms of the configurability they offered (the range of preprogrammed options that the user could draw upon) in relation to the diversity of adopter practices and requests. In our observation of user group meetings, we frequently encountered instances where the majority of users asked for a particular configuration that was not offered by the system.

9.2.4   Localized Adopter Practices Versus Generic Systems

The healthcare context is distinctive in terms of the enormous diversity in specific hospital procedures and individual ways of working. Despite the existence of professional NHS policy guidelines, each NHS hospital is a separate legal entity. It has its own local practices and standard operating procedures. So in performing the day-to-day activities, rather than merely complying with a set of professional guidelines, hospital employees are also expected to abide by the localized operating procedures. This was seen as one of the most significant factors leading to the complexity of HEPMA systems uptake in England. Interviews with users indicated that there were no pre-defined best practices in the health sector because there was still no consensus about what is best. Suppliers, though aware of the differences in localized practices, emphasised the need to introduce standards to the sector.

> *...every NHS trust in the country considers themselves to be different... if you give them a standard OBS* [output based specification]*... they make it unique to them... every question* [on the OBS] *has a nuanced, has a little twist in there... (Comment in supplier event)*

The implementation of generic HEPMA systems foregrounded these variations in practices. Operational differences between hospitals became visible, which had not previously been evident. The lack of standard practices became particularly apparent in implementing systems with higher levels of integration and complexity compared to standalone applications. The diversity of practices was not only hospital-specific. Practices varied between departments and specialties, making it difficult for standard applications to cater for the needs of all wards within a hospital.

9.2.5   'Untamed' Adopter Demands?

Adopters emphasized the particularity of hospital procedures and practices. However their responses highlight the lack of adequate awareness amongst users about the exigencies of packaged applications and in particular the trade-off between the costs of customization versus adapting processes to functionality in the package. This resulted in users having what others portrayed as rather unrealistic, indeed 'untamed', expectations of packaged HEPMA solutions. In this respect, users' expectations from packaged solutions were more in line with what might be expected from bespoke (tailored) information systems. Thus many users expressed a desire for local practices to be directly incorporated into the system.

> *...we are all doing the same job but we are managing the processes differently, so when we implement technologies we all want to implement it in our own way (Adopter Interview, P1)*

...some of the changes we are asking [Product_Name] *for are things that individual Trusts* [hospitals] *do... (Adopter Interview, P4)*

Given these expectations, hospitals felt they should have direct links with the vendor company to develop their specific requirements.

So companies I've worked for before have always had […] a user that partly worked in the Trust [hospital] *and partly worked for them* [in the vendor company] *so that they are a current user. So they knew the problems so that they could take that back to the* [vendor] *company and already start to look at ways of sorting that out. (Adopter Interview, P2)*

Suppliers referred to escalating adopter expectations as "over-aspirational functional specifications" (Comment in supplier event). They also highlighted the need for early alignment of user expectations and actual system purposes and functions.

...aligning expectations if that managed earlier then everyone is on the same page to begin with... (Comment in supplier event)

A further problem arose from insufficient knowledge about what the actual needs of hospitals were. Both users and vendors expressed concerns about uncertainty surrounding users requirements.

...electronic prescribing and medical administrations are quite complex. Until there is kind of more experience or hospitals on these systems it's harder to get some kind of consensus on what are the features and what isn't. (Adopter Interview, P4)

We further noted a lack of knowledge in English hospitals of both HEPMA solutions and of the implementation and use of packaged applications more generally. One issue that, will be the subject of a future paper, concerns the limited circulation of experience in IT procurement and implementation within the NHS. Many of the staff who played a central role in a particular hospital implementation then went back to their health professional role. Apart from a small number who moved over to work for technology suppliers, there was no ready way of carrying forward and exploiting this expertise within NHS professional structures.

9.3   Discussion

Vendors of HEPMA applications are investing significant effort in expanding their market base internationally. Hospitals in England, in turn, appear keen to implement systems that have the potential to deliver the widely anticipated benefits of such systems. We found that despite this willingness from both sides, for the various reasons considered above, progress with implementing these systems in England is proceeding slowly. To understand the underlying reasons we have developed a broader analytical framework based upon this work and our earlier research into the evolution of Enterprise Systems.

9.3.1   Analysing the Long-Term Evolution of Information Infrastructure

The concept of installed based, which unites the contributions in this volume, was coined to capture tensions arising in the development of electronic *Information Infrastructures* (IIs) – defined as systems of (computer-based) systems that support an increasingly wide range of tasks across an ever-more extensive base of users. Efforts to standardize functions around specific existing users and uses may impede the extension of an infrastructure to new users and uses (Hanseth et al. 1996). This concept has informed various development and implementation strategies to prevent lock-in around existing configurations and provide flexibility to allow new functionality to be taken on board (Grisot et al. 2014). The II discussion, however, has largely been at the level of the 'cultivation' of individual organisational information infrastructures.

Our research into the development and implementation of Enterprise Systems (ES) and other corporate information infrastructures (Pollock and Williams 2008) suggests that we need to analyse these developments not just at the level of particular infrastructures and organisations but also across communities of vendors and their adopters (Koch 2007). We have studied the development and implementation of these kinds of highly complex technologies over three decades (Pollock and Williams 2008). This extended timeframe of enquiry has provided insights into both the evolution of these technologies and the arrangements for their development and implementation. In the 1980s, initial attempts to supply what were then known as Computer Aided Production Management (CAPM) systems as COTS packaged solutions were characterized by sharp mismatches between supplier offerings and user needs. Our subsequent research allowed us to observe how these offerings have 'co-evolved' with their user communities. ES Suppliers have learnt how to develop and exploit close links with their adopter communities to develop generic solutions that can be used and be useful across a wide range of adopter organisations. Our insights derive from extending the scope of empirical research not just laterally, across arrays of vendors and adopters etc., but also along an extended 'longitudinal' timescale (Pollock and Williams 2008).

CAPM refers to the set of technologies that resulted from a UK government initiated program during the 1980s. By adding new functions onto existing Manufacturing Resource Planning (MRP II) technologies, CAPM sought to offer integrated packaged solutions to production control and coordination tasks. It was seen as a stepping stone towards Computer Integrated Manufacture (CIM) (Williams 1997; Webster and Williams 1993). In response to the promotion efforts of government (the Department of Trade and Industry, the Science and Engineering Research Council) and other influential actors such as consultants and vendors, a large number of suppliers from different fields were attracted to offer "CAPM" solutions (Clark et al. 1992; Newell and Clark 1990). The availability of government funds encouraged many vendors of MRP II and related systems to project their products under the name CAPM. This resulted in a swarming of supplier offerings around the concept of CAPM, with functionalities being added to existing products to fulfil the expectations of policymakers, pundits and adopter organisations (Webster and Williams 1993). However attempts to implement CAPM packages ran into sharp difficulties which resulted in up to 50% of systems being abandoned. The most immediate features were:

1. An acute lack of fit between the presumptions underpinning the packaged solution and the circumstances of particular adopter organisations; and,
2. The CAPM products launched initially were often still-unfinished with various new functionalities added that were poorly integrated (Webster and Williams 1993).

As a result, would-be adopters found themselves drawn in to an unplanned collaboration with suppliers in a struggle to get these standard packages to work in the adopting organisation's particular circumstances. In this process we saw a more or less radical reworking of the solution, with some functionalities being abandoned and new functions emerging.

The immediate result of this accelerated development and diffusion was the launch of products that were often immature and unstable (Webster and Williams 1993). In the subsequent decade however a new generation of ERP and ES systems emerged, building very directly upon these applications. They incorporated the underpinning philosophy and many technical elements of CAPM and its predecessors – in particular the idea of connecting multiple functions across the enterprise with an integrated and interoperable system – and were also heralded as a stepping stone to CIM (Xue et al. 2005; Pollock and Williams 2008). The concept of ERP began gaining momentum through the 1990s, particularly as firms renewed their systems to avoid anticipated 'millennium bug' problems. A range of successful products emerged. Some (e.g. JDEdwards, Peoplesoft) fell by the wayside as the ES product market restructured, leaving global giants such as Oracle and SAP in dominant positions. As a result we find that today SAP's R3 system has been adopted by the majority of FTSE 100 and Fortune 1,000 firms CIM (Pollock and Williams 2008).

The success of ESs built upon several decades of experience with its predecessor technologies (stock control, production control, Material Requirements Planning [MRP], MRP II) (Williams 1997). There are two crucial features underpinning these developments:

i. Successful suppliers of packaged ES solutions had, over time, elaborated sophisticated *generification* strategies, through which they elicited, aligned, sifted and sorted the diverse requirements of their communities of adopters
ii. Permanent linkages were established within the ES community – in particular through user-clubs linking suppliers and adopter communities (Mozaffar 2016).

The subsequent success of ERP/ES was rooted in the mutual adaptation of both adopter organisation practices/processes and packaged features (Hong and Kim 2002; Leonard 2011).

9.3.2 Analysing the State of the Technology Market/Technology Field

These considerations suggest that if we wish to understand difficulties encountered in HEPMA procurement and implementation, it may be helpful to analyse the evolution and current state of development of the HEPMA market in England, drawing parallels and insights from our studies of the ES technology field.

The idea of the maturation of technology fields can be traced back to classic 1970s studies by Abernathy and Utterback who proposed a three stage model (Abernathy and Utterback 1978). In an initial *experimentation phase*, we see the rapid entrance of diverse and changing products into a new market, the ultimate direction of which is still unknown. As the market and the applications of the technology become better appreciated by suppliers and adopters, in the next, *transitional phase*, the market begins to converge around what is known as a 'dominant design' with broadly comparable characteristics. In the *mature phase*, as dominant designs become established, we find concentration of the market around a smaller number of products with higher performance. The focus of supplier efforts shifts from differentiation to enhancing performance and lowering costs within an existing product paradigm. Similar stage models have been advanced to analyse the cyclical evolution of product markets including the software product life cycle (Agarwal and Tripsas 2008; Fincham et al. 1995). 'Institutionalist' organisation theorists have described the homologous processes by which new 'technological fields' (Pollock and Williams 2011; Swanson and Ramiller 1997, 2004) emerge and take shape by establishing consensus amongst communities of vendors, consultants and adopters. The establishment of a technological field greatly reduces uncertainties about the characteristics of a technology both for vendors and customers. They are coupled with the emergence and stabilisation of classifications of technologies and criteria for their assessment. Here we reject simplified (e.g. technology management) approaches which take for granted the formation of technological fields and their progression, once established, to maturation and seek a more dynamic, processual account of the evolution of technological fields which explores how boundaries and names may be recast and maturation may be reversed by the emergence of new technical solutions or business models (Fincham et al. 1995). In the ES field we saw the emergence of new kinds of *knowledge intermediaries* – industry analysts like Gartner Inc. – which capture and collate community experience to advise adopters about available software products and their vendors. By overcoming the asymmetry of access to information between vendor and adopter this provides the 'knowledge infrastructure' needed for the operation of the IT markets for these complex software products whose capacities and fit to the needs of particular adopter organisations cannot be readily established, for example, by inspection (Pollock and Williams 2011, 2016).

9.3.3   Is the HEPMA Market Replicating the Path of ERP?

Our study of the evolving nature of the HEPMA market in England, exhibits some interesting and insightful parallels with the earlier history of integrated systems in the commercial sector: ERP and its predecessor CAPM Systems. This drew our attention to (i) how vendors developed *generification strategies* to create generic solutions that could bridge to a wide-range of adopter contexts, (ii) the development of multiple webs of relations between vendors and adopters through which knowledge about user requirements and vendor offerings could be exchanged, and (iii) how new knowledge intermediaries emerged to advise adopters in their procurements. We were able to assess the extent to which comparable arrangements had emerged in the UK HEPMA market.

9.3.4   The English HEPMA Market Is Still in an Emergence Stage

The comparison with the ES case suggests that the HEPMA market in England is still in an early stage of emergence/growth. Various suppliers have entered the market with each one having a relatively small number of implementations in progress (Mozaffar et al. 2014). The HEPMA market exhibits a high technical variety in development of products with diverse features and forms. These products originate from different geographical and technical backgrounds and are offered in different forms with dissimilar features and functions. This would suggest that their technological features have not yet become de facto standards or 'dominant designs' (Agarwal and Tripsas 2008; Utterback 1974) in the English market. In this market there is still no accepted architecture, established use practice or evaluation criteria to guide and constrain the efforts of suppliers and adopters (Sheikh et al. 2014). This also contributes to diverse supply strategies and use of numerous terminologies and definitions all of which act as barriers to smooth and rapid adoption.

The lack of shared understanding creates a problem for potential adopters in understanding the options available (Helm and Salminen 2010; Jalkala and Salminen 2010). It also creates uncertainty for vendors about customer requirements. End user requests are typically more diverse than anticipated. Suppliers have difficulties in responding systematically to this diversity (Agarwal and Tripsas 2008; Adner and Levinthal 2001) given this lack of clear 'preferences' (Clark 1985). The market remains in the experimental stage with new products and suppliers still emerging.

Suppliers had adopted different approaches to respond to the diverse needs of the English market. On one end of the spectrum were those suppliers which had already grown and stabilized their products in other national markets. Some offered their international products with only minor modifications to cater for the English hospitals' needs. Others had embarked upon concerted attempts to re-design and develop their applications around the particular needs of English hospitals. When we contrast the HEPMA and ES market today, we can see that HEPMA vendors had not yet developed 'generification strategies' (Pollock and Williams 2008) in relation to establishing mechanisms to decide which of the diverse array of user requirements would be taken on board in their core product but instead tended to respond to requests in an ad-hoc manner. Conversely, since HEPMA systems did not yet incorporate sufficient libraries of common workflows that the user could switch on in configuring the system, rather than by rewriting code, adopter organisations felt compelled to submit customisation requests.

The lack of consensus amongst adopter and vendor communities and domain experts indicates that the technological field is still developing. The field has not yet developed structures and actors to mobilize consensus and set the boundaries of technology (a role carried out in other sectors by industry analysts like Gartner (Pollock and Williams 2011), and by entities such as the Health Information Technology Standards Committee and certifying organisations). These could help reduce procurement uncertainties in various ways: enabling development of generic cases for innovations, creating a space for comparison of different artefacts and suppliers, and helping users come to more realistic and realizable expectations about HEPMA functionalities and its effective use.

9.3.5 Conclusions

We identified several tensions in design and implementation of HEPMA systems in England. The problems can be sorted into six categories: (1) products derived from non-clinical systems proved problematic in England's increasingly patient-centred health system; (2) the process of Anglicization of systems by suppliers from other countries of origin needs to be given sustained attention; (3) the healthcare sector has particularly diverse needs and practices which run counter to the goals of generic applications; (4) current products are limited in configurability in relation to the diversity of adopter requirements which results in escalating customisation requests (5) rather than respond in an ad-hoc manner to proliferating customisation requests vendors need to develop generification strategies (perhaps through user groups) to sift, sort and prioritise these requests to keep control over the strategic development of their product and (6) adopters have little awareness of the exigencies of exploiting COTS solutions resulting in 'untamed' demands from packaged applications.

We conclude that effort to promote HEPMA arguably attracted a range of relatively unfinished solutions into the market prematurely. In this process neither the developers nor the adopting organisation were prepared for the complexities of matching generic products to a diverse adopter context. This echoes elements of previous UK experience with CAPM/ERP systems. We infer that, although policy incentives can be effective in achieving adoption (Aarts and Koppel 2009), they may also have accelerated premature purchase of immature solutions. This suggests a need for a gradual move in the market for such immature technology. So instead of suppliers seeking rapid large-scale implementation of their products, they may need to take a more deliberate and purposeful approach in developing their products for new markets, which will involve partnering with specific institutions until many of the kinks are worked out. Also adopting hospitals need to be more clear and realistic in expressing their needs in relation to packaged applications. Furthermore, more effective mechanisms are required to bridge the gap between the generic standardized technological solutions and the particularity of national and local needs. In order to achieve this, suppliers must not underestimate user diversity. They need to develop strategies to deal with such diversities in the market. At the same time the adopting organisations need to become pre-aligned to these packages and around views within the Health Service of best practice. In short, what is needed is a co-evolution of organisation and technology together. Public policy might usefully be geared towards promoting – and allowing time for – such extended engagement (though competitive public procurement/tendering arrangements may not facilitate this kind of supplier-user engagement) (Lee et al. 2015).

Finally, we suggest that HEPMA is not the final stage in the process of developing health IIs. Though conceived as a discrete, pharmacy technology, HEPMA systems linked the pharmacy to the ward, and went beyond the point of prescription to the administration of medicine throughout and after their hospital stay. As a result HEPMA systems involved a wide range of stakeholders across the hospital junior doctors, consultants, nurses across different specialities, with their various work practices and requirements (a point which becomes crucial when we consider the difficulties catering for diverse 'end-user' requirements). HEPMA moreover became – at least in the historical trajectory of English hospitals - bound up with the integration of a growing range of digital information services (most immediately laboratory results) at the point of healthcare delivery throughout the hospital. Once introduced, these packaged HEPMA solutions became the starting point for the continued extension of systems and their integration with other systems within the hospital and beyond (for example discharge letters to general practitioners). HEPMA systems are becoming core components of hospital health information infrastructures. We suggest that HEPMA has served as a stepping stone to information integrated health care (in a way that parallels the earlier history of enterprise systems in industrial organisations (Fleck 1988)). Our research has identified a range of immediate problems associated with development, procurement and implementation of HEPMA systems in the English healthcare system. Our comparison with the prior experiences with ES allows us to see these as part of a longer-term social learning process (Sørensen 1996). To overcome these challenges, vendors and adopters must understand their current and potential user-base and develop strategies to address the heterogeneities and multiplicities of adopter requirements and practices. This diagnosis in turn provides important lessons for attempts to build health information infrastructures. England, as one of the leading countries in Europe in adoption of such technologies, can be seen as a site of innovation in which the market and products are being shaped simultaneously. Similar patterns in terms of difficulties of HEPMA adoption have been observed in many countries (Mäkinen et al. 2011; Aarts and Koppel 2009). However England is one of the leading countries with the highest rates of HEPMA adoption (Aarts and Koppel 2009; Van Dijk et al. 2011; Schoen et al. 2006), and other countries may benefit from analysis of UK experiences.

The large scale of the NIHR-funded research programme allowed us, rather exceptionally, to study the implementation of a range of supplier offerings in multiple sites and over an extended period. We identified sharp echoes between these, still emerging, experiences and findings from our own personal research conducted over three decades into the evolution of ES solutions. These highlighted the need to go beyond single site snapshot studies of information infrastructure implementation and also examine the development of the component technologies (in this case discrete and integrated packaged HEPMA solutions) amongst closely coupled communities of developers and adopters of particular products and within evolving technological fields (Pollock and Williams 2008, 2016). The need to understand longer-term evolution of products across a community requires us to go beyond (or radically re-specify) the concept of Installed Base. Here we have drawn upon a long-established tradition of work from organisational studies and related perspectives: notably the institutionalist concept of technology field and related work on product life-cycles. These have provided a helpful framework to guide the extension of our detailed ethnographic study beyond single sites and moments to encompass longer-term developments across vendor/adopter communities. Our work here has focused upon the 'community' of vendors, adopters and consultants linked to a particular technology. This does not however imply a 'flat' approach to community which risks portraying the co-evolution of technologies and their adopters as a simple process of joint learning and consensus building. Instead our studies of both ES and HEPMA highlight the overlapping webs of relationship through which these 'communities' are structured and segmented into a complex topology (Pollock and Williams 2016; Mozaffar 2016). Here we find a contradictory process in which diverse players grapple to accommodate goals in tension – for example supplier efforts to standardize technologies and adopter desires to differentiate systems around their particular (local or disciplinary) methods of working. These play out and need to be analysed over multiple cycles of design and implementation.

Acknowledgments We gratefully acknowledge the input from our Independent Programme Steering Committee, which is chaired by Prof Denis Protti, Prof Munir Pirmohamed, Prof Bryony Dean Franklin, Ms. Eva Leach, Ms. Rosemary Humphreys, and Ms. Ailsa Donnelly. We also gratefully acknowledge the input of Mrs. Rosemary Porteous, who transcribed the interviews; and the input of our patient representatives including: Mr. Antony Chuter; Ms. Susan Howe; Mr. Paul Henry; Ms. Jillian Beggs; and Ms. Ember Heselwood. We are very grateful to all participants and to the wider programme team for all their valuable inputs, particularly Ms. Ann Slee, Dr. Jamie Coleman and Dr. Lucy McCloughan.

Collaborators On behalf of the NIHR ePrescribing Programme Team: Dr. Jamie Coleman (Senior Clinical Lecturer, University of Birmingham), Ms. Ann Slee (Honorary Research Fellow, University of Edinburgh), Dr. Ann Robertson (Research Fellow, The University of Edinburgh), Prof Tony Avery (Professor of Primary Health Care, The University of Nottingham), Dr. Laurence Blake (The University of Birmingham), Mr. Antony Chuter (Patient Representative), Dr. Sarah Slight (NIHR Career Development Fellow, The University of Nottingham), Dr. Alan Girling (Senior Research Fellow, The University of Birmingham), Dr. Lisa Lee (Research Fellow, The University of Edinburgh), Dr. Behnaz Schofield (Research Fellow,

The University of Edinburgh), Prof Richard Lilford (Professor of Clinical Epidemiology, The University of Birmingham), Dr. Lucy McCloughan (eHealth Research Manager, The University of Edinburgh), Prof Jill Schofield (Head of School of Economics Finance and Management, University of Bristol), Dr. Zoe Morrison (Lecturer, University of Aberdeen).

Funding This article presents independent research funded by the National Institute for Health Research (NIHR)'s Programme Grants for Applied Research Programme (RP-PG-1209-10099). The views expressed are those of the authors and not necessarily those of the NHS, the NIHR or the Department of Health. It also draws important historical insights from two awards from the Economic and Social Research Council: a fellowship awarded to Neil Pollock 'The Social Study of the Information Technology Marketplace(s)' (RES-063-27-0221) as well as an earlier research grant to Williams, Pollock and Procter (RES-000-23-0466) on 'The Biography and Evolution of Standardised Software Packages'.

References

Aarts J, Koppel R. Implementation of computerized physician order entry in seven countries. Health Aff. 2009;28:404–14.

Abernathy WJ, Utterback JM. Patterns of industrial innovation. Technol Rev. 1978;80:40–7.

Adner R, Levinthal D. Demand heterogeneity and technology evolution: implications for product and process innovation. Manag Sci. 2001;47:611–28.

Agarwal R, Tripsas M. Technology and industry evolution. Chap 1, in Shane, S. (ed). The handbook of technology and innovation management. Hoboken, NJ: Wiley-Blackwell; 2008:1–55.

Ahmed Z, McLeod MC, Barber N, Jacklin A, Franklin JD. The use and functionality of electronic prescribing systems in English acute nhs trusts: a cross-sectional survey. PLoS ONE. 2013; doi:10.1371/journal.pone.0080378.

Avery AJ, Savelyich BS, Sheikh A, Morris CJ, Bowler I, Teasdale S. Improving general practice computer systems for patient safety: qualitative study of key stakeholders. Qual Saf Health Care. 2007;16:28–33.

Bates DW, Kuperman GJ, Wang S, Gandhi T, Kittler A, Volk L, Spurr C, Khorasani R, Tanasijevic M, Middleton B. Ten commandments for effective clinical decision support: making the practice of evidence-based medicine a reality. J Am Med Inform Assoc. 2003;10:523–30.

Bates DW, Leape LL, Cullen DJ, Laird N, Petersen LA, Teich JM, Burdick E, Hickey M, Kleefield S, Shea B. Effect of computerized physician order entry and a team intervention on prevention of serious medication errors. JAMIA. 1998;280:1311–6.

Black AD, Car J, Pagliari C, Anandan C, Cresswell K, Bokun T, McKinstry B, Procter R, Majeed A, Sheikh A. The impact of eHealth on the quality and safety of health care: a systematic overview. PLoS Med. 2011;8:188.

Buntin MB, Burke MF, Hoaglin MC, Blumenthal D. The benefits of health information technology: a review of the recent literature shows predominantly positive results. Health Aff. 2011;30:464–71.

Carter P. Operational productivity and performance in English NHS acute hospitals: unwarranted variations. UK Department of Health. 2015. Available online at: www.gov.uk/government/uploads/system/uploads/attachment_data/file/499229/Operational_productivity_A.pdf.

Clark KB. The interaction of design hierarchies and market concepts in technological evolution. Res Policy. 1985;14:235–51.

Clark P, Burcher P, Bennett D, Newell S, Swan J, Sharifi S. The decision-episode framework and computer-aided production management (CAPM). Int Stud Manag Organ. 1992;22:69–80.

Cresswell K, Coleman J, Slee A, Williams R, Sheikh A. Investing and learning lessons from early experiences of implementing ePrescribing systems into NHS hospitals: a questionnaire study. PLoS ONE. 2013;8(1):e53369.

Crowe S, Cresswell K, Avery AJ, Slee A, Coleman JJ, Sheikh A. Planned implementations of ePrescribing systems in NHS hospitals in England: a questionnaire study. JRSM Short Rep. 2010;1:33.

Fernando B, Savelyich BS, Avery AJ, Sheikh A, Bainbridge M, Horsfield P, Teasdale S. Prescribing safety features of general practice computer systems: evaluation using simulated test cases. BMJ. 2004;328:1171–2.

Fincham R, Fleck J, Procter RN, Scarbrough H, Tierney M, Williams R. Expertise and innovation: information technology strategies in the financial services sector. Oxford: Oxford University Press; 1995.

Fleck J. Innofusion or diffusation?: the nature of technological development in robotics. Edinburgh: University of Edinburgh; 1988.

Grisot M, Hanseth O, Thorseng AA. Innovation of, in, on infrastructures: articulating the role of architecture in information infrastructure evolution. J Assoc Inf Syst. 2014;15:197–219.

Hanseth O, Monteiro E, Hatling M. Developing information infrastructure: the tension between standardization and flexibility. Sci Technol Hum Values. 1996;21:407–26.

Helm S, Salminen RT. Basking in reflected glory: using customer reference relationships to build reputation in industrial markets. Ind Mark Manag. 2010;39:737–43.

Hibberd R, Cornford T, Lichtner V, Venters W, Barber N. England's electronic prescription service: infrastructure in an institutional setting. 2017. (In this volume).

Hong KK, Kim YG. The critical success factors for ERP implementation: an organizational fit perspective. Inform Manag. 2002;40:25–40.

Jalkala A, Salminen RT. Practices and functions of customer reference marketing – leveraging customer references as marketing assets. Ind Mark Manag. 2010;39:975–85.

Koch C. Production management systems: bricks or clay in the hands of the social actors. In: Clausen C, Williams R, editors. The social shaping of computer-aided production management and computer-integrated manufacture. Luxembourg: European Commission; 1997.

Koch C. ERP–a moving target. Int J Bus Inform Syst. 2007;2:426–43.

Lee L, Williams R, Sheikh A. How does joint procurement affect the design, customisation and usability of a hospital ePrescribing system? Health Inform J. 2015;22:828. 1460458215592915.

Leonard DA. Implementation as mutual adaptation of technology and organization. Manag Knowl Assets, Creat Innovs. 2011;17:429.

Mäkinen M, Rautava P, Forsström J, Äärimaa M. Electronic prescriptions are slowly spreading in the European Union. Telemed e-Health. 2011;17:217–22.

McKibbon KA, Lokker C, Handler SM, Dolovich LR, Holbrook AM, O'Reilly, D, Tamblyn R, Hemens BJ, Basu R, Troyan S. Enabling medication management through health information technology. Evidence Reports/Technology Assessments, No. 201, Rockville (MD): Agency for Healthcare Research and Quality (Report No.: 11-E008-EF); 2011.

Mozaffar H. User communities as multi-functional spaces: innovation, collective voice, demand articulation, peer informing and professional identity (and more). In: Hyysalo S, Jensen T, Oudshoorn N, editors. The new production of users: changing innovation collectives and involvement strategies: Abingdon, Routledge; 2016.

Mozaffar H, Williams R, Cresswell K, Morison Z, Slee A, Team AS. Product diversity and spectrum of choice in hospital ePrescribing systems in England. PloS ONE. 2014;9:e92516.

Mozaffar H, Williams R, Cresswell K, Morrison Z, Bates DW, Sheikh A. The evolution of the market for commercial computerized physician order entry and computerized decision support systems for prescribing. J Am Med Inform Assoc. 2015;23(2):349–55. ocv095.

Newell S, Clark P. The importance of extra-organizational networks in the diffusion and appropriation of new technologies the role of professional associations in the United States and Britain. Sci Commun. 1990;12:199–212.

Pollock N, Williams R. Software and organizations. New York: Routledge; 2008.

Pollock N, Williams R. Who decides the shape of product markets? The knowledge institutions that name and categorise new technologies. Inf Organ. 2011;21:194–217.

Robertson A, Bates DW, Sheikh A. The rise and fall of England's national programme for IT. JRSM. 2011;104:434–5.

Schiff GD, Klass D, Peterson J, Shah G, Bates DW. Linking laboratory and pharmacy: opportunities for reducing errors and improving care. Arch Intern Med. 2003;163:893–900.

Schoen C, Davis K, How SK, Schoenbaum SC. US health system performance: a national scorecard. Health Aff. 2006;25:w457–75.

Sheikh A, Cornford T, Barber N, Avery A, Takian A, Lichtner V, Petrakaki D, Crowe S, Marsden K, Robertson A. Implementation and adoption of nationwide electronic health records in secondary care in England: final qualitative results from prospective national evaluation in "early adopter" hospitals. BMJ: Brit Med J. 2011;2010:343.

Sheikh A, Jha A, Cresswell K, Greaves F, Bates DW. Adoption of electronic health records in UK hospitals: lessons from the USA. Lancet. 2014;384:8–9.

Sørensen KH. Learning technology, constructing culture. Socio-technical change as social learning. STS Working Paper 18/96. Trondheim: Center for Technology and Society, Norwegian National University of Science and Technology; 1996.

Swanson EB, Ramiller NC. The organizing vision in information systems innovation. Organ Sci. 1997;8:458–74.

Swanson EB, Ramiller NC. Innovating mindfully with information technology. MIS Q. 2004;28:553–83.

Utterback JM. Innovation in industry and the diffusion of technology. Science. 1974;183:620–6.

Van Dijk L, De Vries H, Bell D. Electronic prescribing in the United Kingdom and in the Netherlands. Prepared for: Agency for Healthcare Research and Quality US Department of Health and Human Services. 2011. p. 540.

Webster J, Williams R. Mismatch and Tension: Standard Packages and Non-standard Users in P. Quintas (ed.), Social dimensions of systems engineering: People, Processes, Policies and Software Development. Hemel Hemstead: Ellis Horwood; 1993:179–96.

Westbrook JI, Reckmann M, Li L, Runciman WB, Burke R, Lo C, Baysari MT, Braithwaite J, Day RO. Effects of two commercial electronic prescribing systems on prescribing error rates in hospital in-patients: a before and after study. PLoS Med. 2012;9:e1001164.

Williams R. The social shaping of a failed technology? Mismatch and tension between the supply and use of computer-aided production management. In: Clausen C, Williams R, editors. The social shaping of computer-aided production management and computer-integrated manufacture. Proceedings from a COST A4 workshop in Gillelege, Denmark. Luxemburg: Office for Official Publications of the European Communities; 1997.

Wolfstadt JI, Gurwitz JH, Field TS, Lee M, Kalkar S, Wu W, Rochon PA. The effect of computerized physician order entry with clinical decision support on the rates of adverse drug events: a systematic review. J Gen Intern Med. 2008;23:451–8.

Xue Y, Liang H, Boulton WR, Snyder CA. ERP implementation failures in China: case studies with implications for ERP vendors. Int J Prod Econ. 2005;97:279–95.

Pollock N, Williams R. How industry analysts shape the digital future? Oxford: Oxford University Press; 2016.

Open Access This chapter is distributed under the terms of the Creative Commons Attribution-NonCommercial 2.5 International License (http://creativecommons.org/licenses/by-nc/2.5/), which permits any noncommercial use, duplication, adaptation, distribution and reproduction in any medium or format, as long as you give appropriate credit to the original author(s) and the source, provide a link to the Creative Commons license and indicate if changes were made.

The images or other third party material in this chapter are included in the chapter's Creative Commons license, unless indicated otherwise in a credit line to the material. If material is not included in the chapter's Creative Commons license and your intended use is not permitted by statutory regulation or exceeds the permitted use, you will need to obtain permission directly from the copyright holder.

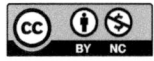

Medication Infrastructure Development in Germany

Stefan Klein and Stefan Schellhammer

10.1 Introduction

In principle, the advantages of the digital transformation of the German healthcare system have been recognized by stakeholders and policy-makers. The need to move forward has been emphasized by governmental and representative bodies. Funding has been allocated to finance pilot projects and infrastructure development.

The electronic health card has been and continues to be the flagship of German ehealth initiatives. Its vision is nothing less than to replace most of the manual, paper-based communication processes by secure, digital pathways. Thereby, the initiative aims for providing a nationwide infrastructure on which in the future numerous applications can be build. It is essentially conceived as the entry ticket into the German healthcare system for every health insurance beneficiary.

Yet, so far, the development of the ehealth card in Germany is characterized by delays and significant reductions in the functional scope compared to the original plans. For instance, electronic prescriptions are not any more considered as a priority application. While the government pushes the project further, it remains uncertain when and in what form the first applications will materialize.

Some argue that the "project's sheer size, scale and complexity" is a major cause for its current state (Drews and Schirmer 2015 p. 12). An iterative approach combined with a more balanced economic distribution of costs and benefits is suggested as a more promising way (ibid.). While we do not deny that such arguments are worth to consider, we would like to suggest the notion of "installed base of opposition" in order to make sense of the difficulties plaguing German ehealth initiatives. We have developed and used this concept to trace the development of a rather focused, albeit scalable ehealth project over the last 10 years. The clear focus of the initiative on medication management for

S. Klein (✉) • S. Schellhammer
University of Münster, Leonardo-Campus 11, 48149 Münster, Germany
e-mail: stefan.klein@uni-muenster.de; stschell@wi.uni-muenster.de

© The Author(s) 2017
M. Aanestad et al. (eds.), *Information Infrastructures within European Health Care*, Health Informatics, DOI 10.1007/978-3-319-51020-0_10

polypharmacy patients not only implies significantly fewer stakeholders (patients, doctors, nursing homes, pharmacies) but also allows for a tangible definition of economic benefits as well as improvements to quality of care. The initiative aims to improve medication compliance for polypharmacy patients by providing patient specific medication packs functioning as dose administration aids, called automated drug (or dose) dispensing (ADD). The involved work process is not entirely new but close to the existing practice of blistering pharmacies or blister centres. Especially nursing or care homes and polypharmacy home care patients have been targeted as customers. The initiative aims to automate and informate this process to achieve economies of scale and to reduce errors due to manual blistering.

Ideally, the weekly production of individualized medication packs would be built on key components of a general information infrastructure such as e-prescriptions, consolidated medication plans, and electronic communication between doctors, pharmacists, ADD operators and health insurance providers in order to be able to operate most efficiently. Thus, ADD would benefit from and nicely tie into an existing information infrastructure like the one envisioned by the electronic health card, but it may very well function without such a basis.

In this chapter we will show that this well-focused initiative suffered the same fate as the wider electronic prescription in Germany: It does not feature anymore in the discourse of ehealth applications. In our analysis, we were struck by the lack of an open and substantive discourse among the involved stakeholders. Given the cooperatist and consensus oriented governance of the German health care system, a resistance that ranges from a lack of open discourse to outright blockade is disturbing. Therefore, we come to the conclusion that the slow and cumbersome progress of infrastructure development in the German healthcare sector can be explained by the existence of an installed base of opposition. This interpretation does not bode well for the latest attempt by the government to jumpstart the digital transformation of the German health care sector.

Methods
In order to capture the public discourse about medication infrastructure development, research for this paper started with the collection and analysis of newspapers, reports, press releases, position papers, blogs, presentations and studies of the health-care community. These documents have been complemented by legal documents and international academic literature, dealing with medication compliance, ADD etc. Moreover, we have interviewed researchers involved in the study of ADD in Germany and Finland, representatives of Kohl Medical, as well as members of the blister community, pharmacists and doctors. An earlier version of this paper was shared with a representative of Kohl Medical for validation purposes. One of the authors gave an invited talk about the European landscape of ADD at a Blister conference in order to solicit further feedback.

10.2   One Step Forward Two Steps Back: The Situation of eHealth in Germany

In 2003, plans to modernize the German healthcare system by eHealth technology were put in place as part of a law by the federal government. In particular it was envisioned that: "From 1 January 2006 all 72 million customers of the health insurance companies in Germany [...] which give access to state health care, should be using a "health card" with a microchip. [This] should make 700 million handwritten prescriptions redundant" (Tuffs 2004, p. 131).

Now, more than 10 years after the envisioned starting date, the system is still far from being operational. In fact, in December 2015 the German parliament passed the so-called "ehealth law" incorporating a roll-out plan to ensure the operation of the electronic health card system by 2018. Although the system has been reduced in its functional scope and now features a step-wise approach including financial incentives to spur adoption, it is still unclear whether the new starting date will be met.

In the following we will briefly revisit the history of the "most extensive e-health communication project in the world" (Tuffs 2004, p. 131).

The initial plans, which passed into law in 2003, listed various functional properties for the electronic health card: Apart from providing data to identify the insured person, it should include data required for the European Health Insurance Card (EHIC) and allow for electronic prescriptions. Furthermore, the card was supposed to support a number of additional applications, such as the use of medical data for emergency treatments, a digital form of communication between physicians and patients (doctor's or referral letters), data necessary for medication safety, an electronic patient record, and information about the donation of organs (§ 291a SGB V).

The initial starting date (of 2006) had to be abandoned in 2005. Instead, a number of field tests were conducted in seven test regions in 2007 and 2008 (Elmer 2014). The introduced solution caused substantial problems partially leading to an extension of the test phase and partly even to the termination of the tests. As a reaction to the failed pilots, the German Medical Association repeatedly positioned itself against the current concept of the eHealth card (Bundesärztekammer 2008).[1] Furthermore, in 2009, the private insurances retracted from the project.

In response to these developments the government decided to put the project on hold for review after the election in 2009 (Neumann 2009). This led to a re-organization and re-start of the project in 2010. In particular, the stakeholders agreed to reduce the initial scope of the card to just three initial applications: (1) basic patient and insurance data (2) introduction of an emergency data set, and (3) secure communication between health care professionals (VFA 2014). Since then, the introduction of electronic prescriptions has largely disappeared from the political agenda. In 2010 a representative survey among physicians showed that e-prescription is perceived as the application of the health card, which is viewed most skeptically (Institut für Demoskopie Allensbach 2010, p. 19)

---

[1] The German Medical Assembly documented their critical stance also in the memoranda of subsequent years.

Since 1 January 2015 the electronic health card is the exclusive credential to receive medical treatments. About 97% of all insured patients have received the card (GKV Spitzenverband 2015). Yet, so far even the basic functionality is not online. Because of the newly introduced picture of the patient alongside the stored basic patient data it is mostly seen as an expensive way to curb insurance fraud. Also this basic functionality is facing resistance as doctors do not regard cross-checking the identity and insurance of a patient as their genuine task but as an administrative burden that is passed on by health insurance companies (Bundesärztekammer 2015). Even the first field test of the online patient data seems to be delayed again, jeopardizing the subsequent phases (Borchers 2015).

In December 2015 a new law called "law for secure digital communication and applications in healthcare" has passed the German parliament. It essentially sets clear guidelines and deadlines to ensure the implementation of the ehealth card without further delay (Stafford 2015). For instance, until 1 October 2016 a paper-based medication plan has to be made available for patients, who need at least three medications. In 2018 this is supposed to work electronically. As of 2018, emergency health information can be stored on the ehealth card, if the patient wishes. The online verification and updating of patient data is conceived as one of the first applications to be available nationwide. After the implementation, foreseen until mid-2018, the law specifies 1 July 2018 as a deadline after which doctors who do not participate will incur a 1% reduction of their reimbursement (Bundesregierung der Bundesrepublik Deutschland 2015).

The specific deadlines, milestones, and sanctioning mechanisms as well as financial incentives mentioned in the law suggest a clear roadmap capable to overcome the stalled implementation process. Yet, the reactions to the initial draft of the law raise doubts as to whether the optimism of the federal government in regard to the impact of the law is justified (Bundesärztekammer 2015; Schersch 2015).

10.3   Case Background

10.3.1 Medication Management for Polypharmacy Patients

Comprehensive medication management for polypharmacy patients (Lochner et al. 2011) has been recognized as a key area of health care in need of improvement and innovations: it affects a growing number of patients, has huge financial implications and ties into broader issues such as patient health and medication safety, medication records, coordination across different medical specialists, and cooperation between medical doctors and pharmacists.

Medication safety and compliance are major issues in the management of medication for polypharmacy patients. Polypharmacy patients are patients who regularly have to take four or more distinct types of medication. They are typically suffering from diseases such as coronary heart disease, congestive heart failure, hypertension, or diabetes mellitus. Given the sheer number of medication and over-the-counter drugs (OTC) taken, there is a high risk of critical interactions. Adverse drug reactions and critical interactions among medicines can often be identified and resolved before the actual administration of the drug takes place. However, accurate identification of risks relies on comprehensive information about the current and past medication regime of the patient. Medication safety addresses specifically adverse drug reactions and critical interactions among medicines. Compliance or adherence[2] focuses on the patients' behaviour in particular in long-term medication therapies.

The response to this set of problems varies across different health care systems. Yet, there is a broad consensus about the key components of a solution (Haefeli et al. 2012):

1. A comprehensive patient medication record to document a patient's medication.
2. A control for critical interactions based on the medication record.
3. Monitoring of the medication effects over time.
4. Dose administration aids to support patients and their helpers to follow the medication regime (dosage and timing).

While we will be looking specifically into dose administration aids throughout this chapter, they are only one component of a comprehensive medication management (Royal Pharmaceutical Society 2013) that typically requires components (1–3) as a prerequisite.

10.3.2   Automatic Dose Dispensing (ADD) as a Key Component for Medication Management

Adherence is in particular a problem for chronically ill elderly patients, who constitute the largest segment of polypharmacy patients. The use of dose administration aids, such as the 7×4 pill box or the weekly blister wallet, is regarded as good practice to support compliance (Corlett 1996): the medication plan is translated into separate physical compartments marked with the assigned day, time and filled with the respective medication. So the physical presence of the medication functions like a reminder to take the assigned medication, a materialized logic of compliance. However, from the patients' or caretakers' point of view, filling pill boxes, is a tedious and therefore error-prone process (Lauterbach et al. 2007). Hence, provisioning of dose administration aids is mandated for specific patients in a number of countries including Australia, Austria, Denmark, Switzerland and The Netherlands based on the assumption of enhanced safety, improved medication adherence, reduced cost and time efficiency (Bell et al. 2013).

Automatic dose dispensing (ADD), the industrial production of patient-specific dose administration aids for solid oral medicines, has been introduced in primary

---

[2] Adherence is the broader concept, which encompasses acceptance (redeeming the prescription), persistence (continuing the medication therapy) and compliance (following the prescriber's instructions) (Düsing 2006, 11). Throughout this chapter we will use adherence and compliance synonymously.

care for home-dwelling elderly patients in a range of countries, such as Denmark, Finland, The Netherlands, Norway and Sweden (Cheung et al. 2014). ADD builds on and extends established practices of arranging medicines in pill boxes, e.g. the widely used 7×4 pill box has twenty eight separate compartments for pills. Each compartment may contain several pills, which are to be taken at the same time during a day (morning, noon, afternoon, evening). Those aids, blisters packs, blister wallets or collections of sachets, also provide information about patient, medication and schedule for administering the medication. From a patient's perspective, ADD replaces the 7×4 pill box by sachets or blister packs, each of which contain the pills of the pill box compartments. These blisters are produced and sealed on an industrial level according to industrial quality standards (GMP – good manufacturing practice). Thus, ADD substitutes the manual administration of medication, dose administration aids filled by patients, their careers or pharmacists, or blisters produced manually or (semi-)automatically by pharmacists or regional blister centres. ADD is typically provided across regions or nationwide, it is a way of scaling up the production and provisioning of blisters for quality and efficiency reasons.

10.3.3 Attempted Infrastructure Innovation

Given the prevalence of national regulation in health care, we have been studying the public discourse about improving medication management in Germany over the course of 10 years. There has been a broad consensus about the need to improve the safety of medication therapy. Since 2007 a series of action plans to improve the safety of medication therapy have been established and executed (AkDÄ 2007), see also (World Alliance for Patient Safety 2008) and specifically to address the risks and costs of non-compliance (ABDA and KBV 2011a; Arzneimittelinitiative Sachsen-Thüringen 2014; Ärztliches Zentrum für Qualität in der Medizin (ÄZQ) 2011; Bierwirth and Paust 2004; Braun and Marstedt 2011).

Pharmacists and operators of blister centres have been lobbying for the official recognition of the advantages of blistering, i.e. the provision of patient specific dose administration aids in form of blister packs, for years. However, their success and impact has been quite limited. Within the Federation of German Associations of Pharmacists (ABDA) they appear to be regarded as a small special interest group of pharmacists focusing on servicing care homes.

We will be investigating specifically the introduction of industrial automatic dose dispensing (ADD) as an infrastructure innovation in the German healthcare system.

10.4 Case Presentation

10.4.1 From Semi-automated Packaging to Industrial Scale ADD

In 2000 the first care homes in Germany started to introduce patient-specific blisters packs to their patients ("Patienten-individuelle Verblisterung in Deutschland – eine Bestandsaufnahme," 2010). Over the next 16 years a number of pharmacies

(28 according to the BlisterBlog (http://verblistern.info/blog/) de facto perhaps two or three times as many) and regional blister centers (29 according to the BlisterBlog (http://verblistern.info/blog/)) has commenced their operation to package pills manually or semi-automatically into blister cards or tubular bags. Two associations (BPAV, BVKA) have been founded to represent the interests of these organizations.

10.4.2 The Design of the ADD Pilot Infrastructure

In 2005, the regulatory preconditions for the industrial production of patient-specific blisters have been established in principal, however, eligibility criteria, rules for reimbursement and the collaboration between doctors and pharmacists in reviewing medication plans had not been included. Subsequently, two industrial ADD operators – 7×4 Pharma and AvidiaMed[3] – have set-up production sites and run trials. The blistering facilities of 7×4 Pharma had been designed to produce weekly blister packs for polypharmacy patients at a national scale, i.e. up to 100.000 patient specific blisters per day. In parallel a number of blister centers have been set-up by pharmacies at a regional level, which produce blisters for a small number of participating pharmacies. Moreover, a number of pharmacies offer the (manual) production of dose administration aids as an additional, usually complimentary service.

While there are numerous options of how to design ADD, 7×4 Pharma had opted for key design features for their pilot: They used blisters instead of sachets, in order to increase the quality of the medication packs. 7×4 Pharma covers a dispensing range or assortment of 400 standard, generic and proprietary substances (Kohl 2010, p. 10). 7×4 Pharma operated as a service provider for pharmacies, in collaboration with general practitioners and specialist doctors instead of direct deliveries to care homes and home care patients. They designed a process flow (Fig. 10.1), which illustrates the direct collaboration with doctors, pharmacists and wholesalers and the indirect involvement of patients and insurance providers. Three components of medication management, specifically medication information management are crucial for the operation of ADD:

- Electronic information exchange akin with *electronic prescription* between ADD operator, physician and pharmacy. ADD assumes up to date comprehensive information about all of patient's prescriptions in order to be able to provide a comprehensive blister of all oral medicines.
- Based on the prescriptions, a consolidated and comprehensive patient *medication plan* is created.
- A *medication list*, typically based on active ingredients identifies standard medication and possible substitutes. The medication list can help to deal with the complexity and multiplicity of medicines.

---

[3] As 7 × 4 Pharma was the first, most prominent and indeed most controversial attempt to establish ADD in Germany, we have focussed on their case.

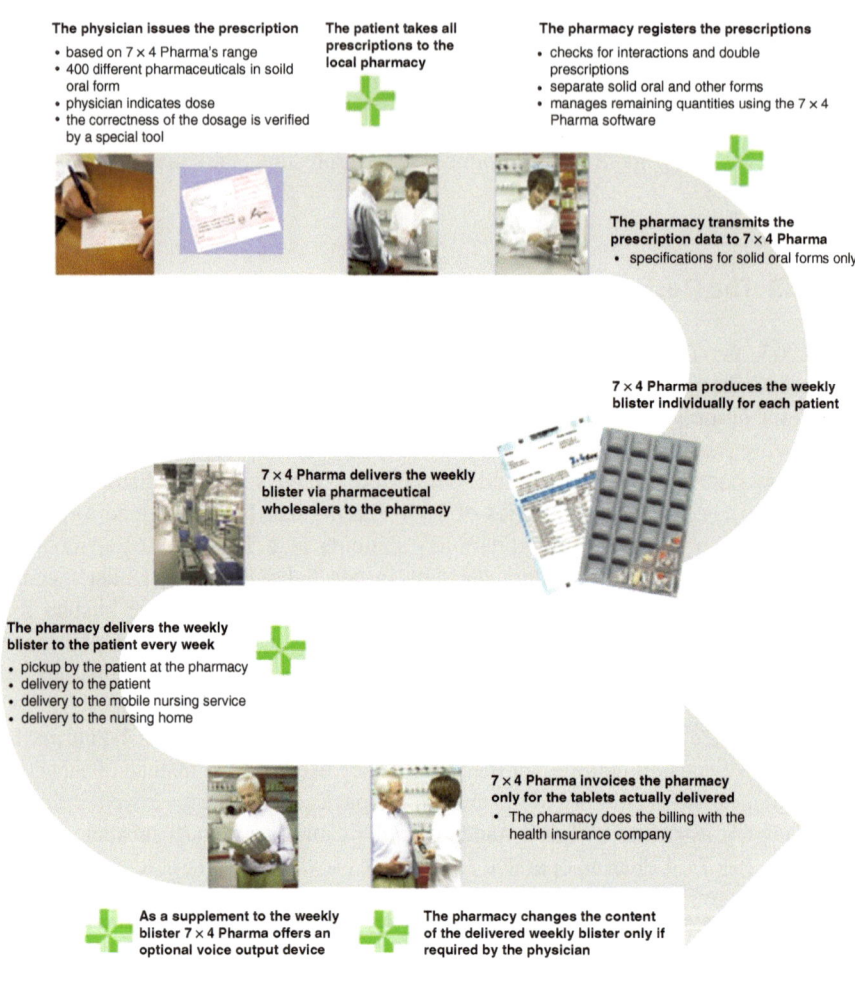

The physician issues the prescription
- based on 7 × 4 Pharma's range
- 400 different pharmaceuticals in soild oral form
- physician indicates dose
- the correctness of the dosage is verified by a special tool

The patient takes all prescriptions to the local pharmacy

The pharmacy registers the prescriptions
- checks for interactions and double prescriptions
- separate solid oral and other forms
- manages remaining quantities using the 7 × 4 Pharma software

The pharmacy transmits the prescription data to 7 × 4 Pharma
- specifications for solid oral forms only

7 × 4 Pharma produces the weekly blister individually for each patient

7 × 4 Pharma delivers the weekly blister via pharmaceutical wholesalers to the pharmacy

The pharmacy delivers the weekly blister to the patient every week
- pickup by the patient at the pharmacy
- delivery to the patient
- delivery to the mobile nursing service
- delivery to the nursing home

7 × 4 Pharma invoices the pharmacy only for the tablets actually delivered
- The pharmacy does the billing with the health insurance company

As a supplement to the weekly blister 7 × 4 Pharma offers an optional voice output device

The pharmacy changes the content of the delivered weekly blister only if required by the physician

Fig. 10.1 ADD process flow (Kohl 2010, p. 11)

Yet none of these had been formally introduced or regulated in Germany in 2005, and none of these are in place to this day.

The creation and exchange of these documents implies an adjustment of existing practices and involves – apart from the ADD operator – patients, physicians, pharmacies, pharmaceutical wholesalers, caretakers or nursing homes and health insurances as illustrated in Fig. 10.1.

- Physicians use the 7×4 Pharma software to issue prescriptions based on the medication list.
- Patients take all their prescriptions to one pharmacy.
- The pharmacy registers and checks the prescriptions for critical interactions, dosage and double prescriptions, e.g. pain killers prescribes independently by different specialists. The pharmacy passes the consolidated prescriptions to the ADD operator.

- A pharmaceutical wholesaler delivers the blisters to the pharmacy.
- The pharmacy is invoiced by 7×4 Pharma based on the number of tablets delivered.
- The pharmacy charges the insurance providers.

10.4.3 Debates About ADD in Germany

Between 2004 and 2007 a number of studies – commissioned by Kohl Medical AG, 7×4 Pharma's parent company – have been published, which examined different facets of ADD and provided the rationale for industrial ADD at a national level (Glaeske 2007; Lauterbach et al. 2004a, b, 2006, 2007).

In 2006, Wille and Wolf (2006) published a study – commissioned by the association of research active pharmaceutical companies (VfA) – on the costs and benefits of secondary blisters, which contradicted the studies by Glaeske, Lauterbach et al. and concluded that ADD is neither cost efficient nor effective.

Meanwhile, in 2009, the 7×4 Pharma facility went live (Hollstein 2009). Subsequently pilot studies – based on industrial ADD as well as regional blistering – have been conducted in collaboration with health insurance providers in order to assess the effects of ADD in life settings.

At the beginning of 2011, the results of two pilot studies have been published. One was based on industrial ADD (Leker and Kehrel 2011), the other was based on blisters produced by pharmacies (Neubauer 2011; Neubauer and Wick 2011) in cooperation with health insurance providers. The studies provide evidence that ADD contributed to improvements of both medication safety and compliance. Moreover they postulated cost saving of up to 31 € per patient per week (Neubauer and Wick 2011).

In spring 2011, the Federation of German Associations of Pharmacists (ABDA) and the National Association of Statutory Health Insurance Physicians (KBV) published a proposal for improved medication supply in Germany, which addressed the same issues of compliance of polypharmacy patients and medication supply (ABDA and KBV 2011b). While the proposal can be seen as complementary to ADD, it refrains from even mentioning the issue of drug administration.

In August 2011, the association of statutory physicians and the association of pharmacies for the state of Brandenburg (Landesapotheker- und Landesärztekammer Brandenburg 2011) issued a position paper, which assessed and rejected ADD. The association of patient individual blister companies (BPAV 2011) issued a critical and angry rebuttal. The association of pharmacies supplying nursing homes (BVKA Schumbach 2013a) has also articulated critique against ABDA's blockade of ADD.

In November 2011 7×4 Pharma's production of blisters was discontinued. It had become obvious by then that the regulator was not inclined to fill the gap left in the 2005 law due to the coordinated resistance of ABDA and KBV (Schumbach 2013b). Hypothetically speaking, had the regulator provided reasonable rules for eligibility for patient-specific blisters and for reimbursement of the blister production and the requisite medication review, it could have triggered the development and extension of the information infrastructure and thereby making blistering a viable model. The fact that the

ABDA and KBV concept paper (ABDA and KBV 2011b) has been published in 2011 and that 7×4 Pharma was sold during the same year may be more than a coincidence.

In mid 2013, the second industrial provider, AvidiaMed (2013), closed its ADD operation. A pilot study based on the ABDA-KBV proposal (Arzneimittelinitiative Sachsen-Thüringen 2014), initially scheduled to start at the end of 2013, has been delayed by a year (Ziegler 2013).

10.4.4 Status in 2016: Slow Diffusion and Persistent Opposition

About 7,5 Mio patients in Germany take five or more medication regularly (Hillienhof 2015). While the two national ADD initiatives have been terminated, local and regional blister initiatives have continued and are gradually extending their operations. In 2011 about 25% of home care facilities use and pay external blister providers (Rauers 2011). The economic logic for blistering is a combination of quality assurance and outsourcing of preparing the medication for patients: the external production of blisters can usually be done at a lower cost than the preparation of pill boxes in the care homes.

The diffusion of blistering among home care patients is much lower. It is not established as a practice and is rarely recommended by doctors or pharmacists. The daily practices of taking medication is not in scope of a broader debate. Eligibility and reimbursement have not been clarified by the regulator and when pharmacies provide blistering as a free service for their patients, they risk being sued for price dumping (Wessinger 2014).

To this day, there is a strong and outspoken opposition in Germany against blistering by the associations of doctors (KBV), pharmacists (ABDA) and the research active pharmaceutical manufacturers (VfA) industry, and (therefore) not actively pursued by the regulator.

Despite clarifying the legal status of patient specific blisters and the required license for the production in 2005, no subsequent clarification of eligibility, division of responsibilities and reimbursement have been provided by the regulator, which leaves providing blisters for care homes as one of the few economically viable options.

Core ehealth information infrastructure components, notably electronic prescription and electronic patient medication plan, upon which blistering could be more easily extended, have not yet been introduced.

There is neither a public discourse nor research about the benefit and risks of dose administration aids for elderly polypharmacy patients. The official statements against blistering are categorical and do not even leave space for a nuanced reflection of design options.

All this has led to the widespread perception that the issue is "dead" and does not require any further consideration. Notably, even the word "blistering" is largely avoided in the public discourse, except for the dedicated blister community, which seems like a marginalized minority. There are no significant research programs or projects on how to support elderly people in managing their medication. The discussion what should be covered by medication management is still ongoing (Dartsch 2013).

10.5   Analysis

The field of medication management with the goal to improve medication safety and compliance addresses a complex ensemble of diverse practices, health care governance and regulation as well as technology (codes, standards and artefacts, such as electronic patient health cards). The case underscores that infrastructure evolution is happening over extended periods of time, at a large scale and deeply embedded in practices (Reimers et al. 2012). It highlights not only the role of the installed base, but also the need for aligning the scope of initiatives (from local or regional to national) and the "availability" or state of the installed base at the appropriate level as a prerequisite for infrastructure innovation.

10.5.1 Deficiencies in Installed Base

As an attempted infrastructure innovation, the 7×4 Pharma initiative has been aimed at scaling – from a local or regional level to a national level – and extending existing practices of blistering, building and initiating an evolution of technical components (information infrastructure) and regulatory adjustments. It can be seen as a bold move to create facts that might have engendered a momentum of transformation.

However, it became obvious that neither the necessary supporting practices, such as the compilation, review and sharing of prescriptions and patient medication plan, nor the underlying information infrastructure (electronic prescriptions and digital mediation plans, electronic communication between physicians and pharmacies and software supported review of medication plans), nor the supporting regulation (rules for eligibility and reimbursement) had emerged at a national level.

There is still no mechanism in place to share medication records among health care professionals on a routine basis. Even though each health care professional is in principal obliged to control for critical interactions, there is no clear division of labour between pharmacists and doctors regarding the monitoring of medication effects over time. Both professions regularly rely on the vigilance of patients and their helpers. New routines, roles and linkages between doctors, patients, pharmacists, the blister operator and the health insurance provider were developed during the pilot project, but did not spread beyond the pilot and did not persist once the pilot was terminated. In other words, the installed base of local and regional practices and initiatives, locally deployed information systems and existing regulation of blistering, were not suitable for or not aligned with the goals of building a national infrastructure.

Obviously, 7×4 Pharma had been aware of the situation and has made major efforts throughout the pilot project to initiate a rudimentary information infrastructure development themselves. They provided software for medication review, the exchange of prescriptions and medication plans to physicians and pharmacists, and suggested ways of collaborating with the clearly articulate goal to improve the quality and efficiency of patient care. The design of the pilot study and the research based on the pilot (Leker and Kehrel 2011) were in line with the principles of benefits assessment as articulated by the G-BA[4] and the regulation about pilot projects in health care (§§ 63–65 SGB V). Still the lack of both, regulatory adjustments and standards has inhibited the proliferation of these practices that have been developed during the pilot.

One might interpret it as a bootstrapping approach, which – however – assumed that it would be sufficient to jumpstart the development dynamics, which would then convince the decision making bodies, the Federal Joint Committee (G-BA) and regulating authorities, to take over.

10.5.2 An "Installed Base of Opposition"

7×4 Pharma encountered what we would describe as an **installed base of opposition.** This opposition is multi-faceted and driven by different rationales. We have identified four key concerns:

1. 7×4 Pharma and its parent company, Kohl Medical AG,[5] have been perceived as a competitor constituting a new entrant into the health care market (Bellartz 2006).
2. The proposal of a mandatory medication list, i.e. the assortment of 400 medicines for blistering, has drawn critique from the doctors association (KBV).
3. The association of research active pharmaceutical manufacturers (VFA) funded research to proof the ineffectiveness of ADD and has been quite outspoken in its critique.
4. Innovations of the IT infrastructure, such as electronic prescriptions and electronic medication plans, and a wider dynamics of innovation have been critically reviewed by KBV.

The 7×4 Pharma design proposal caused predictable concerns or outright resistance across a large set of actors in the health care system:

1. The existing blister community (pharmacies and blister centres) inevitably perceived 7×4 Pharma as competitor and the ADD pilots as potentially disruptive innovation, even though they shared an interest in regulatory amendments in favour of blistering.

As blistering is particularly relevant for pharmacies who deliver to care homes and nursing homes, home care providers and polypharmacy patients, many pharmacies

---

[4]For more information about the mandate of the G-BA: http://www.english.g-ba.de/legalmandate/procedures/methods/evidence/

[5]Kohl Medical AG also owns kohlpharma, the largest European importer for medication.

see themselves as not really affected by the issue. ABDA as a pharmacy association appears to have decided to speak for the latter group rather than for the former. Even though the 7×4 Pharma proposal goes to great pains to emphasize and indeed strengthen the role of the pharmacists (Kohl 2010), there still may be a concern about potential disintermediation, i.e. direct delivery of blister packs to the patients.

Opponents of blistering aimed to undermine the credibility of 7×4 Pharma's ADD initiative, which provided a prominent and relatively easy target given the specific design proposals, in particular the positive list, and the position of Kohl Medical AG. Speculative concerns, such as the risk of a monopoly of 7×4 Pharma, or even conspiracy theories about the intended vertical control of the medication market by Kohl were two examples of the employed tactics (Bellartz 2006). By aiming at ADD, they indirectly also undermined the credibility of the regional blister centres. The opposition appears to follow distinct tactics of focussing on controversial design issues while not engaging in any dialogue about possible design improvements, and creating their own initiative, which could be regarded as a red herring, while avoiding the issue of blistering, and causing or accepting delays. The official statements about blistering by physician and pharmacist associations (Landesapotheker- und Landesärztekammer Brandenburg 2011) have been criticized as one sided, bloating risks and obstructing blistering, without recognizing the facts of widely established practices of blistering and using dose administration aids in Germany and – more widespread – internationally (BPAV 2011; Schumbach 2013a). We have not found evidence of a willingness of ABDA and KBV to recognize the need for dose administration aids and to engage in a dialogue about improvements of the design of ADD or blistering in general in order to better address patients' needs or to suggest or conduct further research to clarify the contested issues. The benefits of patient specific blisters, if properly administered, have been shown by several studies (Leker and Kehrel 2011; G. Neubauer and Wick 2011), yet these results seem to be "inconvenient truths", which are refused and opposed.

2. Many doctors and their association (KBV) are against, what has been referred to as the positive list, a mandatory list of medication that can be provided by 7×4 Pharma,

Since 2006 insurance companies can and do negotiate discounts with pharmaceutical manufacturers (Bundesministerium für Gesundheit 2006). This could pose a potential conflict with the mandatory list of medication suggested by 7×4 Pharma.

3. The association of research active pharmaceutical manufacturers (VfA), which commissioned an academic study aiming directly at 7×4 Pharma's initiative, had strong reasons for their opposition. If ADD would be introduced in Germany as suggested by 7×4 Pharma, they would have a lot to lose: (a) control over which medication is dispensed to the participating polypharmacy patients, (b) according to the pilot results, less medication would be discarded because of the

provision in weekly blister packs instead of larger retail packages, (c) medication in blisters can be provided at a lower price (Pradel 2015), (d) eventually the ADD operators may be able to procure medication in large packages for the use in blister automats – like in Finland – rather than the current retail packages. The widely cited study (Wille and Wolf 2006), whose content was reiterated by VfA itself (Verband Forschender Arzneimittelhersteller e.V. (VFA) 2009) proved to be very effective in discrediting the efficiency and effectiveness of patient specific blisters based on conceptually derived claims, yet without providing primary empirical evidence. In that way the study would not qualify as evidence according to the standards of the Federal Joint Committee (G-BA).

4. There is widespread reservation or even open resistance against electronic prescription among doctors (Franke 2010; Institut für Demoskopie Allensbach 2010). While the implementation of the medication plan is welcomed in principle, specific concerns still remain (Hillienhof 2015) and the responsibilities regarding compiling and reviewing a comprehensive medication plan are not clear yet (ABDA – Bundesvereinigung Deutscher Apothekerverbände 2015).

We suspect that the concern, the discussion about patient specific blisters might open a pandora's box of subsequent, uncontrollable changes in the health care system, is a key reason for the opposition. In a description of his research on his web site, Neubauer states that based on the insights of the ADD pilot projects, he will be exploring possible improvements of the health care system at large.[6]

Based on the prevalent opposition, the regulator decided not to take any action in favour of blistering (Schumbach 2013b): implementation issues of the 2005 regulation such as eligibility for blistering, reimbursement of costs, roles and responsibilities for aggregating and checking medication plans, let alone the underlying IT infrastructure for e-Prescription and electronic medication plans were left open.

10.6 Discussion

In this section we will be looking at different lenses and interpretations of the notion of installed base as well as the German health care system's propensity to innovation. The case provides different insights on the emergence of infrastructures and the related installed base.

First, it illustrates the various, interconnected facets of the installed base: constellations of practices, specifically of an integrated medication management, health care regulation and governance, and technology: "there is a historicity stemming from the manner sediments of earlier solutions, entrenched routines, prevailing perceptions and social institutions constitute and solidify existing practices." (Aanestad et al. 2005, p.5, see also Aanestad and Jensen 2011, p.162). The introduction of ADD would imply a transformation and extension of practices of medication

---

[6] See: project description "Patient individual secondary pharmaceutical blister packs in care homes" on http://ifg-muenchen.com/arzneimittel-und-medizinprodukte/

management (consolidation of prescriptions, creating and reviewing the medication plan) and related information sharing practice (between specialist doctors and the GP, GP and pharmacy, pharmacy and ADD operator), practices of distributing medication and practices of invoicing and reimbursing medication. This transformation will create uncertainties as to who – physician or pharmacist – will be in charge, what will be the basis of reimbursement (if any) and how will the coordination between physician or pharmacist be organized. Moreover, the proposals for ADD relate to entrenched opposition of doctors and pharmacists. Doctors fear to lose control over their choice of medication, something which is already happening to some degree as a result of health insurance policies. Pharmacists fear to lose revenue as a result of new business models (Online pharmacies) or new entrants (ADD operators), who might try to bypass community pharmacies.

This illustrates, *second*, the possibly inhibiting role of an installed base of practices, which are not open for discourse, experimentation and innovation, instead seem to focus more on caring for their own economic interests, retaining control and perpetuating the status quo. In particular the national doctors' and pharmacists' associations (KBV and ABDA) appear to be entrenched in politics and lobbying for the majority of their members. The blatant unwillingness even to engage in a dialogue about blistering is striking.

Third, it shows the difficulties of scaling a medication infrastructure before the relevant installed base has been scaled as well or is at least ready for scaling. This includes a momentum of technical innovations and related norms and practices. In this way, the installed base does not only highlight the temporal dynamics of infrastructure development and evolution, but the installed base also becomes a platform and indeed background upon which novel or specialized infrastructures can be built or scaled.

Turned around, this might suggest an expectation that the successful scaling of an infrastructure, specifically ADD, might spur and accelerate the adjustment and adaptation of the underlying installed base and cause a political momentum and reorientation. 7×4 Pharma's goal was to convince the regulator to take action and provide the necessary steps by delivering a proof of concept (pilot installation) with participation of patients, doctors, pharmacists, insurance companies and academics. Insurance companies aided by academics acknowledged the effectiveness of the solution and were meant to provide the necessary credibility.

Conclusion

We have interpreted the ADD initiatives in Germany as attempts to scale scattered local and regional practices of blistering and establish a national infrastructure. The analysis of the failure of these initiatives revealed a lack of an appropriate or even appropriately flexible installed base in terms of established practices of physicians and pharmacists as well as cooperation between them, enabled by regulation and technology, specifically a patient information infrastructure encompassing electronic prescription and patient medication plans.

While both national-level initiatives can also be seen as bootstrapping attempts to foster the development of the bespoke installed base, they encountered categorical opposition and resistance. While in particular in the case of the association of the pharma manufacturers (VfA), the opposition can be explained by obvious economic interests, the resistance of physician and pharmacy associations is less obvious. Both also represent members who are not only in favour of, but are actually producing and distributing blisters to their patients.

The tactics of opposition seem to suggest a profoundly negative attitude, which is not even open to discourse and reasoning. It is astounding that the international examples of practice, critical discourse and research about dose administration aids as integrated part of medication management dose are not actively considered.

A justification for the resistance to infrastructure innovation might reflect prior experience of government initiated large scale health care infrastructure projects, such as the electronic patient health card. Especially the health card appears as a typical example of a megaproject (Flyvbjerg et al. 2003), which encountered huge resistance, delays, cost overruns and in the end achieved much less then has been promised at the start. Given this experience, an attitude of hesitation becomes understandable.

The governance structure of the German health care system is based on cooperatist consensus building and decision making prior to regulation. The Federal Joint Committee (G-BA) is the decision-making body of the joint governance of physicians, dentists, hospitals and health insurance providers in Germany (www.english.g-ba.de). The G-BA has an innovation fund, which will be available as of 2016 in order to facilitate and study new forms of medical care. Pilot projects for medication safety for multimorbid patients are among the suggested initiatives. This initiative might be read as an admission that innovative forms of care require more attention in Germany.

10.7   Appendix: List of Acronyms

ABDA	Federation of German Associations of Pharmacists
ADD	Automatic dose (or drug) dispensing (ADD), the industrial production of patient-specific dose administration aids, e.g. blister packs, typically for solid oral medicines for a defined period, e.g. 7 days.
AkdÄ	Drug Commission of the German Medical Association
Blistering	The provision of patient specific dose administration aids in form of blister packs.
BPAV	Bundesverband Patientenindividueller Arzneimittelverblisterer e.V. (national association of producers of patient specific blister packs).
BVKA	National Association of Pharmacies supplying care homes or nursing homes.
GB-A	The Federal Joint Committee (G-BA) is the highest decision-making body of the joint self-government of physicians, dentists, hospitals and health insurance funds in Germany. [http://www.english.g-ba.de/]
KBV	National Association of Statutory Health Insurance Physicians
VfA	Association of Research Active Pharmaceutical Manufacturers

References

Aanestad M, Jensen T B (2011). Building nation-wide information infrastructures in healthcare through modular implementation strategies. The Journal of Strategic Information Systems, 20(2), 161–176.

Aanestad M, Monteiro E, Kimaro H, Macombe E, Macueve G, Mukama F, Muquingue H, Nhampossa J, Lungo J. Strategies for development and integration of health information systems: coping with historicity and heterogeneity (No. 5/2005). Oslo. 2005. Retrieved 06 Jan 2017 from http://folk.uio.no/systarb/wp/052005.pdf.

ABDA – Bundesvereinigung Deutscher Apothekerverbände. Kiefer: Medikationsplan im E-Health-Gesetzentwurf ist Etikettenschwindel. ABDA Pressemitteilungen. 2015. Retrieved 14 Sept 2015, from http://www.abda.de/pressemitteilung/artikel/kiefer-medikationsplan-im-e-health-gesetzentwurf-ist-etikettenschwindel/.

ABDA, KBV. Zukunftskonzept Arzneimittelversorgung. 2011a. Retrieved 31 May 2016, from http://www.abda.de/fileadmin/assets/Pressetermine/2011/ABDA_KBV/Zukunftskonzept_07_10_2011_KBV_ABDA_Homepage.pdf.

ABDA, KBV. Zukunftskonzept Arzneimittelversorgung – Gemeinsames Eckpunktepapier. Berlin. 2011b. Retrieved 31 May 2016, from http://www.kbv.de/html/2947.php.

AkDÄ. Aktionsplan Arzneimitteltherapiesicherheit (AMTS). 2007. Retrieved 31 May 2016, from www.akdae.de/AMTS/Aktionsplan/.

Arzneimittelinitiative Sachsen-Thüringen. ARMIN – Die Arzneimittelinitiative Sachsen-Thüringen. 2014. Retrieved 21 Mar 2015, from http://www.arzneimittelinitiative.de/grundlagen/.

Ärztliches Zentrum für Qualität in der Medizin (ÄZQ). Sichere Arzneimitteltherapie. 2011; doi:10.6101/AZQ/000002.

AvidiaMed. Pressemeldung: Körber fokussiert Kernaktivitäten der Sparte Pharma-Verpackungssysteme. 2013. Retrieved 06 Jan 2017, from http://www.koerber.de/cn/medien/aktuelle-meldungen/meldung-liste/article/koerber-fokussiert-kernaktivitaeten-der-sparte--pharma-verpackungssysteme.html.

Bell JS, Johnell K, Wimmer BC, Wiese MD. Multidose drug dispensing and optimising drug use in older people. Age Ageing. 2013;42(2013):556–8.

Bellartz T. Apothekenmarkt – Die Expansion des Edwin Kohl. Pharmazeutische Zeitung online. 2006. Retrieved 06 Jan 2017, from www.pharmazeutische-zeitung.de/index.php?id=849.

Bierwirth R, Paust R. Compliance und empowerment in der Diabetologie. Bremen: UNI-MED; 2004.

Borchers D. Elektronische Gesundheitskarte: Feldtest muss verschoben werden. Heise online. 2015. Retrieved 31 May 2016, from http://www.heise.de/newsticker/meldung/Elektronische-Gesundheitskarte-Feldtest-muss-verschoben-werden-2763723.html.

BPAV. Entgegnung des BPAV auf das gemeinsame Positionspapier der Landesapotheker- und Landesärztekammer Brandenburg vom August 2011. 2011. Retrieved from http://www.blisterverband.de/.

Braun B, Marstedt G. Non-compliance bei der Arzneimitteltherapie: Umfang, Hintergründe, Veränderungswege. In: Böcken J, Braun B, Reipschläger U, editors. Gesundheitsmonitor 2011. Gütersloh: Bertelsmann Stiftung; 2011. p. 56–76.

Bundesärztekammer. Beschlussprotokoll des 111. Deutschen Ärztetages vom 20. bis 23. Mai 2008 in Ulm. Berlin. 2008. Retrieved 31 May 2016, from http://www.bundesaerztekammer.de/aerztetag/beschlussprotokolle-ab-1996/111-daet-2008/.

Bundesärztekammer. Beschlussprotokoll des 118. Deutschen Ärztetages in Frankfurt am Main vom 12.05. bis 15.05.2015. Berlin. 2015. Retrieved 31 May 2016, from https://www.pa-deutschland.de/files/beschlussprotokoll2015.pdf.

Bundesministerium für Gesundheit. Gesetz zur Verbesserung der Wirtschaftlichkeit in der Arzneimittelversorgung (AVWG) tritt zum 1. Mai 2006 in Kraft. Pressemitteilung. 2006. Retrieved 20 Sept 2015, from http://www.bmg.bund.de/presse/pressemitteilungen/2006-02/arzneimittelversorgungs-wirtschaftlichkeitsgesetz-tritt-in-kraft.html.

Bundesregierung der Bundesrepublik Deutschland. Entwurf eines Gesetzes für sichere digitale Kommunikation und Anwendungen im Gesundheitswesen. Berlin, Germany. 2015. Retrieved 06 Jan 2017, from http://www.bmg.bund.de/fileadmin/dateien/Downloads/E/eHealth/150527_Gesetzentwurf_E-Health.pdf.

Cheung K-C, van den Bemt PMLA, Bouvy ML, Wensing M, De Smet PAGM. Medication incidents related to automated dose dispensing in community pharmacies and hospitals – a reporting system study. PLoS ONE. 2014;9(7):e101686.

Corlett AJ. Caring for older people: aids to compliance with medication. BMJ. 1996;313(7062):926–9.

Dartsch D. Serie AMTS: Medikationsmanagement hier und anderswo. Pharmazeutische Zeitung Online. 2013. Retrieved 31 May 2016, from http://www.pharmazeutische-zeitung.de/index.php?id=50085.

Drews P, Schirmer I. The failed implementation of the electronic prescription in Germany – a case study. In Proceedings of the 23rd European Conference on Information Systems. Münster. 2015. p. 1–15.

Düsing R. Medikamentöse Therapie mit verblisterten Arzneimitteln: Möglichkeiten und Chancen. Bonn. 2006. Retrieved 31 May 2016, from http://www.kohlpharma.de/_data/mediapool/download_daten_assist/1171892367_070125_Duesing-Studie.pdf.

Elmer A. Großprojekt Elektronische Gesundheitskarte. IM+io, (03), 20–26. 2014.

Flyvbjerg B, Bruzelius N, Rothengatter W. Megaprojects and risk – an anatomy of ambition. Cambridge: Cambridge University Press; 2003.

Franke N. Elektronische Gesundheitskarte: Ärzte lehnen E-Rezept ab. Pharmazeutische Zeitung Online 35. 2010. Retrieved 31 May 2016, from http://www.pharmazeutische-zeitung.de/index.php?id=35100.

GKV Spitzenverband. Das Wichtigste über die elektronische Gesundheitskarte. 2015. Retrieved from https://www.gkv-spitzenverband.de/media/dokumente/presse/publikationen/Flyer_eGK_2015.pdf.

Glaeske G. Analyse der Verordnungen in einer GKV-Population im Hinblick auf die Eignung für eine individuelle Verblisterung. 2007. Retrieved 31 May 2016, from www.7x4pharma.de/_shared/p_file_download.php?locale=de&files_id=2803.

Haefeli WE, Hoppe-Tichy T, Seidling H. Abschlussbericht – best practice strategien in Europa als Grundlage für die Optimierung von Arzneimittelverordnung, anwendung und das Therapiemonitoring in Deutschland. Heidelberg: Universitätsklinikum Heidelberg; 2012. Retrieved 4 January 2017 from https://www.bundesgesundheitsministerium.de/fileadmin/Dateien/Publikationen/Gesundheit/Bericht/Abschlussbericht_BestPractice_AMTS_20160226_deutsche_Abb.pdf

Hillienhof A. KBV fordert Änderungen am geplanten Medikationsplan. Berlin: Deutsches Ärzteblatt; 2015.Retrieved 06 Jan 2017, from http://www.aerzteblatt.de/nachrichten/63578/KBV-fordert-Aenderungen-am-geplanten-Medikationsplan.

Hollstein P. Kohl gibt Startschuss für 7×4-box. APOTHEKE ADHOC. 2009. Retrieved 06 Jan 2017, from http://www.apotheke-adhoc.de/nachrichten/nachricht-detail/kohl-gibt-startschuss-fuer-7x4-box/?L=0%3Ft%3Ft%3Ft%3Ft%3Ft%3Ft%3D1?t=1.

Institut für Demoskopie Allensbach. Der Einsatz von Telematik und Telemedizin im Gesundheitswesen: Ergebnisse einer Repräsentativbefragung. eHealth-Report: Institut für Demoskopie Allensbach. Allensbach. 2010. Retrieved 06 Jan 2017, from http://www.bundesaerztekammer.de/fileadmin/user_upload/downloads/pdf-Ordner/Telemedizin_Telematik/Telemedizin/eHealth_Bericht_kurz_final_1_.pdf.

Kohl E. Patient compliance and treatment success individualised blister packs using the 7×4 box as an example. 2010. Retrieved 06 Jan 2017, from http://www.costeff.eu/_shared/p_file_download.php?files_id=70.

Landesapotheker- und Landesärztekammer Brandenburg. Positionspapier: Qualitätsgesicherte Arzneimitteltherapie und Arzneimittelversorgung von Patienten, die in unterstützenden Wohnformen (Heimen) betreut werden. 2011. Retrieved from http://www.laekb.de/50ueberUns/20Beitraege/90Archiv/70Archiv2011/110509_Positionspapier110818.pdf.

Lauterbach KW, Gerber A, Lüngen M. Internationale Erfahrungen mit der Verblisterung von Arzneimitteln. Köln. 2004a. Retrieved 06 Jan 2017, from https://www.7x4-pharma.com/_shared/p_file_download.php?files_id=2798.

Lauterbach KW, Gerber A, Stollenwerk B, Lüngen M. Verblisterung von Arzneimitteln für Bewohner von Alten-und Pflegeheimen und in der häuslichen Pflege: Beschreibung und Bewertung eines Pilotprojekts (September 2004 bis Dezember 2005) Verblisterung von Arzneimitteln. Köln. 2006. Retrieved 06 Jan 2017, from www.7x4pharma.de/_shared/p_file_ download.php?files_id=2801&locale=de.

Lauterbach KW, Lüngen M, Gerber A. Nutzung der Verblisterung von Arzneimitteln im Rahmen von Disease-Management-Programmen. Köln. 2004b. Retrieved 06 Jan 2017, from https:// www.7x4-pharma.com/_shared/p_file_download.php?files_id=2797.

Lauterbach KW, Lüngen M, Gerber A, Kohaupt I, Büscher G. Quantifizierung der Fehlwurfrate beim Stellen fester oraler Darreichungsformen in drei Pflegeheimen. Köln. 2007. Retrieved 06 Jan 2017, from https://www.7x4-pharma.com/_shared/p_file_download.php?files_id=2799.

Leker J, Kehrel U. Abschlussbericht der Studie zur patientenindividuellen Arzneimittelverblisterung in Berliner Pflegeeinrichtungen Struktur des Berliner Pilotprojektes (Präsentation). 2011. Retrieved 06 Jan 2017, from http://www.wmscdn.de/uploads/9758/9758.pdf.

Lochner S, Buitkamp M, Kirch W. Polypharmazie – wie beurteilen Patienten die Medikamentenverschreibung der Ärzte? In: Böcken J, Braun B, Reipschläger U, editors. Gesundheitsmonitor 2011. Gütersloh: Bertelsmann Stiftung ; 2011. p. 77–92.Retrieved 06 Jan 2017, from http://gesundheitsmonitor.de/studien/detail/?tx_itaoarticles_pi1[article]=169&tx_ itaoarticles_pi1[action]=show&tx_itaoarticles_pi1[controller]=Article&cHash=9064ed16fc59 25bcca27a905a5c86f73.

Neubauer G. Patientenindividuelle Arzneimittel-Verblisterung für Bewohner in Pflegeheimen – Bericht zum Modellprojekt der AOK Bayern. Berlin. 2011. Retrieved 06 Jan 2017, from www. bvka.de/Veranstaltungen/Neubauer%20BVKA%20Berlin%2024-10-11.pdf.

Neubauer G, Wick A. Patientenindividuelle für Bewohner von Pflegeheimen (PIVP) Zusammenfassung der wichtigsten Ergebnisse des Modellprojekts der AOK Bayern. 2011. Retrieved 06 Jan 2017, from http://www.wmscdn.de/uploads/9756/9756.pdf.

Neumann P.. Rösler stoppt die elektronische Gesundheitskarte. Die Welt. 2009, November. Retrieved 06 Jan 2017, from https://www.welt.de/politik/deutschland/article5267140/Roesler-stoppt-die-elektronische-Gesundheitskarte.html.

Patienten-individuelle Verblisterung in Deutschland – eine Bestandsaufnahme. Der BlisterBlog – Patientenindividuelle Arzneimittelverblisterung. 2010. Retrieved from http://verblistern.info/ blog/.

Pradel J. BGH glaubt nicht an Stückel-Boni. Apotheke Adhoc. 2015, August 11. Retrieved 06 Jan 2017, from http://www.apotheke-adhoc.de/nachrichten/apothekenpraxis/nachricht-detail-apothekenpraxis/verblisterung-bundesgerichtshof-bgh-erlaubt-rabatte-fuer-rx-teilmengen/.

Rauers J. Pflegeheime setzen Apotheken unter Druck. Apotheke adhoc. 2011. Retrieved 06 Jan 2017, from http://www.apotheke-adhoc.de/nachrichten/nachricht-detail/pflegeheime-setzen-apotheken-unter-druck/?t=1.

Reimers K, Johnston RB, Klein S. Evolution of inter-organizational information systems on long timescales: a practice theory approach. In: Vaidya K, editor. Inter-organizational information systems and business management: theories for researchers. Hershey: IGI Global; 2012.

Royal Pharmaceutical Society. Improving patient outcomes The better use of multi – compartment compliance aids. 2013. Retrieved 06 Jan 2017, from http://www.rpharms.com/support-pdfs/ rps-mca-july-2013.pdf.

Schersch S. E-Health-Gesetz: Apotheker in der Nebenrolle. Pharmazeutische Zeitung Online. 2015. Retrieved 06 Jan 2017, from http://www.pharmazeutische-zeitung.de/index. php?id=58157.

Schumbach K.. Blisterapotheken: ABDA mauert. Apotheke adhoc. 2013a. Retrieved 21 Aug 2013, from http://www.apotheke-adhoc.de/nachrichten/nachricht-detail/bvka-tagung-steinweg-verblistern-muss-honoriert-werden/.

Schumbach K. Kein Honorar für Verblisterung. Apotheke adhoc. 2013b. Retrieved 30 Aug 2013, from http://www.apotheke-adhoc.de/nachrichten/nachricht-detail/verblisterung-hennrich-verblistern-ist-kein-thema/?tx_ttnews%5BsViewPointer%5D=1&cHash=0315a0f1b 5a6f6b6e67fcad1417b375c.

Stafford N. Germany is set to introduce e-health cards by 2018. BMJ. 2015;h2991.

Tuffs A. Germany plans to introduce electronic health card. BMJ. 2004;329:131.

Verband Forschender Arzneimittelhersteller e.V. (VFA). Industrielle Neuverblisterung von Arzneimitteln. Berlin. 2009. Retrieved 06 Jan 2017, from www.vfa.de/download/pos-neuverblisterung.pdf.

VFA. Die elektronische Gesundheitskarte: Was sie kann und was sie noch können soll. 2014. Retrieved 06 Jan 2017, from http://www.vfa-patientenportal.de/patienten-und-versorgung/was-sie-kann-und-was-sie-noch-koennen-soll.html.

Wessinger B. Apotheker begrüßen Blister-Dumpingverbot. Apotheker Zeitung. 2014. Retrieved 06 Jan 2017, from https://www.deutsche-apotheker-zeitung.de/daz-az/2014/az-46-2014/apotheker-begruessen-blister-dumpingverbot.

Wille E, Wolf M. Neuverblisterung von Arzneimitteln. Gutachten im Auftrag des Verbandes Forschender Arzneimittelhersteller e.V. (VFA) Endbericht. 2006. Retrieved 06 Jan 2017, from http://www.vfa.de/pm20060627.

World Alliance for Patient Safety. Summary of the evidence on patient safety: implications for research. edited by Ashish Jha. Geneva. 2008. Retrieved 06 Jan 2017, from http://www.who.int/patientsafety/information_centre/20080523_Summary_of_the_evidence_on_patient_safety.pdf.

Ziegler J. Politik: Mit neuem Namen: ABDA/KBV-Modell startet im Januar: DAZ.online. DAZ.online. 2013. Retrieved 06 Jan 2017, from http://www.deutsche-apotheker-zeitung.de/politik/news/2013/10/11/abdakbv-modell-startet-im-januar/11211.html.

Open Access This chapter is distributed under the terms of the Creative Commons Attribution-NonCommercial 2.5 International License (http://creativecommons.org/licenses/by-nc/2.5/), which permits any noncommercial use, duplication, adaptation, distribution and reproduction in any medium or format, as long as you give appropriate credit to the original author(s) and the source, provide a link to the Creative Commons license and indicate if changes were made.

The images or other third party material in this chapter are included in the chapter's Creative Commons license, unless indicated otherwise in a credit line to the material. If material is not included in the chapter's Creative Commons license and your intended use is not permitted by statutory regulation or exceeds the permitted use, you will need to obtain permission directly from the copyright holder.

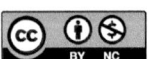

Part III

Governmental Patient-Oriented eHealth Infrastructures

Joan Rodon Modol

11.1   Introduction

This chapter presents the genesis and evolution of the public patient portal called Carpeta Personal de Salut[1] (CPS) of Catalonia, Spain. Our account of the CPS covers the period 2008 to 2015. The CPS gives citizens secure and confidential access to their health data (generated in the public health system). The case narrative shows how the installed base was gradually extended with new partners and services aiming to increase the value and usefulness of the infrastructure in order to attract more users. The reminder of the chapter is structured as follows. In the next two sections, we present the Catalan healthcare model and the installed base of IT systems. This is followed by our narrative of the case. Next we discuss the implications of our findings.

11.2   The Catalan Healthcare Model

The Spanish National Health System comprises both the Central Government Administration and the autonomous regions. The former is in charge of the (1) health basic principles and general coordination; (2) foreign health affairs and international relations and agreements; and (3) legislation on pharmaceutical products. Each autonomous region is responsible of health planning, public health, and healthcare services management. The Health System of the autonomous region of Catalonia involves four main actors: the Catalan Department of Health (DoH); the CatSalut (the Catalan Health Service); health providers; and citizens. The DoH is in charge of establishing health policies and maintaining levels of quality in delivery by creating a health plan, determining a healthcare budget, and accrediting

---

[1] Personal Health Folder.

J.R. Modol
ESADE Ramon Llull University, Av. Torreblanca 59, 08172 Sant Cugat del Vallès, Spain
e-mail: joan.rodon@esade.edu

© The Author(s) 2017   173
M. Aanestad et al. (eds.), *Information Infrastructures within European Health Care*, Health Informatics, DOI 10.1007/978-3-319-51020-0_11

providers. The CatSalut is the public insurer that is responsible for planning, purchasing, and assessing health services according to the needs of the population. The CatSalut establishes service policies in line with the health policies defined by the DoH. The Catalan territory is divided into seven health regions. Each region is structured in turn in health sectors, which bring together the so-called basic health areas formed by neighbourhoods or districts in urban areas, or one or more municipalities in rural areas. The health providers are those organizations that the CatSalut contracts to provide care services. Each health provider has a multiannual contract with the CatSalut that is revised on a yearly basis and includes health objectives, activity, economic amount, rates (pricing), invoicing system, and evaluation system.

The provision of healthcare is done by multiple contracted providers having different ownership: public companies – the Catalan Health Institute (ICS) is the biggest one–, consortia, municipal foundations and private foundations (see Table 11.1). The provision of healthcare is organized into four main levels: primary care; specialized or hospital care; socio-sanitary care; and mental health. Primary care is the gatekeeper and responsible for coordinating the patients' care along the care continuum. Since the primary healthcare reform (in 1985) primary care has evolved from a predominantly curative care model (upon demand from the user population and the work of individual healthcare professionals) to a model that focuses simultaneously on preventive healthcare, curative healthcare, rehabilitative care and the promotion of community health. This transformation was structurally achieved through the creation of basic health areas and the gradual introduction of primary care teams. Nowadays, there are 369 primary care centres, around 77% of them being managed by the public provider ICS.

Specialized or hospital care acts as a consultant of primary care and is responsible for more complex care. There is a public network of hospitals distributed over the territory following the schemes of population distribution. The model of hospital has changed in recent years, progressing from a traditional model of a more closed centre that provides conventional inpatient care, emergencies and an outpatient department, to a centre with a greater outpatient focus, with significant roles for ambulatory major and minor surgery, day hospital and home hospitalization. Nowadays there are 69 hospitals (the ICS manages 8 of those hospitals). Around 79% of the specialized care is managed by non-public providers.

Table 11.1 Ownership of healthcare facilities

Type of center	Public		Non-public	
	Property (%)	Management (%)	Property (%)	Management (%)
Specialized/hospital care	25,94	21,43	74,06	78,57
Primary care	95,40	87,72	4,60	12,28
Mental care	28,87	27,38	71,13	72,62
Long-term care	68,63	62,75	31,37	37,25

Source: Catalan Department of Health

11.3   The Installed Base of IT Systems

The multi-provider nature of the Catalan healthcare model had always given providers autonomy in the management of centers and freedom in selecting, building and managing their health IT (HIT) systems. Historically there had been no guidelines regarding the HIT systems that health providers should have in place. So, the Catalan health system traditionally had a completely decentralized governance model for IT. This led to a situation with more than 60 different HIT systems for primary care and hospital care without any kind of integration, and heterogeneity among providers in terms of the level of adoption of HIT.

For instance, in the case of hospital care there are multiple HIT systems supporting different clinical protocols, messages, catalogues, etc., meaning that each provider has to build multiple interfaces for the same purpose (to interact with other providers). Major providers have HIT systems based on SAP.[2] For instance, ARGOS is a SAP-based HIT developed by IBM that runs in the 8 hospitals of the ICS and some other hospitals.

At the level of primary care, there are several HIT systems (e.g., eCAP, OMI-AP, GO-WIN, SIAP-Win); eCAP is the dominant one. eCAP was developed in 2000 by clinicians of the Catalan Health Institute (ICS). The motives for the development of eCAP were: the existence of three different HIT systems for primary care within ICS; provider lock-ins; and interoperability issues among those HIT systems. More than 80% of primary care centers run eCAP. Moreover, the Health Plan 2011–2015 (HealthPlan 2011) proposed making available eCAP to all the other providers in 2012 aiming at having a common HIT system for all primary care providers. However, by that time there were multiple versions of eCAP reflecting the diverse rollouts of eCAP in the territory. In addition, eCAP had more than 20 databases and each patient's data were stored in several databases. Further, eCAP had a strong physical architecture meaning that professionals were aware of the server they connected each time they run an application.

11.3.1 The Shared Electronic Medical Record of Catalonia

Overall, the multiplicity and heterogeneity of HIT systems, data models and standards, and working processes turned into a problem as the DoH defined efficiency, continuity of care and integrated care as priorities in the successive health plans since early 2000s. The implementation of these priorities required standardizing and sharing information within and across health providers. This motivated the DoH to build and rollout the Historia Clínica Compartida (HC3), a Shared Electronic Medical Record, in 2008. The purpose was that any healthcare professional could access data about her patients regardless which providers had generated the data. The HC3 interconnected all the electronic health record systems (EHR) of the healthcare providers operating in the Catalan public health system. The HC3 was

---

[2] http://go.sap.com/solution/industry/healthcare.html

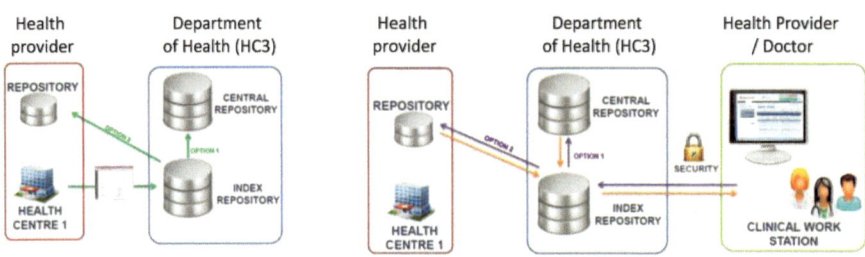

Fig. 11.1 Information management processes of the HC3

neither conceived as the sum of the EHRs of the health providers nor as a way to replace the existing EHR of providers, but as an infrastructure that would organize the access to health data stored in the EHRs of health providers and in some databases of the DoH (Marimon-Suñol et al. 2010). The HC3 consisted of a central node working either as an index or a repository of documents that would give access to all doctors (through a web browser) to the information coming from the EHRs of the diverse providers (see Fig. 11.1).

The information displayed in the doctors' browser came from (1) health providers: primary care (diagnoses, healthcare reports, immunizations, and chronic patient labels), specialized care, long-term care and mental care (discharge report, emergency reports, specialized outpatient clinic reports), and diagnosis procedures (pathology and laboratory reports, radiology image, imaging diagnosis reports, interventions); and (2) the DoH: medical activity database (diagnoses, procedures), prescribed/dispensed drugs (electronic prescription), and advanced directives. The HC3 provided a set of tools for direct messaging between health professionals to facilitate their cooperation.

The interconnection of healthcare providers' systems to the HC3 was regulated through an agreement between providers and the DoH (AgreementForHC3 2009). That agreement established the commitments of parties as well as the technical requirements. Moreover, the CatSalut promoted providers adoption of HC3 by means of economic incentives (defined in the annual contracts with providers) related with the publishing of documents. By the end of 2011, 96.5% of primary care centers and 85.5% of hospital care were connected to HC3 (CatSalutReport 2011).

The HC3 grew with new users, functional requirements (e.g. types of health data, identification codes, interconnection of the HC3 with the Spanish Shared Electronic Medical Record and with the European Patients-Smart Open Services), and technological requirements (e.g. compression of data, new security layers, HL7 messages). Moreover, the Health Plan for the period 2011–2015 (HealthPlan 2011) defined a project, within the line of action number 9 called "Sharing information, transparency, and assessment", to transform the HC3 from a repository of health data into a network of information and services that facilitated the integration of providers. All this involved extending the HC3 with new sources and formats of data, access modes and services, and standardizing the patient trajectory

Table 11.2 Evolution of HC3

	Repository of health data (2008–2011)	Network of information and services (2012–2015)
Source of data	Repository of health data from primary care	Repository of health data from primary, hospital, socio-sanitary and mental care
Format of data	Document-oriented database (stores PDF documents, or a link to the document in the provider EHR)	Structured data about diagnosis, immunizations, spirometry, patient trajectory, etc.
Access	Access through web-browser	Access through web-browser and integration with clinical work stations
Services	Static view of the patient data	Extension of HC3 with a messaging platform to include the patient trajectory and the management of the clinical protocols for the ten chronic pathologies prioritized in the (HealthPlan 2011)

and the management of clinical protocols across providers (Carrau et al. 2013) (see Table 11.2).

Overall, although HC3 respected the installed base of HIT systems, its evolution influenced some of its components. On the one hand, the HealtITPlan (2012) suggested that eCAP (the dominant HIT system at primary care) became the unique system of primary care. First, that would create efficiencies (e.g., any change is implemented once and replicated everywhere; having a unique data model for all the primary care). Second, the strategy of integrated care defined in the HealthPlan (2011) was built around primary care, thus having a unique common system for primary care was supposed to be aligned with the vision of integrated care and continuity of care. On the other hand, in specialized care there are multiple HIT systems. Yet the fact that the major health provider (ICS) runs ARGOS (developed by IBM), and that IBM is a central actor in the definition of the new messaging platform (that extends the HC3) might be catalysts for the reduction of the number of HIT systems in specialized care. Next section presents the story of the Catalan public-oriented portal which was built on the achievements of the HC3.

Method

Data was collected from three main sources: semi-structured in-depth face-to-face interviews (37 interviews), participant observation (the author registered for the CPS on 2011 and has used it intermittently during 2011, 2012, 2013 and 2015; workshop attendance; and informal conversations), and archival data (press documents, reports, meeting minutes, and videos), aiming at data triangulation (Yin 2003). Conducting the interviews was organized in three stages between 2011 and 2015: (1) from March to June 2011 (17 interviews); (2) from March to June 2013 (10 interviews); and (3) from December to October 2015 (10 interviews).

We identified interviewees by referral from other subjects. All the interviews were recorded and immediately transcribed and analyzed next two the archival data and other observations. In that sense, data collection and analysis took place iteratively.

With the data gathered, we constructed an initial timeline of events for the evolution of the CPS. We then wrote a rich chronological case story that put at the forefront the role of the installed base. We organized the case narrative into three stages covering the period 2008–2015.

11.4   Case Narrative

11.4.1 Phase 1: Genesis and Pilot (2008–2011)

The Catalan Department of Health (DoH) launched the project of the Carpeta Personal de Salut[3] (CPS) in 2008 as part of the execution of the Catalan health IT strategic plan for the period 2008–2011 (HealthITPlan 2008).[4] The leader and sponsor of the CPS was the coordination of Health IT of the DoH. With the CPS they wanted to promote responsibility and participation of citizens in matters of their own health (preventive actions and self-care); to have a secure environment for citizens to interact with health system, providers and professionals; and to improve the health care quality and coordination between different care areas, levels and professionals. Following existing regulations about the information rights and autonomy of the patient (InformationRightsAct 2000; PatientAutonomyAct 2002), the health data displayed in the CPS would come from the HC3 (Cerdà-Calafat et al. 2010). The HC3 was the main source of data of the CPS (see Fig. 11.2). The CPS would be a module of the HC3, acting as a web-browser based viewer for citizens to the data generated in the public health system.

Another line of action of the health IT strategic plan, related with the development of the CPS, was the diffusion of digital certificates among citizens in order to interact with the health system. Following the regulations about the protection of personal data (DataProtectionAct 1999; DataProtectionDecree 2007), CPS management decided that citizens would use their personal identification code[5] and a digital certificate to access the CPS. Data transfer would be (https) encrypted with 128-bit

---

[3] Carpeta Personal de Salut means Personal Health Folder.

[4] The HealthITPlan (2008) was part of the Health Plan for the period 2006–2010, which for the first time defined IT as a strategic lever of the health system. The HealthITPlan (2012) defined the project of the CPS as part of the strategic line "Facilitate and orient the access of citizens to information and service for self-care".

[5] The DoH gives each citizen of Catalonia an individual health card which contains data fields such as personal identification code (which corresponds to the code of the insured citizen), the name and surname, the social security affiliation number, type of insured (level of coverage), the expiration data. All these data fields are coded in a magnetic stripe.

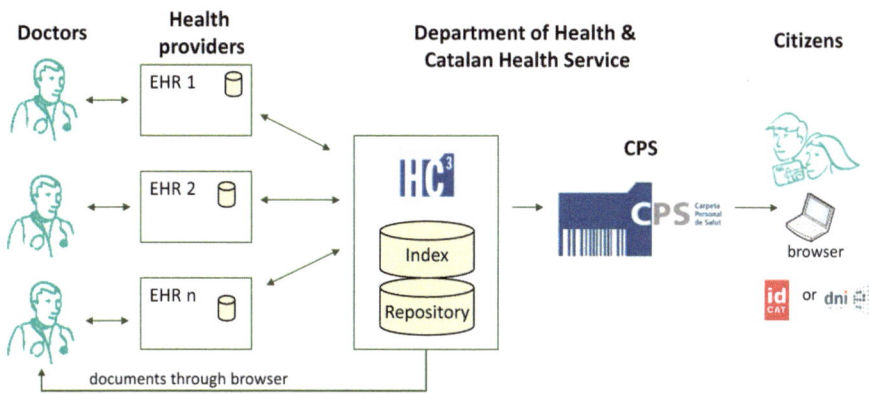

Fig. 11.2   Architecture showing the relation between HC3 and CPS

key. There would be two types of valid digital certificates: the one issued by the Catalan Certification Agency (CATCert[6]) called idCat, and the one embedded in the National Identity Number (DNI electronico). To obtain the first type of digital certificate citizens would have to first fill an online form, next they would have to physically visit a registration agency where their identity would be checked and they would be given a password. Citizens later would use that password to download the digital certificate from the website of the CATCert. In short there would be three actors involved in the registration process: the citizen, the CATCert which would act as a Certificate Authority, and the organization which would accredit the identity of the citizen. During authentication, CPS would check in the database of insured citizens (of the CatSalut) that the personal identification code corresponded with the identity number contained in the digital certificate, and that the citizen had the right to access data.

In 2009, the sponsors of the CPS run a first pilot with a group of 90 citizens working in the health sector of Calella aiming to test the usability, the adequacy of the data, and identify new requirements. The users were employees of the City Council of Calella and of the main health provider operating in the health sector.[7] Users assessed the CPS satisfactorily: 97% of users evaluated the CPS as something useful or very useful, with 73% of them evaluating the navigation through the CPS as good or very good, and 92% of the users evaluating the language used as appropriate or very appropriate (Saigí et al. 2012). After this pilot, CPS management decided to roll out the CPS on July 2010 with the 21,000 citizens of the health sector of Calella. This release of the CPS included two main types of services: health data from HC3 (e.g. diagnosis, vaccines, and reports such as ambulatory care, hospital

---

[6] The CATCert is a governmental agency that was set up in 2002 in order to implement and rollout the digital signature in all the Catalan governmental institutions and provide services to those organizations ensuring that the electronic transactions fulfill the legal guarantees.

[7] The name of the provider is the Corporació de Salut del Maresme i la Selva (http://www.salutms.cat).

emergencies, and hospital admission) and access to some administrative services that the Catalan Government already offered (e.g. http://web.gencat.cat/en/tramits/index.html).

The rollout involved the cooperation and engagement of several local actors in the territory who were close to citizens: the health provider operating in that health sector; the city council that was in charge of communicating to the public; and other local organizations (one of which issued the digital certificates). The leader of CPS qualified such a rollout strategy as "low profile": "we started with this very limited concept of a personal health folder in the sense that it was a collection of documents that were already in the shared electronic medical record [HC3]". The sponsor considered that it was important to adopt a strategy that minimized conflict with professionals since the CPS entailed profound changes in the role and relationships between doctors and patients, and between doctors themselves.

Following this territorial rollout strategy, the CPS was extended to two additional health sectors where the same health provider operated. The CPS was also extended to 1,500 blood donors (from throughout Catalonia). Yet by that time the usage of CPS was still marginal; on December 2011, 88,727 citizens had access to the CPS, but only 365 had accessed it 1,282 times (CatSalutReport 2011).

11.4.2 Phase 2: Opening the CPS (2012–2013)

The health IT strategic plan for the period 2012–2015 (HealthITPlan 2012)[8] defined an strategic line "Deploy a multichannel network to communicate and interact with citizens" involving seven concrete actions on the CPS: (1) boost an strategy that promotes citizens self-care; (2) extend the CPS to all the citizens of Catalonia; (3) increase the functionalities of the CPS; (4) include the medication plan into the CPS; (5) include value-added services into the CPS; (6) promote the access to the CPS through different channels; and (7) promote the diffusion of digital certificates among citizens.

In accordance with these actions, by early 2012 the CPS was extended to other health sectors in Catalonia where other providers operated. Secondly, they built a mobile web app to access the CPS. They also extended the CPS with new reports (e.g., laboratory test results and imaging reports) and new information services from other systems of the DoH (e.g. the medication plan from the electronic prescription system) (see Fig. 11.3). In March 2012, the DoH launched the web-portal Canal Salut,[9] which provided information to citizens in order to promote healthy lifestyles, strengthen the ability of citizens to make informed decisions about their own health

---

[8] While HealthITPlan (2008) putted the focus on the need to build technical/hard infrastructure, HealthITPlan (2012) changed the focus an emphasized the need for service infrastructure. This change in focus was aligned with two lines of action of the HealthPlan (2011): line of action 2 "A system that is more focused on chronic patients", and line of action 9 "Sharing information, transparency, and assessment".

[9] Canal Salut means Health Channel, http://canalsalut.gencat.cat

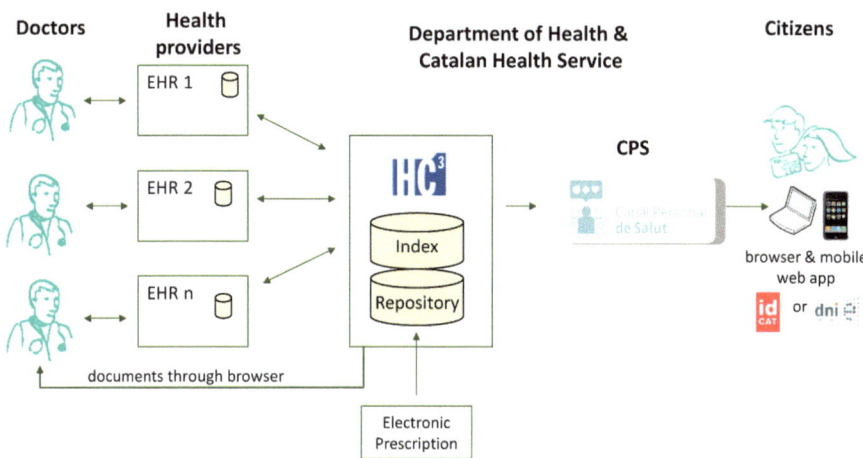

Fig. 11.3 Extension of the CPS architecture

care, and improve citizens' access to health services, among others. By the end of 2012,[10] the DoH announced the deployment of CPS to everyone in Catalonia (about seven million people), and the name of the CPS was changed from Carpeta Personal de Salut (Personal Health Folder) to Canal Personal de Salut (Personal Health Channel) to emphasize the idea of interactivity and communication between patients and professionals.

Until then the CPS had mainly worked as a viewer of the HC3. This was a constraint since the CPS mainly offered content (general reports and health records) to patients but not services. In addressing this constraint, by mid-2012 the CPS managers decided to open CPS to third-party services that were not owned by the DoH. With this opening strategy CPS management aimed to leverage on the installed base of services of third-parties (e.g. health providers, software vendors, pharmaceuticals) and on the latter's capacity to keep innovating on new services. Furthermore, this opening strategy added value to the CPS without requiring the DoH to increase the budget of the CPS. To implement this strategy, TICSalut[11] set up an interoperability framework that defined the conditions for third-party devices, systems and services to interoperate with CPS (InteropFramework 2012). Companies that wanted patients to access their services through CPS would have to fulfil certain conditions in order to obtain the interoperability recognition. Accordingly, under this interoperability framework, the ownership and control of the services of the CPS started to separate. The DoH would gave up the ownership of the new services

---

[10] By that time, there was the appointment of a new coordinator of Health IT at the DoH who also became the leader of the CPS.

[11] TICSalut is an agency, constituted in 2006, within the DoH that works to promote the development and use of IT in the field of health, acts as an observatory for new trends, innovation and monitoring of emerging initiatives and provides services for the standardization and accreditation of products.

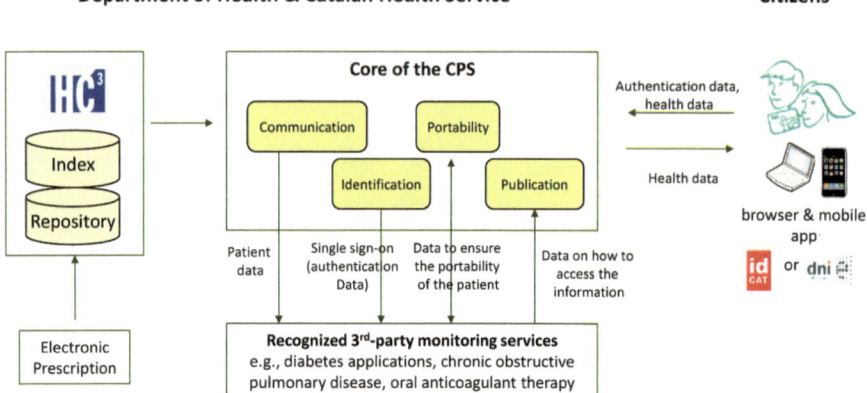

Fig. 11.4 Extension of the CPS to incorporate the interoperability framework

but not their control (e.g., the DoH had the right to decide which new services would be offered).

In the case of systems and services, the interoperability framework consisted of four profiles (see Fig. 11.4): identification (in order to guarantee a single sign-on from the citizen for the CPS and the third-party service); communication (so that third-party services can access relevant patient information stored in HC3); publication (the third-party publishes a set of services that citizens will see in CPS; patients can access those services directly by means of a service embedded in CPS or an URL); and portability (a set of conditions to ensure that personal health data stored by the third-party service can be moved, if the citizen desires, to other third-party services). Each of these profiles defined a set of messages that CPS and the third-party services should exchange. With the deployment of the interoperability framework, the DoH would not develop new services but would partner with those third-party providers who offer their services through CPS. The DoH would control the content and the application of the interoperability framework.

The DoH started by targeting firms providing services for monitoring diabetes (in 2012), and the management of chronic obstructive pulmonary disease and oral anticoagulant therapy (in 2013). In the case of the services for monitoring diabetes, CPS management exploited the fact that the ICS was making a tender for the supply of test strips for the following years.[12] The DoH asked the ICS to include compliance with the interoperability framework as a bid condition. From that moment, the interoperability framework became an obligatory passage point for providers of devices for the treatment of diabetes who wanted to access the public health system. These services for tele-monitoring diabetes provided three main types of functionalities: patients recording and tracking of blood glucose readings and other informa-

---

[12]The providers of test strips – usually pharmaceutical companies such as Sanofi, Roche – also provide the other devices for the treatment and control of the disease – e.g. glucometers, insulin pens, and the software application for patient to self-monitor their disease.

tion, health professionals monitoring the status of patients, and information exchange between patients and health professionals. Yet the fact that these services could be accessed through the CPS did not add additional value because the CPS was merely an additional channel to access those monitoring applications. Moreover, neither health professionals nor patients received any incentive to go through the CPS. So the fact that these three types of services got the interoperability recognition, did not mean that patients and health professional would immediately abandon their direct access to those services in favor of the CPS.

For providers of those services it was a way to stay close to the DoH. Moreover, CPS management realized that the providers would not easily update their services to new releases of the CPS' APIs. One of those providers argued that they had already done an effort to adapt their application to the CPS for the first time, but they could not keep the pace of updates required by the CPS because decisions about service changes were not made in the local office in Catalonia, but in the headquarters office which was abroad. In short, the CPS was not able to revert the existing practices of the health professionals, diabetes patients, and providers of diabetes monitoring services, and the relationships between health professionals and those providers.

11.4.3 Phase 3: Scaling the CPS (2014–2015)

By mid-2013 the adoption level of the CPS was still unsatisfactory – e.g., until May 2013 only 4,664 citizens had accessed the CPS since its inception; on average there were less than 1,000 accesses per month; reports and diagnoses were the top searched information services (Gallego 2013). CPS management considered that its low rate of adoption and use was due to the lack of use of digital certificates among citizens and the associated registration and authentication processes. These processes were cumbersome and complicated for citizens, particularly, taking into account that some health providers (e.g., ICS) already offered online services for patients (e.g., booking appointments) with much simpler authentication procedures (e.g., code of the citizen's health card). However, the CPS' registration and authentication processes had been implemented following the recommendations of the Catalan Data Protection Authority (APDCat[13]) in 2009. By mid-2012 CPS management asked again the APDCat about the need for a digital certificate. This time the APDCat reinterpreted the need for a digital certificate and suggested that a username and password were sufficient (ElectronicDataAccess 2012). So, removing the digital certificate would simplify the registration and authentication processes and this in turn, would make the CPS more attractive for citizens.

---

[13] The APDCat was created in 2002, and its Statute regulated in 2003. It is an autonomous and independent authority whose competences in the public sector data are registration, control, inspection, sanction and resolution, and also the adoption of proposals and instructions. http://www.apd.cat/en

The changes to the registration and authentication processes were as follows. First, registration would take place at the primary care center of the citizen, where she would have to physically visit to request the access to the CPS. At the primary care center they would check the identity of the citizen through national identify number and the identification code of individual health card, and the citizen would sign an authorization form. Then the citizen would receive an SMS with a PIN code that she would use in the registration process and an email with a link to complete the registration process. In this last step of the registration process, the citizen would choose an 8-digit password. The access to the CPS would take place through the personal identification code plus the national identity number plus the 8-digit password (so there was no need for a digital certificate). Second, citizens' usernames and passwords would be managed by the CatSalut; the CATCert would not be involved in the registration and authentication process.

On October 2014, a pilot was launched in 33 primary care areas. As a result of the positive outcomes of the pilot,[14] on May 2015 they started the deployment of the new registration and authentication processes to the rest of primary care areas of Catalonia. On August 2015 more than 25,000 citizens had accessed the CPS (Solans 2015).

In parallel, the CPS was renamed again from Canal Personal de Salut (Personal Health Channel) to Cat@Salut La Meva Salut (Cat@Salut My Health). This change aimed to increase the involvement of citizens and strengthen its diffusion, use and awareness. Accordingly, the user interface of the CPS was also adapted so that the access to data was simpler and more intuitive.

Within the context of the HealthITPlan (2012) the DoH created in 2013 a working group that defined a non-face to face care model for the Catalan health system (NonF2FCareModel 2014). The model, which put the CPS at its core, included the functional requirements, the agents and the interactions among agents, the contents, and the communication channels. The goal was to transform the CPS into a dynamic and proactive environment rather than a passive one. This required integrating non-face to face care into the existing clinical working stations, and giving recognition to the non-face to face activity of health professionals as part of their duties. One of the services defined by the non-face to face care model was eConsultation (a non-face-to-face, secure consultation service between citizens and health professionals). With eConsultation, citizens can send (through the CPS) at any time a request to the health professional (doctor or nurse), receive email notifications when the professional responds the request, check the response at the CPS, and see a record of all the queries. This service is integrated with the clinical workstation of professionals. This service has been integrated into the CPS and is being piloted at nine primary care centers of Barcelona, which are operated by three health providers[15] running the eCAP workstation, from July 2015 to October 2015. Moreover, three additional services of the ICS got the interoperability recognition (e.g., online booking appointment, change of doctor, international vaccination).

---

[14] Monthly accesses more than tripled (Solans 2015).

[15] The three health providers are ICS, PAMEM and CAPSE.

On February 2014, the TICSalut, commissioned by the DoH and the Department of Social Welfare and Family, collaborated with the mHealth Competence Center of the Mobile World Capital Barcelona[16] in the development of the Mobility Master Plan for Health (mHealthPlan 2015). The goal of the mHealthPlan (2015), which the DoH approved on February 2015, was to boost the mobility of health and social services as a lever to improve the health and welfare of people and contribute to the sustainability of the system. The mHealthPlan (2015) identified the lines of action and projects of the HealthPlan (HealthPlan 2011) and the non-face to face care model (NonF2FCareModel 2014) that could incorporate mobility.

As part of the implementation of the mHealthPlan (2015), the TICSalut worked on a health apps marketplace[17] that would match the demand (the public health system, patients and rest of citizens, social and health professionals) and supply (health and social care providers, IT vendors, pharmaceutical companies, insurance companies, and medical equipment vendors) of health and social services. A core component of the marketplace would be the accreditation process which aimed at generating trustworthy apps through a quality certificate. The accreditation process assesses four main aspects of apps: (1) design and usability (assessment of the user experience); (2) content and functionality (assessment of the quality and utility of content); (3) confidentiality and security of data (assessment of the management and processing of data); and (4) technological requirements (assessment of the reliability and adaptability requirements).

The accreditation process comprises six steps: (1) an app developer requests a accreditation for an app; (2) the developer does a self-assessment of the app; (3) if the app meets a minimum criteria then the developer can ask to provisionally include it in the marketplace (with the status "pending accreditation"); (4) an accreditation committee does a complete and detailed assessment of the app; (5) if the app passes this assessment it gets the quality certificate; and (6) the app is finally published in the marketplace as accredited; the marketplace acts as a portal with information about health apps accredited and redirects users to the corresponding Android and/or iOS market in order to download the app.

Initially they conceived three main types of apps to be prescribed by health and social care professionals: core apps (public-owned apps that exchange data with existing systems of the DoH); non-core apps having the exchange capacity (publicly or privately owned apps that exchange data with the CPS); and non-core apps not having the exchange capacity (privately owned apps that do not exchange data with the CPS).

From mid-2015 TICSalut started working on the design of another core architectural component of the marketplace: the Digital Health Platform (see Fig. 11.5).

---

[16] The mission of the mHealth Competence Center is to promote the improvement of the welfare and health of citizens by personalizing services based on mobile technology. The director of the mHealth Competence Center is the former executive president of TICSalut.

[17] By the end of 2013 the TICSalut started conceptualizing a marketplace of health apps with different degrees of certification and validation where patients could find apps recommended by doctors (RepTICSalut 2013).

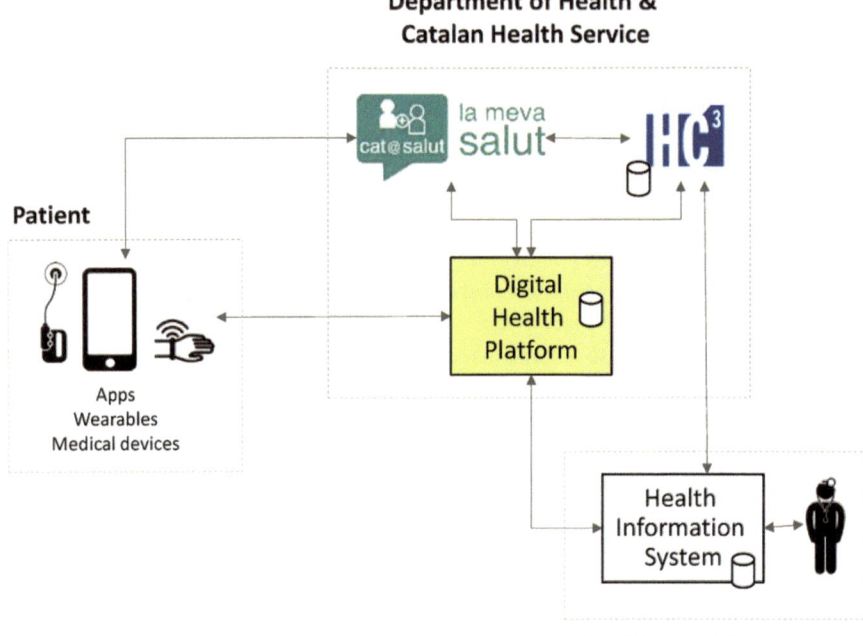

Fig. 11.5 Relationship between the Digital Health Platform and other components

Those apps (and later wearables and medical devices) that are accredited will be allowed to store and/or retrieve information from the Digital Health Platform. So the Digital Health Platform will act as a repository of patient-generated health data and in turn, it be interoperable with the CPS, HC3 and/or health information systems of health providers. Patients will access the content of the Digital Health Platform through the CPS. In other words, the Digital Health Platform will give the public health system access to health data generated by patients outside the public health system.

11.5 Analysis and Discussion

Our account has shown how the CPS was built on an installed base. It started as a web-browser viewer of a subset of citizens' health data stored in the systems of the public health system, and has gradually turned into an information infrastructure as new relations with other systems, services, actors, regulations, practices, and so on, have been established. Table 11.3 summarizes the evolution of the CPS according to several dimensions (goal, users, services, authentication mode, access mode, regulations) for each of the three phases.

Table 11.3 Evolution of the Catalan public patient portal

	Phase 1: genesis and Pilot of the CPS (2008–2011)	Phase 2: opening the CPS (2012–2013)	Phase 3: scaling the CPS (2014–2015)
Name	*Carpeta Personal de Salut* (Personal Health Folder)	*Canal Personal de Salut* (Personal Health Channel)	*Cat@Salut La Meva Salut* (Cat@Salut My Health)
Goal	View health data	Promote communication between patient and professional	Promote e-health services around the mobile
Users	Pilot in Calella (21,000 citizens) with the only health provider operating in that town. Afterwards it was extended to nearby towns (e.g. Malgrat de Mar, Lloret de Mar, Palafolls) were the same provider operated, Blood donors (1,500). There was 90,000 citizens with access	The rollout was gradually extended from 2012. It was organized into 3 phases: (1) 0.35 million citizens; (2) around 1,5million citizens; and (3) all Catalonia (7million)	All citizens insured by the CatSalut (around 7 million) Not only health but also social services

(Continued)

Table 11.3 (Continued)

	Phase 1: genesis and Pilot of the CPS (2008–2011)	Phase 2: opening the CPS (2012–2013)	Phase 3: scaling the CPS (2014–2015)
Services and functionalities	Health data from HC3: personal data, diagnoses, vaccines, and reports such as ambulatory care, hospital emergencies, and hospital admission	+	+
		Medication plan (a system which is not part of HC3)	Recognized services: Online booking appointment of the ICS (22/12/2014); Change of doctor of the ICS (22/12/2014); International vaccination of the ICS (1/12/2014)
		Promotion of health (push to citizens) through the web-portal Canal Salut	eConsultation (pilot July 2015)
	Access to the virtual procedures office to do some request with the health service	Anticipatory wills	Waiting list for the surgical processes (surgical process, status, center, data of inclusion, surgery forecast, average time at the waiting list, maximum time guaranteed by the CatSalut)
		New reports (Laboratory test results, imaging reports)	Integrated with other external sources (e.g. other regions' reports, other systems of the DoH)
		Patients' agenda/schedule at primary care	Development of the apps marketplace
		My controls (recognized tele-monitoring services and devices):	Digital health platform
		Diabetes: Emminems (Roche, 23/8/2012), MedicalGuard (Grupo Pulso, 22/6/2012), Diabetic (Sanofi, 22/6/2012)	Tracking claims and request of health certificate
		Oral anticoagulant therapy: TAOnet (Roche, 26/08/2013), G.O.T.A (Isaza Distribuciones Técnicas, 8/8/2013)	Interconnect with patients' social media platforms
		Spirometer for chronic obstructive pulmonary disease: DATOSPIR 120 i 110 (A,B,C,D) (Sibelmed, 31/5/2013); DATOSPIR 600 (D,T,F) (Sibelmed, 31/5/2013); DATOSPIR MICRO (A,B,C) (Sibelmed, 31/5/2013); DATOSPIR Touch (Easy,Diagnostic) (Sibelmed, 31/5/2013)	

Authentication	Two digital certificates: idCAT (Windows and Linux) + eDNI	+ Two digital certificates: idCAT (Windows and Linux) + eDNI	+ New authentication process: username and robust password; idCAT for Android; Pilot: biometric signature on tables (at Hospital of Campdevànol) and mobile identity (with 25 users)
Access mode	Browser (laptop, desktop)	Browser (laptop, desktop) and mobile web app	Browser (laptop, desktop) and mobile web app; wearable; medical device
Regulations and other expressive components that consolidate the CPS	Information rights and autonomy of patients; Protection of personal data; Health plan 2006–2010; Health IT strategic plan 2008–2011	Health Plan 2011–2015; Health IT Strategic Plan 2012–2015; Interoperability framework developed by TICSalut	ElectronicDataAccess (2012); NonF2FCareModel (2014); Mobility master plan for health (mHealth.cat); Accreditation process developed by TICSalut; Health plan 2016–2020; Government Agreement (25/2/2014) to create the integrated health and social care plan (SocialHealth 2014)

The underlying vision for the building of the CPS has been the idea of self-care and preventive care – i.e., that citizens become more autonomous, responsible and participative in matters concerning their own health. The realization of this vision requires reconfiguring multiple of the existing relationships and the creation of new ones. For instance, since patients will have more information about their own health, their relation with professionals, who are used to have control over the access to the patients' data, will probably change; the relationship between patient and the government is expected to become less paternalistic; the responsibilities boundaries among professionals will most likely shift; and since the CPS will become a new channel for the provision of health services, the public administration will have to reconsider the payment criteria for those services to health professionals and providers.

Accordingly, the effects of realizing this vision are multiple and complex, and beyond the control of any single actor in the health system. For the sponsors of the CPS that meant that they had to engage with indeterminacy and uncertainty, and with multiple possible alternatives. Furthermore, since many of the services could not be specified in advance, their decisions and choices had to be exploratory and adaptable. At the beginning of the project, the sponsors of the CPS took refugee into something known and safe; they decided to tie the CPS' architecture, project organization and development team, and budget to the ones of the Public Shared Electronic Medical Record (HC3). So the CPS started simple, without a big architectural blueprint and complex anticipatory design; the CPS was launched as a web-browser viewer (a module) of the HC3. Since then the CPS has gradually grown in terms of users and services.

A catalyst for that growth has been the building of specific gateways that interconnect the existing socio-technical components with new ones. For instance, the choice of authentication and registration procedures in which CPS' sponsors interpreted existing regulations in a way that maximized the security and confidentiality and by doing so, avoided opposition of professionals who were concerned about it and stimulated adoption from citizens; the interoperability framework, the app accreditation process, and the Digital Health Platform.

Those gateways have encouraged certain effects. First, the interoperability framework and the app accreditation process, for instance, have constituted the base on top of which third-parties can develop new services which add value to existing patients as well as attract new ones to the CPS. Another effect of these two gateways is the changing role of the public administration (DoH and CatSalut) in the provision of certain services. For instance, the DoH does not own those new services but accredits them; in that respect, the public administration keeps the control over the kind of services offered through the CPS. Likewise, with the building of the Digital Health Platform, they are able to leverage the potential of patient-generated health data to grow the existing infrastructure and at the same time, that opens new opportunities for both sides: app developers as well as the public health system.

Overall, this chapter suggests that in order to cope with the conditions of indeterminacy and uncertainty characterizing the building of patient-oriented information infrastructures, designs must always be incomplete, open and connectable so as to be able to respond to new possibilities.

Acknowledgements This research was funded by the program "Internacionalització de la Recerca dels grups de recerca de la URL, un programa impulsat per la Universitat Ramon Llull amb la col laboració de l'Obra Social 'la Caixa".

References

AgreementForHC3. Conveni tipus per implantar la Història Clínica Compartida a Catalunya (HCCC), Department of Health, Catalan Government. 2009.

Carrau E, Labordena MJ, González M. La Historia Clínica Compartida de Cataluña. Soc Esp Inform Salud. 2013;97:8–11.

CatSalutReport. Memòria del CatSalut 2011, Generalitat de Catalunya, Departament de Salut. 2011.

Cerdà-Calafat I, Continente-Gonzalo M, García-López C, Guanyabens-Calvet J. Carpeta personal de salud. Med Clín. 2010;134(1):63–6.

DataProtectionAct. Ley Orgánica 15/1999, de 13 de diciembre, de protección de datos de carácter personal, BOE n° 298 of December 14th 1999, Spanish Government. 1999.

DataProtectionDecree. Real Decreto 1720/2007, de 21 de diciembre, por el que se aprueba el Reglamento de desarrollo de la Ley Orgánica 15/1999, de protección de datos, BOE n° 17 of January 19th 2008, Spanish Government. 2007

ElectronicDataAccess. CNS 29/2012: Accés electrònic a dades de salut sense certificat electronic", Autoritat Catalana de Protecció de Dades, viewed 1 December 2015. 2012. http://www.apd.cat/media/dictamen/ca_461.pdf.

Gallego C. iSalut: Sessió tècnica. Pla de Salut de Catalunya 2011–15. El model d'atenció a la complexitat: Gestió Clínica del PCC i MACA, viewed 1 December 2015. 2013. http://www.uch.cat/index.php?md=documents&id=6513&lg=cat.

HealthITPlan. Pla Estratègic SITIC per a l'Àmbit de la Salut a Catalunya 2008–2011, Catalan Department of Health. 2008.

HealthITPlan. Pla Estratègic SITIC per a l'Àmbit de la Salut a Catalunya 2012–2015, Catalan Department of Health. 2012.

HealthPlan. Health plan for Catalonia 2011–2015, Generalitat de Catalunya. Department of Health. 2011, Catalan Ministry of Health, http://salutweb.gencat.cat/ca/el_departament/pla_de_salut_2011_2015/.

InformationRightsAct. Llei 21/2000, de 29 de desembre, sobre els drets d'informació concernent la salut i l'autonomia del pacient, i la documentació clínica, DOGC n° 3303 of January 11th 2001, Catalan Government. 2000.

InteropFramework. Marc d'interoperabilitat – Carpeta Personal de Salut. Oficina d'Estàndars i Interoperabilitat (OFSTI), Generalitat de Catalunya, viewed 1 December 2015. 2012. http://www.gencat.cat/salut/ticsalut/html/ca/dir3613/marcinteroperabilitatv1_6.pdf.

Marimon-Suñol S, Rovira-Barberà M, Acedo-Anta M, Nozal-Baldajos MA, Guanyabens-Calvet J. Historia Clinica Compartida en Cataluña. Med Clin. 2010;134(1):45–8.

mHealthPlan. Pla Mestre de Mobilitat (mHealth.Cat), Catalan Department of Health. 2015.

NonF2FCareModel 2014, Model d'atenció no presencial en el sistema sanitari de Catalunya 2013–16, Catalan Department of Health

PatientAutonomyAct. Ley 41/2002, de 14 de noviembre, básica reguladora de la autonomía del paciente y de derechos y obligaciones en materia de información y documentación clínica, BOE n° 274 of November 15th 2002, Spanish Government. 2002.

RepTICSalut. Report 2013, viewed 1 December 2015. 2013. http://www.ticsalut.cat/media/upload//arxius/ticSalt2013ANG.pdf.

Saigí F, Cerdà-Calafat I, Guanyabens-Calvet J, Carrau E. Los registros de salud personal: El caso de la Carpeta Personal de Salud. Gac Sanit. 2012;26(6):582–4.

SocialHealth. Agreement GOV /28/2014 of February 25th, to create the Integrated Health and Social Care Plan (PIAISS), viewed 1 December 2015. 2014. http://www.gencat.cat/salut/botss/html/ca/dir3609/doc35966.html.

Solans O. HC3 i La Meva Salut – D'Un repositori d'informació a un instrument estratègic dins del
    model d'atenció integrada centrat en les persones, viewed 1 December 2015. 2015. http://jor-
    nadestic.aificc.cat/storage/presentacions-taules/04-La-meva-salut.pdf.
Yin RK. Case study research: design and methods. Thousand Oaks: Sage; 2003.

Open Access This chapter is distributed under the terms of the Creative Commons Attribution-
NonCommercial 2.5 International License (http://creativecommons.org/licenses/by-nc/2.5/),
which permits any noncommercial use, duplication, adaptation, distribution and reproduction in
any medium or format, as long as you give appropriate credit to the original author(s) and the
source, provide a link to the Creative Commons license and indicate if changes were made.

The images or other third party material in this chapter are included in the chapter's Creative
Commons license, unless indicated otherwise in a credit line to the material. If material is not
included in the chapter's Creative Commons license and your intended use is not permitted by
statutory regulation or exceeds the permitted use, you will need to obtain permission directly from
the copyright holder.

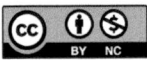

The Norwegian eHealth Platform: Development Through Cultivation Strategies and Incremental Changes

Miria Grisot, Polyxeni Vassilakopoulou, and Margunn Aanestad

12.1 Introduction

This chapter presents the approach followed for the development of the Norwegian national solution for patient-oriented eHealth services (here called HealthNorway). Our research interest is twofold: first, on understanding the initial design decisions and initial evolution in relation to the installed base of existing digital capabilities, and, second, on understanding how HealthNorway was further developed after the initial launch in relation to the long term vision of offering comprehensive and readily available health services to citizens. Drawing from the case, we identify different approaches for infrastructural development in the form of proactive cultivation strategies related to extending, complementing and creating substitutes within the installed base.

The remainder of the chapter is structured as follows: we provide first a brief overview of the Norwegian health system and its digital infrastructure; we then introduce our case and present key activities, concerns and decisions for HealthNorway

M. Grisot (✉)
Department of Informatics, University of Oslo, Postboks 1080, Blindern, 0316 Oslo, Norway
e-mail: miriag@ifi.uio.no

P. Vassilakopoulou
Department of Information Systems, University of Agder,
Postboks 422, 4604 Kristiansand, Norway

Department of Informatics, University of Oslo, Postboks 1080, Blindern, 0316 Oslo, Norway
e-mail: polyxenv@uia.no

M. Aanestad
Department of Informatics, University of Oslo, Postboks 1080, Blindern, 0316 Oslo, Norway

UIT The Arctic University of Norway, Postboks 6050, Langnes, 9037 Tromsø, Norway
e-mail: margunn@ifi.uio.no

© The Author(s) 2017
M. Aanestad et al. (eds.), *Information Infrastructures within European Health Care*, Health Informatics, DOI 10.1007/978-3-319-51020-0_12

development. Afterwards, we analyse the different approaches that were followed for relating to the installed base. We conclude by discussing our findings.

12.2 Norwegian Healthcare

12.2.1 Overview of the Norwegian Healthcare Model

Norway has a predominantly public healthcare sector, where the National Insurance Act guarantees every citizen access to healthcare services paid by the state. Inpatient hospital care is free, while there are consultation fees for physician visits and out-patient treatment, and payment for prescription drugs up to a limit. The patients have free choice of hospitals, but General Practitioners (GPs) serve as gatekeepers for referrals to hospitals or specialists. The specialist healthcare including hospitals and psychiatric care is governed by the Ministry of Health, through four regional Health Authorities established in 2002 (Region West, South-East, Middle and North). These authorities govern also the ICT investments in clinical and administrative systems within their region.

Primary healthcare is offered at the municipal level; GPs, antenatal and postnatal care, immunization and care for the sick and elderly at home or in nursing homes. The municipalities' autonomy is strong, and they make their own ICT investments. In 2008, the Coordination reform, has targeted the less than optimal collaboration between specialist and primary healthcare, primarily through regulatory and financial instruments, but also by supporting standards for electronic communication between the actors. Many physicians (specialists and GPs) run private practices and purchase ICT solutions independently. The government, through the Directorate of Health (from now on referred to as the Agency), has in the last few years taken a more pro-active role in developing national e-health solutions, such as e-prescription, a national summary care record, and web-based health services for citizens. Lately, the e-health related units of the Agency were detached from the overall organization and formed the "e-Health Directorate" which was established on 1.1.2016.

12.2.2 The Digital Infrastructure for Healthcare in Norway

In Norway all GPs offices, hospitals and nursing homes have Electronic Patient Record systems (EPRs). The communication across organizations is supported by a dedicated secure network called Norwegian Health Network (NHN). NHN was established in 2004 by the Regional Health Authorities. NHN was created by harmonizing and consolidating previous existing regional broadband networks, and by pursuing national standards for electronic communication in the health sector. Initially, NHN was used to connect hospitals and gradually it was expanded to GPs, community health centres, nursing homes and recently also pharmacies. All parties sending or receiving electronic communication have their own listing in the National Register of Electronic Addresses.

Over the years, nationally coordinated initiatives sought to shift the health sectors' communication from paper and telephone to electronic communication across the NHN. The exchange of information is currently supported by using standardized messages, for example for referrals and discharge summaries, requisitions and test results, and electronic prescriptions. It should be noted that NHN is a network dedicated to the health providers, and not intended to include communication with the patients.

In November 2012 the white paper "One citizen, One record" was issued by the Government. The strategy identified three main aims: (i) healthcare professionals shall have easy and secure access to patient-and user information; (ii) citizens shall have easy and secure access to user friendly and secure health care services online; (iii) data should be registered automatically and made available for quality improvement, monitoring, governance and research. Against this vision, a number of challenges were also identified such as under-utilized technological possibilities, many independent entities, and many systems with little integration across systems.

Method

Data were collected via three main sources: interviews with informants from the Directorate of Health and technology providers; analysis of project documents, reports, strategy and policy documents; and observations of meetings and workshops in the context of the Digital Dialogue project. Fieldwork was conducted in the period August 2013–December 2014. The data gathered were organized by constructing the event timeline, and by writing the case narrative with attention to main events and decisions taken. The concept of installed base has guided our analysis of the data and directed our focus to how existing socio-technical arrangements have influenced the development of HealthNorway.

12.3 Case Narrative

12.3.1 Phase 1: Rationale for the Development of HealthNorway and Launch

The creation of HealthNorway started with a Government mandate in the Spring of 2010. The mandate pointed to the existence of many patient-oriented initiatives and webpages related to health, both private and public, but to the lack of a national-level, comprehensive initiative. Hence, HealthNorway was initiated with the aim to provide secure digital services, quality checked information on diseases and treatments, and to help citizens perceive services as available and comprehensive (Norwegian Ministry of Health and Care Services 2012). The Norwegian Government envisioned that HealthNorway will strengthen the citizen's role in healthcare by making it easier to find and choose health providers, providing access to personal health information, and by offering services self-service and self-help.

A procurement process started in the summer of 2010 and an agreement was signed in October 2010 with a technology provider. It was made explicit that the Government required a fast pace for HealthNorway. A manager from the technology provider's side recalls: *"It was very high-speed process because the Minister of Health set a politically defined date for launch and that was the 15th of June 2011"*.

Work on the development of HealthNorway started in the autumn of 2010. At that point, in order to meet the deadline of June 2011, it was considered realistic to adopt the simplest of a number of alternative concepts presented and aim for an information oriented portal. The underlying idea was that patients/citizens should be able to find consistent and quality checked definitions of illnesses and treatments in the information pages. The realization of this concept required substantial work in gathering material from the different health service actors and agreeing on common definitions. Reaching consensus among hospitals and other competent centers in the health sector was especially difficult for certain illnesses and diseases. Furthermore, it was decided to use as main information sources material written in English which not only required translation to Norwegian but also adaptions to convey information on the specific treatments used in Norway. On top of these challenges, the information content had to be expressed in a way that would be understandable by everyone and this created the need to involve professional writers.

Technically, HealthNorway was built upon an off-the-self platform which made possible its swift launching in June 2011. The Agency kept both the ownership and the management of HealthNorway and soon after the initial launch a new organizational unit dedicated to HealthNorway was created within the Agency. One of the Agency managers explained how work was organised: *"our main job is to develop HealthNorway. Everybody works on the whole of it especially the ones working with user experience, they work not in silos but as a whole group, but our budgets are organized by projects, and we have resources allocated to these different projects, but we are still working on finding a good model where we make sure that we cannot focus just on this project but we need to see the whole system for the user, and the users want that"*.

12.3.2 Phase 2: Strategy Beyond the Initial Launch

After the launch of HealthNorway, a process started to define a new strategy toward 2017 aiming at describing the vision and action plan for further development. A manager from the technology provider's side recalls: *"then we started to look into what kind of services we think we should develop on our own, what have other countries developed, what works or doesn't work, and we tried to get as much input from patients and services as we could, so we have a road map for the next five years"*. The strategy team received input from a range of stakeholders. They organized workshops inviting participants both within and outside the Agency, from patient organizations, to health professionals from different hospitals, and professionals working with health and communication. A manager recalls: *"we tried to recruit a broad group of people, and we started out with open questions, so now we have this portal, the Minister of Health has released it, it's out there, so what should*

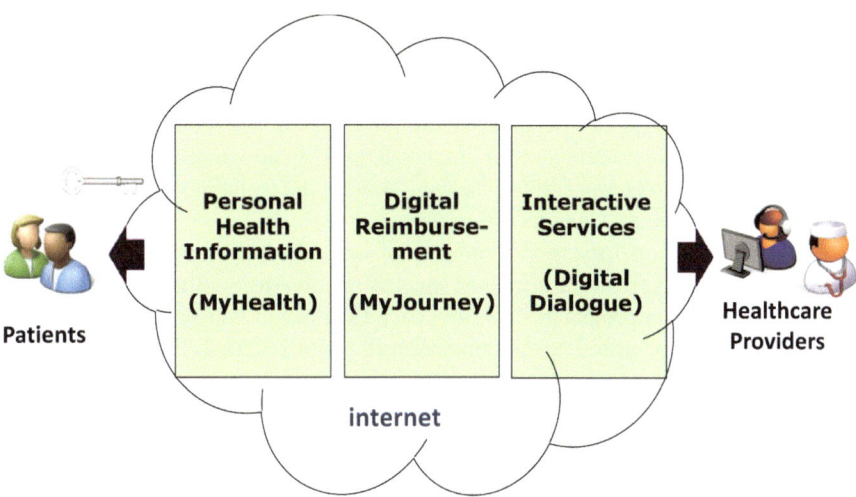

Fig. 12.1   Three priority areas for the extension of HealthNorway

we fill it with now, what do you need?". Thus, the development of the services on HealthNorway started as an open process.

During the fall of 2011, the strategy team planned the work for two main dimensions: information content and electronic services. It was agreed that the priority should be on designing new citizen-oriented services in line with the main strategic political goals to *"reinforce patient- and users- role by making the everyday experience of healthcare easier and at the same time contribute to increase quality and effectiveness of health services"* (quote from the strategy plan). The strategy was ready in February 2012, it described the services to develop and how HealthNorway will fulfil the requirements and expectations of citizens while at the same time addressing health policy objectives.

From March 2012, the strategy plan was implemented starting with a pre-study (March–June 2012) where the feasibility of three different services was assessed: My Health Information (later called My Health), My Patient Journey (for health-related reimbursable travel expenses), and secure messaging services between patients and healthcare providers (later called Digital Dialogue). The three service areas were considered as having a relatively high degree of maturity, potentially substantial benefits and acceptable implementation complexity in relation to other services outlined in the strategy plan. Figure 12.1 presents the three priority service areas, which are described in the following three subsections.

12.3.3 Access to Personal Health Information

According to the pre-study, "MyHealth Information" was a service area that would give citizens access to their personal health information. This service area was identified in the strategy for HealthNorway as well as requested by patients' and health professionals' organizations. The service aimed to offer citizens unified access to personal health information, independently of when and where information was produced (e.g. GP office visit, hospital stay, prescription). The pre-study team mapped different types of personal health information, and identified which information would be more relevant for citizens to access and would give more benefits (e.g. discharge letters, referrals, tests results). Also the team identified constrains in relation to e.g. ethical, legal, technical aspects.

The pre-study also mapped a number of ongoing local initiatives developing solutions for giving patients access to specific health information and met with key respective actors: a project at the University Hospital of North Norway (UNN) in Tromsø for online access to patient records (pilot in 2012–2013), a portal for patient – hospital communication that was already in use at Oslo University Hospital (OUH), a solution in use at Diakonhjemmet hospital in Oslo for sending electronically discharge letters to patients, a portal supporting communication between hospital, users and relatives at Sunnaas rehabilitation hospital, and a solution used by a private medical laboratory for giving on line access to laboratory test results. These were organization-based projects aimed to give patients access to specific health information. The HealthNorway team also looked at international experiences related to sharing health information with patients. A case considered interesting in the context of public healthcare was the national health portal in Denmark.

In addition to these solutions, a number of ongoing national initiatives were identified which aimed to give access to specific health information such as Summary Care Records, active prescriptions "My Prescriptions", vaccination "My Vaccines" records, and expense reports "My Expenses". These solutions had at the time of the study different levels of maturity. The Summary Care Record was planned to start piloting in September 2013, while My Prescriptions, My Vaccines, and My Expenses were already in use. These solutions provided access to information residing at national-level data repositories. In the pre-study it was decided that for the short term, MyHealth Information would include the existing services (e.g. My Prescriptions) and also the Summary Care Record for users in the pilot area. The pre-study also indicated the need to consider the prospect to incorporate local (mostly hospital-based) ongoing initiatives. Such local initiatives were the one by UNN for providing access to the patient records, and the OUH initiative that supports patient access to discharge letters.

Another key consideration of the pre-study was the fulfilment of the legal conditions for offering access to personal health information. It was decided to allow citizens themselves to "opt-in" on a voluntary basis for accessing electronically personal health information (through an individual consent). Furthermore, security level 4 would be required. This is the highest security level defined in the "Framework for Authentication and Non-Repudiation in Electronic Communication in and with the Public Sector" which is maintained by the Agency for Public Management and eGovernment (DIFI) and contains overall guidelines for public agencies when it comes to security for electronic communications.

The pre-study concluded that the services were to be developed over time and it advised to start with services most readily available, where information elements are structured and standardized.

Digital Support for Reimbursing Health Related Travel Costs

The second service area presented in the pre-study was "Patient Travel". This service aimed to simplify the administrative process of requesting reimbursements for travelling to health services. In Norway patients have the right to reimburse all expenses related to travelling "to and from" health service providers, including both primary care and specialists, and for travels to and from rehabilitation services. There are significant volumes of reimbursement claims processed annually so the simplification of the related processes can contribute to substantial cost reductions for the government and service improvement for the citizens. The process in place was paper-based and with very high daily volumes of letters to be processed manually. Every day the central office would receive about 100 kg of post and send out a similar amount. After each travel, patients would fill a paper form, attach a certification of their visit, receipts and relevant documentation, sign and post to the national center for patient travels. After the processing of their reimbursement claim, they would receive a letter with the decision in the mail, and the sum would be transferred to their bank account. This process made reimbursements slow and complex.

The aim of "Patient Travel" was to create an online electronic form for requesting reimbursement and make the service both more efficient for the public administration and more accessible to patients. The long term goal defined was to have a mechanism in place that would trigger reimbursements automatically without the need of having patients to proactively claim the funds that they are entitled to receive. The pre-study concluded that a pre-project had to be initiated in order to identify the legal, economical, functional and technical requirements for the digitization of the current process and the development of the new electronic service.

Digital Communication Between Patients and Healthcare Providers

An overall mapping of services that could make use of secure digital communications between patients and healthcare providers was included in the pre-study. The intention was to make everyday life easier for patients, and to a certain degree also for health providers. A key requirement defined was the user-friendliness of the new services and the assurance that they will be intuitive, clear and adapted to different individual needs.

The pre-study focused on asynchronous communication between patients and their health providers in cases where a patient-provider relation was already established, for instance between patients and their General Practitioner (GP). It indicated also that secure message services should initially target primary care: *"The reason is that user-initiated communications will intervene significantly in the work processes, organization and ICT support, and that this seems more complex for hospitals than for primary care. For contracted specialists it will be considered to implement certain dialogue on an equal footing with primary care"* (quote from the pre-study). The services considered were the ones judged as generic and applicable to different health provider groups and different health institutions. The study clearly stated: *"processes around appointments, e-consultation and document/form exchanges are generic processes that can be transferred from one area to another"*.

It was concluded that communication services will be developed first for supporting GP-patient interactions. Specifically, the pre-study specified the need to develop the following electronic services: renewal of prescriptions, appointment reservation and dialogue messages. In addition, the pre-study identified the need to create a storage solution for the messages of the dialogue service. If messages were to be stored only in the GPs' Electronic Patient Record systems (EPRs) it would be difficult to ensure uninterrupted accessibility by patients. Another aspect discussed in the pre study was how to make patients' messages available to GPs and what would be the role of the EPR vendors in setting up the services. The pre-study stated that it was not yet clear how HealthNorway would relate to private actors, such as vendors, but it recognized the importance to enter in dialogue with them for defining an integration strategy between HealthNorway and existing systems used by health personnel.

Different options were considered. One possibility was to link the HealthNorway with the existing private eHealth portals already used by several GP offices for their communication with patients. Some of these solutions had functionality for booking appointment, and renewing prescriptions and medical certificates. These solutions and their users – GPs, administrative personnel in the GP offices, and patients – could be a possible installed base for the new services. Technically, this would require to redirect users from HealthNorway to the private portals. It was decided not to opt for this solution and instead to link the healthcare providers' side with HealthNorway via the existing GPs' EPR systems.

One reason for this decision was that although all GP offices have an EPR system, not all of them offer electronic services to their patients (Vassilakopoulou and Grisot 2014). A participant of the pre-study from the Agency recalls: *"It was a large discussion about how could it actually be possible to use what was already in the market and how would actually turn out before the citizens. (...) how would the user experience be in that case, and how would the security be"*. It was considered best if HealthNorway created an equal right and opportunity for all regardless of where they lived, or the kind of system their doctor had. Another reason was that the future plan for HealthNorway was to provide a comprehensive interface for patients to access organized information from multiple different sources. This comprehensive interface would gradually support the creation of a timeline as organizing principle for messages, prescriptions, certificates, appointments, diagnoses, and discharge letters in one place. Thus, it was important to not redirect to third parties in order to avoid missing pieces of the overall communication history. Furthermore, redirecting to third parties would

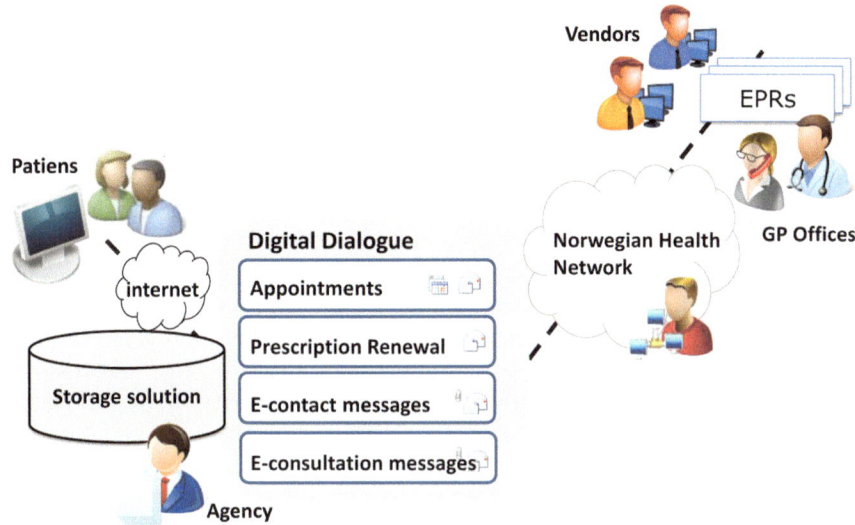

Fig. 12.2 Digital communication between patients and GP offices

harm the uniformity of the user experience and would create complications in security handling.

The decision to link the healthcare providers' side with the patients via the existing GPs' EPRs created the need to work with the EPR vendors and enroll them in the project. However, it was not certain that all EPR vendors would be willing to participate. Some were small vendors who provided EPR systems to GPs but not patient portals. One pre-study participant recalls that for them this was a "*fantastic opportunity to join, to hop on the boat*". But other vendors had their own patient portal and questioned "*how should we earn money in this market, because what's happening now is that we have our patient portal, with other services that you say that you want to develop we have them in place already, it's not big, we have them spread all over, but now you want us to just blend in with the others and that you just take over the portal side*". It was realized that having to rely on EPR vendors' collaboration was a major risk but it was decided that the expected benefits justified the risks. Figure 12.2 presents the overall arrangement decided for the digital communication between patients and GP offices.

12.3.4 Phase 3: Mature Services and Further Development Through Alliances

In August 2013, the secure service MyHealth was launched. By logging-in citizens could access the following main services: My Expenses, My GP, and My Prescriptions. Additionally, a number of other simpler services were offered such as electronic forms for ordering the European health insurance card and submitting notifications of experienced drug side effects. The highest security level for patient authentication was ensured using three alternative and already existing eID solutions: BankID (the Norwegian Banking Sector's common digital authentication and online signing solution), Buypass (jointly owned by Norway Post and Norwegian Lottery) and Commfides (a private solution). At a later point, other functionalities were added, for instance a service called "About me" where citizens could access their personal and contact information from the central National Registry and the GP Registry.

In November 2013, access to the Summary Care Record was added to MyHealth for the inhabitants of the pilot area. This service was the result of a project run by the Agency with the aim to support health personnel in emergency situations with access to patients' core medical information. The Summary Care Record contains key patient health information entered by GP/attending physician, and it retrieves prescription history, and information from national registries (e.g. the history of admissions and hospitalizations in the specialist health service is retrieved from the Norwegian Patient Registry (data from 2008)). In MyHealth, citizens can access the record, see the access log, register new information such as primary contact person, and disease history (structured selections), or they may opt out of the record entirely.

During autumn 2013 and the first semester of 2014, HealthNorway was redesigned, and in June 2014 relaunched with a new interface supporting mobile use. It was also migrated to a new version of the underlying technical platform, with a new search engine. This was important for improving usability and also, for ensuring the long-term evolvability of the platform.

In the same period, two local initiatives aiming for patient-oriented services started. Both initiatives were aligned with two priority areas of HealthNorway – providing personal health information and providing interactive services between patients and health providers – and contributed to its further development.

The first initiative was taken by UNN (University Hospital of North Norway in Tromsø) that decided to offer patients access to their hospital records. A survey revealed that most patients requesting copies of their hospital records would like to have them electronically. A project to develop a "proof of concept" solution for online access to patient records was launched in March 2012. The project was managed and financed by UNN and was implemented in close collaboration with the software company that provides the EPR for hospitals in the North Region. The EPR provider developed a solution for extracting data from medical records based on the specifications provided by UNN and also, based on the national recommendations provided by the Agency. From March 2014, the North Regional Health Authority took over the project. The online record access service was tested with 500 end-users and soon after testing it was made available to all residents of North Norway (in December 2015). The new electronic service allows patients to electronically retrieve health record documents from public hospitals in North Norway. Since 2015, the service can be accessed by patients through the secure HealthNorway interface.

The second initiative was a project initiated by the West Regional Health Authority who wanted to facilitate message exchanges between hospitals and patients. This was motivated by the need to reduce the number of appointment "no-shows" improving the utilization of available resources. In 2012 there were 82,000 missed scheduled appointments in the Western Region resulting in a significant waste of resources. In September 2013, the Agency endorsed the initiative and started a project to provide electronic support for the communication between patients and hospitals aiming for better coordination between the two parties. The project delivered a new electronic service for patients that have appointments at hospitals in the Western Region. These patients can have an overview of their appointments, confirm their attendance and send messages to the hospital (e.g. for changing the appointment time or even deciding to cancel the appointment altogether). Additionally, patients can check the status of their referrals for specialist services within the hospitals in the Region. For each referral they can check when it was received by the hospital, if it is still being processed or if a time slot has already been allocated to the. This service was offered in HealthNorway in 2015. By endorsing and including the two regional initiatives, HealthNorway is gradually becoming a universal interface to patient oriented electronic services in Norway.

In 2014 the Agency collaborated with the Norwegian National ICT (NICT) which is the interest body for information and communication technologies in the specialist healthcare sector formed by the four Regional Health Authorities. The collaboration aimed to the identification of citizens' needs for digital services in specialized care. The objective was to obtain insights for further developing HealthNorway and making it an entry point for both primary and specialized digital health services. The result was an extensive mapping and analysis of users' needs involving health personnel, citizens and management bodies of the health regions. The analysis ended up with the identification of 11 priority service areas (for example, services for supporting hospital appointment booking including preparation and follow-up after visits, services for providing an overview of visited health providers). This work informed the formulation of a strategy for digital specialist health services for citizens up to 2020, and led to the formation of a specific project on digital citizen services for the specialist sector (named the DIS) which started in January 2015. The project is expected to launch new electronic services in 2017.

In Fig. 12.3, we provide an overview of key milestones in the evolution of HealthNorway. Additionally, in Fig. 12.4, we present the time series of users per month from July 2011(right after the portal launch) till August 2016. HealthNorway managed to attract users' interest over the years and the monthly number of users is now about 1,4 million (the total population of Norway is approximately 5 million).

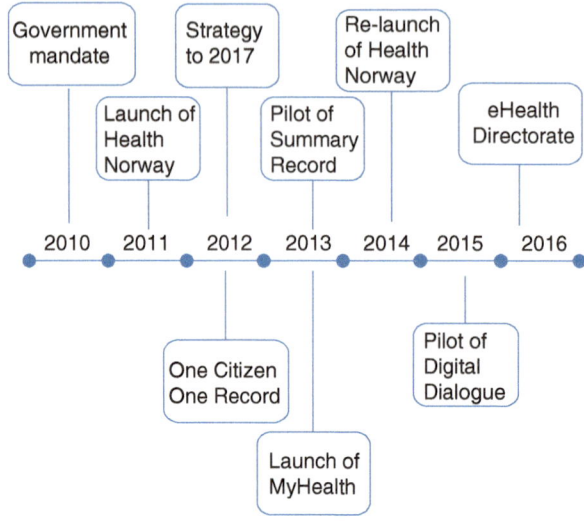

Fig. 12.3 Key milestones in the evolution of HealthNorway

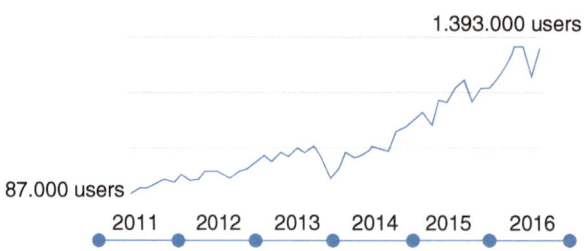

Fig. 12.4 Users per month from HealthNorway launch till Aug 2016

12.4 Analysis

In the paragraphs that follow we analyse how the installed base influenced the evolution of the portal, and how designers have engaged in "cultivation" strategies (Dahlbom and Mathiassen 1993; Ciborra 1997; Ciborra and Hanseth 1998). The installed base consists of various existing information systems, work and information practices, legal frameworks, standards and institutional conventions which relate to patient-oriented electronic health services. When faced with the installed base, the team building HealthNorway took different strategic decisions on what to "grow" in the new eHealth solution and what to redesign and substitute. This process stretches in time. The development of HealthNorway is not an "one-off" effort but entails a long lasting process of continuous launching of new services and further refinements. Thus, HealthNorway's services, contents and architecture were not fully specified and designed beforehand, but gradually grew by taking into account the overall government aims for patient oriented electronic services, the desires of the prospective users (citizens and healthcare providers) and the opportunities and limitations of the healthcare milieu. This process developed according to different reasons as for instance the qualities (e.g. scalability) and levels of maturity of existing components.

The strategy after the initial launch was to grow by adding relevant electronic services. Specifically, three service areas were identified and prioritized: (i) access to personal health information, (ii) travel reimbursements, (iii) digital dialogue with health practitioners. The Agency approached the design of these new services first by mapping existing technologies and information practices, and making sense of the existing institutional arrangements. In our analysis we interpret the ways the three service area were grown, as the enactment of strategies to deal with different aspects of the installed base.

In the case of access to personal health information, My Health, the pre-project team mapped a set of already existing projects, some of which had already implemented solutions on national level for giving access to selected personal health information, and were accessible via various health providers' websites. For instance, ePrescription was rolled out on a national scale and citizens could see their active and old prescriptions. On a different website, it was possible to log-in and change GP. The approach here was to include in HealthNorway services that were already developed in projects run previously by the Agency itself or by other public health organizations. In addition, the strategy was to create an area – My Health - where types of access to personal health information could be easily added, and which would work as central access point for citizens. Following this strategy, after the launch, My Health was gradually enriched by offering even services which were not yet nationally scaled and were only offered to citizens in specific geographical areas. Thus, the Agency developed My Health by including existing services which acted as a strong installed base to build on. This approach allowed reaping benefits in the short term. Indeed, this service area was launched relatively swiftly and made available in August 2013. The Agency followed the more long-term strategy to gradually complement the installed base of existing services by adding new services according to the long-term visions of offering access to comprehensive personal health information.

In the case of "Patient Travel" the aim was to simplify the administrative process of requesting reimbursements for travelling to health services. In this case the installed base consisted of existing work, communication and information practices and of a paper-based system (citizens sending forms to the reimbursement office). In this case, the Agency decided for a digitization of the existing arrangement, adding brand new digital capabilities to the installed base that could serve as substitutes the traditional paper-based capabilities with the aim to eventually phase them out. The core idea was that an online electronic form would be made available for citizens requesting reimbursement to facilitate the transition from purely paper-based processes to digital supported ones. Digitization processes are seldom straightforward transpositions of pre-existing non-digital arrangements. The participants in the pre-study were aware of the possible complications and they defined as a next step the analysis of the legal, economical, functional and technical requirements. Indeed, this service area is the least developed today (January 2016). The digitization necessitated changes in the corresponding regulations that were adopted by the

Norwegian Parliament in June 2015. These changes included the legal ratification of electronic claims submission for the patients that choose to do so, a new provision that stipulated that patients do not have to provide travel evidence as this would be retrieved from the registries and a new rule for covering a standard mileage allowance instead of the cost of cheapest scheduled public transport. It is envisaged that the electronic service will be made available in HealthNorway in 2016.

In the case of secure digital communications between patients and healthcare providers the task was to design and create a novel service, which would complement other existing modes of communicating such as visits and phone conversations. In this scenario, the team had different options for the development of the service. The team examined existing web-based services that some GP offices already offered, for instance for requesting appointments or renewing prescriptions. However, this base was considered weak because it was heterogeneous (many different and diverse websites), not secure enough (not all private eHealth portals in the market had implemented the security level required by law), and the user experience was evaluated as becoming too complicated and fragmented in a scenario where the national portal would redirect to the each GP's own page. Alternatively, the approach adopted was to work with the installed base of EPRs in use in the GP offices (all GP offices in Norway have an EPR system), and extend them to support the dialogue service. In this case the installed base included also the capabilities and knowledge of EPR vendors about GP office practices. However, this entailed a complex coordination effort. Indeed, the development of this service proved challenging and it necessitated the development of a sensitivity to the constraints and singularities of all the actors enrolled and the emerging interdependencies (Grisot and Vassilakopoulou 2015). As of early 2016, the new communication services are being piloted and it is expected that they will be fully launched soon.

Overall, the analysis of how the installed base has influenced the evolution of HealthNorway in the three different service area, show that the Agency engaged in different ways with the existing installed base, by complementing, creating substitutions, and expanding it. Overall, the analysis shows some key characteristics of cultivation strategy. First, in building HealthNorway, the Agency has deliberately engaged with the existing technology and institutional arrangements in place, and has built alliances for bringing together the efforts of distributed actors. Second, HealthNorway has expanded by orientating towards the satisfaction of concrete needs in order to motivate prospective users to adopt the new services. Third, overall changes have been incremental, exploratory and gradually intervening on various level (architecture design, user experience, technical platform) while keeping a coherent vision.

12.5   Discussion and Conclusion

In this chapter, we explored the different approaches employed for advancing the development of the Norwegian patient oriented healthcare portal (HealthNorway) that was initially launched with a limited functionality. The aim for HealthNorway is to eventually become a single, national point for patient oriented electronic health services. This aim created the need to engage with the installed base in a variety of ways and with different purposes.

We identified that the overall strategy employed entailed starting with concrete needs, capitalizing on what is already in place and proceeding in an incremental and exploratory way. This seems to be a prudent strategy. Prior information infrastructures' literature has indicated that the successful development of information infrastructures such as the Internet, mobile phone platforms and healthcare-specific arrangements has been achieved by following similar strategies (Hanseth and Lyytinen 2010; Aanestad and Jensen 2011; Aanestad and Hanseth 2002). Our findings are specific to processes for advancing the development of infrastructures that are already in place, nevertheless, they are congruent with recent findings by Grisot et al. (2014) that identified three different types of infrastructure innovation: in, of, on infrastructures. Innovations of infrastructures are about implementations of totally new infrastructures, innovations in infrastructures concern replacements/modifications of an infrastructure's existing components without changing the architecture and innovation on infrastructures concern additions of new components on top of what exists. Similarly, in our case, complementing the installed base entails finding ways to realize some of its latent potential by embracing capabilities already developed by others and linking to them. This is an approach that can yield benefits in the short term. Creating substitutes within the installed base entails creating new working arrangements and this involves encountering and handling sociotechnical complexity. Hence, this approach requires the dedication of efforts for a considerable length of time. Finally, extending the installed base entails complex coordination and enrolling efforts for the multiple actors that control distributed information infrastructure resources.

Acknowledgments This research was part of the Responsive Architectures for Innovation in Collaborative Healthcare Services (REACH) project, funded by Norwegian Research Council, VERDIKT program (project nr. 213143). We are grateful to the members of the team working on Helsenorge.no who participated in the study.

References

Aanestad M, Hanseth O. Growing networks: detours, stunts and spillovers. In: Cooperative systems design. A challenge of the mobility age, Proceedings of the Fifth International Conference on the Design of Cooperative Systems (COOP 2002), Saint Raphaël, France, 4–7 June 2002. Amsterdam: IOS Press; 2002. p. 38–49.

Aanestad M, Jensen TB. Building nation-wide information infrastructures in healthcare through modular implementation strategies. J Strateg Inf Syst. 2011;20:161–76.

Ciborra C. De profundis? Deconstructing the concept of strategic alignment. Scand J Inf Syst. 1997;9:2.

Ciborra C, Hanseth O. Toward a contingency view of infrastructure and knowledge: an exploratory study. Proceedings of the International Conference on Information Systems, Helsinki, Finland, December 13–16. Association for Information Systems. 1998.

Dahlbom B, Mathiassen L. Computers in context: the philosophy and practice of systems design. Cambridge, MA: Blackwell Publishers; 1993.

Grisot M, Vassilakopoulou P. The work of infrastructuring: a study of a National eHealth Project. ECSCW 2015: Proceedings of the 14th European Conference on Computer Supported Cooperative Work, 19–23 September 2015, Oslo, Norway. Springer; 2015.

Grisot M, Hanseth O, Thorseng A. Innovation of, in, on infrastructures: articulating the role of architecture in information infrastructure evolution. J Assoc Inf Syst. 2014;15:197–219.

Hanseth O, Lyytinen K. Design theory for dynamic complexity in information infrastructures: the case of building internet. J Inf Technol. 2010;25:1–19.

Norwegian Ministry Of Health And Care Services. Stortingsmelding nr. 9: Én innbygger – én journal. Digitale tjenester i helse- og omsorgssektoren. 2012.

Vassilakopoulou P, Grisot M. Infrastructures for patient-centeredness: connecting novel and existing components to serve strategic agendas for change. European Conference on Information Systems – ECIS 2014. Tel Aviv; 2014.

Open Access This chapter is distributed under the terms of the Creative Commons Attribution-NonCommercial 2.5 International License (http://creativecommons.org/licenses/by-nc/2.5/), which permits any noncommercial use, duplication, adaptation, distribution and reproduction in any medium or format, as long as you give appropriate credit to the original author(s) and the source, provide a link to the Creative Commons license and indicate if changes were made.

The images or other third party material in this chapter are included in the chapter's Creative Commons license, unless indicated otherwise in a credit line to the material. If material is not included in the chapter's Creative Commons license and your intended use is not permitted by statutory regulation or exceeds the permitted use, you will need to obtain permission directly from the copyright holder.

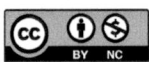

Building National Healthcare Infrastructure: The Case of the Danish e-Health Portal

13

Tina Blegind Jensen and Anne Asmyr Thorseng

13.1 Introduction

Sundhed.dk facilitates patient-oriented digital services which provide access to and information about the Danish healthcare services. Since its launch in 2003, sundhed.dk provides several functionalities such as quality assured health information, access to medical records and medication, and an overview of the Danish healthcare system. Sundhed.dk creates linkages between existing data sources, opens up data sets to new user groups, and facilitates communication between healthcare providers and citizens. The portal also ensures further development not only by providing a secure infrastructure, search optimization, and user interfaces, but also by supporting the development of new services.

Sundhed.dk has earned good reputation and high standing in the healthcare sector internationally. Health authorities from other countries, that wish to build similar solutions, have approached sundhed.dk for advice and best practice (Sundhed.dk 2014a). However, the positive reputation and high level of maturity of sundhed.dk has not been established overnight. Thus the assumption by other countries of simply copying the code, the user interface, and the technical infrastructure is far too simplistic if they wish to attain what Denmark has achieved with respect to e-health services for citizens. Other infrastructural resources in place, including existing systems, regulations, communication standards, as well as organizational structures in the Danish healthcare sector, have played a vital role in establishing the national

T.B. Jensen (✉)
Department of IT Management, Copenhagen Business School,
Howitzvej 60, 2000 Frederiksberg, Denmark
e-mail: blegind@cbs.dk

A.A. Thorseng
Department of Informatics, University of Oslo,
Gaustadalléen 23 D, Blindern, 1080 Oslo, Norway
e-mail: athorseng@gmail.com

© The Author(s) 2017
M. Aanestad et al. (eds.), *Information Infrastructures within European Health Care*, Health Informatics, DOI 10.1007/978-3-319-51020-0_13

209

e-health infrastructure (Thorseng and Jensen 2015). Consequently, the design, development, and implementation of an e-health initiative such as sundhed.dk, that has become an integrated part of a national infrastructure, becomes relevant to study.

In line with the aim of the book, this case chapter provides insights into the role of the installed base – i.e., pre-existing technologies, regulatory frameworks, data resources, and organizational arrangements – in the evolution of sundhed. dk. In particular, we argue that the main reasons for the current positioning of sundhed.dk have been its ability to (1) collate and assemble existing data resources, (2) repurpose and enhance current data sources in the health sector, and (3) engage a multiplicity of stakeholders. We argue that these activities represent three ways of capitalizing on the installed base that has led to the evolution and current situation of the e-health portal. At the same time, we show how these three modes come with a number of challenges for sundhed.dk in its pursuit of further innovation.

The rest of the chapter is organized as follows. We start out by introducing the Danish healthcare sector to set the context for sundhed.dk. Further, we describe the development of sundhed.dk, its purpose, as well as its current organization. Based on this description, we analyze how the organization behind the e-health portal succeeded in establishing a national healthcare infrastructure by assembling existing data resources, repurposing current healthcare services, and mobilizing key stakeholders. We conclude the chapter by providing some thoughts on the future for sundhed.dk.

Method

The empirical material for this chapter stems from 13 semi-structured interviews conducted between March and October 2014 with staff at the central office of sundhed.dk as well as with partners from the regions, ministry, and other health authorities in Denmark. In addition, we have included documents in the form of press releases, official papers, internal documents, and online information. Three representatives from the sundhed.dk office have read the chapter and verified its content before publication.

13.2 The Danish Healthcare Sector

Denmark is like other Scandinavian countries known for its comprehensive welfare system. Denmark provides free and equal access to public healthcare services to its relatively small population of 5.6 million inhabitants. Accordingly, access to all public hospitals as well as general and specialized practitioner services is financed through general taxes. Dentists, out of hospital medicines, as well as some therapies are provided under co-payment or private models on a case basis. The public healthcare system is organized in primary healthcare and the hospital sector. Primary healthcare deals with general health problems and consists of general practitioners

(GPs), practicing specialists, dentists, physiotherapists, nursing homes, dental care for children, and preventive health schemes. The hospital sector handles medical conditions that require specialized treatment and intensive care. Patients are referred to the hospital by their GP unless it is acute illness or accident. Patients have the right to choose between all public hospitals for treatment, and since 2002, they also have the right to choose a state financed treatment at a private hospital if waiting times are exceeded.

The healthcare system in Denmark is predominantly public and government-controlled through comprehensive legislation and annual budgetary allocations. The Ministry of Health has a coordinating and supervisory role, but operational responsibilities are embedded in a decentralized administrative structure consisting of 5 regions and 98 municipalities (Pedersen et al. 2012). The regions are responsible for the everyday operation of hospitals and primary care. At a national level, the interest organization – Danish Regions[1] – coordinates the common interests of the five regions and negotiates the annual financial framework for the regions with the government, as well as with the private practicing sector. The municipalities are in charge of public health, homecare, nursing homes, school health service, rehabilitation, and social services. The ambition is to provide a healthcare system that is efficient, of high quality, and that enables free choice of provider by its citizens. In 2015, the annual government healthcare expenditures amounted to 150 billion DKK (equivalent to 20 billion euros).

The Danish healthcare sector relies heavily on information technology for the provision of healthcare. More than 95% of the Danish population have access to the internet, and broadband penetration is among the highest in Europe (Danish Regions 2010). A unique personal identifier (CPR number) is issued to all Danish citizens at birth, and citizens can obtain a secure web-ID (NemID) free of charge to access public sites with e-services. Denmark is a small country in terms of population and geographic area; yet, it is at the forefront in the digitalization of medical information and in electronic healthcare record management. Centralized databases store medical information of Danish citizens, including hospitalization information and prescription history. GPs, hospitals, and pharmacies are electronically connected to handle patient records, e-prescriptions, lab results, discharge letters, and electronic referrals to hospitals and specialists (Protti and Johansen 2010). In 2014, 97% of laboratory test results were delivered online, and 100% of prescriptions were transmitted to pharmacies electronically.

The high level of digitalization of the Danish healthcare sector can be explained partly by the early development of communication standards[2] initiated in the mid-1990s for the common communication flows between medical practices, hospitals, and pharmacies, as well as the secure Danish Healthcare Data Network. In addition, over the last decade, the Danish government has initiated and sponsored a number

---

[1] Danish Regions is the interest organization for the five regions in Denmark.

[2] MedCom was established in 1994 as a public funded, non-profit cooperation. It facilitates the cooperation between authorities, organizations, and private firms linked to the Danish healthcare sector.

of initiatives to increase the digitalization of its healthcare services. National health-care digitalization strategies have been published since 1996 to set the agenda for e-health initiatives. One such initiative is the Danish national e-health portal, sund-hed.dk, which provides access to and information about patient-oriented digital ser-vices in the Danish healthcare sector. Next, we describe the purpose of sundhed.dk, its evolution, as well as its current organization. This description serves as back-ground information for analyzing how sundhed.dk managed to capitalize on its installed base to become what it represents today.

13.3   Case Narrative: Sundhed.dk

13.3.1 Purpose of Sundhed.dk

The purpose of sundhed.dk is to consolidate relevant information from all parts of the healthcare service and establish an electronic gateway for citizens and health-care providers to the Danish healthcare system. The ambition is to empower patients by offering insight into and transparency of healthcare services, as well as to offer healthcare professionals easy access to clinical information about their patients. Since its launch in 2003, the objective of sundhed.dk has been to obtain better coor-dination across healthcare services by providing a government-controlled entry to health information across a relatively decentralized healthcare system. At a strategic level, the ambition is to encourage a common strategy, investments, and solutions for the healthcare services at a national level and to integrate healthcare services on the internet (Sundhed.dk 2016).

Sundhed.dk is at the forefront of governmental e-health portals (Sundhed.dk 2014b), and it serves as a unified hub for electronic communication between patients and healthcare providers. The portal is sector-wide in terms of its governing struc-ture as well as the several national and regional solutions it encompasses. The e-health portal is presented as a central component for patient-oriented digital ser-vices in the national healthcare digitization strategies (The Danish Government et al. 2008, 2012).

Internationally, sundhed.dk is recognized for its provision of patient-oriented digital services at a national level. Other countries turn to the central office of sund-hed.dk to learn from their experience. However, the development of sundhed.dk – as we know it today – was built step-by-step over a number of years, as we describe next.

13.3.2 Timeline of Sundhed.dk

In 2001, the Association of County Councils in Denmark and the Ministry of Interior and Health initiated the work of establishing a common public e-health portal. The various stakeholders in the healthcare sector agreed on the prospect of establishing a common infrastructure and a shared system across municipalities and

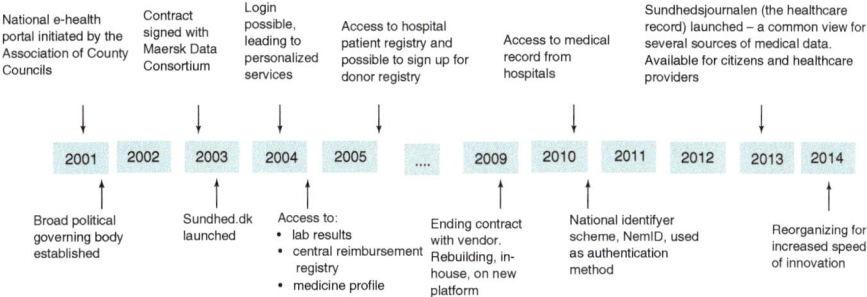

Fig. 13.1 Timeline of main events

regions all over Denmark. Figure 13.1 shows the timeline of the main events that led to and further triggered the development of sundhed.dk.

A broad political governing body, consisting of The Association of County Councils, The Ministry of the Interior and Health, The Greater Capital's Hospital Association, as well as Copenhagen and Frederiksberg Municipalities, was established to support the start of the e-health portal. One of the first tasks for the board of directors was to prepare a tendering process. Due to the scope and complexity of establishing the common infrastructure, it was decided to carry out the tender as a contest, which was launched in spring 2002. The winner of the contest was Maersk Data Consortium consisting of LEC, ACURE, PLS/Ramboll and Bysted with whom the central office of sundhed.dk signed a contract in the beginning of 2003. An analysis of the needs and the development of the first version of the e-health portal was carried out before its launch in December 2003.

In the initial phase of sundhed.dk, the purpose was to add quality-assured medical information that would serve both citizens and healthcare providers. Information about waiting lists at certain hospitals soon became available on the portal. At the beginning of 2004, the functionality of sundhed.dk was expanded with services that require login with a digital signature. A first attempt was made with electronic access to lab results for healthcare providers by connecting to a subset of lab systems already in use in Denmark. From 2004, patients were able to view their electronic medicine profile online. The prescription solution built on an already existing solution called "Medicine Profile" provided by the Danish Health and Medicine Authorities. Later, in 2014, this solution was phased out and replaced by a new solution for prescription handling called "Common Medicine Card" provided by the Danish Public Health Institute. An electronic guidance to the healthcare service was established and it was possible to search for healthcare providers, i.e., GPs, physiotherapists, and psychologists, based on location and availability. Finding their GP on sundhed.dk, patients would be directed to the GP website to initiate booking of appointments and conducting email consultations. Since vendors of booking and email-consultation solutions already had a strong market position, the partners of sundhed.dk agreed to directing patients to the GPs' own sites, where they could access their GP's solution for booking and e-consultation.

By 2005, patients were able to access the Danish National Patient Registry in which all treatments performed in the hospital sector were listed. This registry, created in 1977, contains personal data about all patients admitted to hospital since 1977, and from 1995 also out-patients registrations (Lynge et al. 2011). Additionally, based on the Central Reimbursement Registry, information about all treatments a patient had received in the public health service were accessible to the patient. By 2006, doctors in 11 out of 19 counties could check online lab results via sundhed.dk. By the end of 2007, the portal had about 170,000 unique users every month.

In April 2009, sundhed.dk was launched on a new technical platform, which meant that the central office gained more control over the portal and reduced costs by being independent of external consultants and developers. This process was described by staff as "*taking the portal home*" (head of staff, sundhed.dk). Subsequently, a development department now did most development of services in-house, while external consultants were approached to develop standalone services. Apart from smaller developments, there were two major initiatives in this period. One initiative was to make medical records from public hospitals available so that patients would be able to see parts of their medical record such as treatments, diagnoses, and notes made by the healthcare personnel. The e-record was created to ensure information sharing across regions and hospitals; for example, if a patient from Copenhagen were admitted to another region of the country, doctors would now have access to data from previous treatments. The e-record was thus a read-only repository that supplemented the local electronic healthcare information with information from other areas. An important milestone for sundhed.dk, in 2010, was managing access to the portal via NemID. Citizens could now use the same authentication method as banks and other public Danish agencies. This meant that single sign-on was enabled and users needed to remember only one password. In 2015, approximately four million Danes had a NemID account (NemID 2014) and could thus potentially log onto sundhed.dk.

Another major initiative in this period was the healthcare record (sundhedsjournalen) launched in 2013. This initiative enabled a 'one-stop-view' for both patients and healthcare providers with access to medical data such as records stemming from the e-record described above, medicine data, and other critical health information.

13.3.3 Sundhed.dk Organization

Sundhed.dk is organized around key stakeholders in the healthcare sector. It consists of a secretariat (i.e., the central office which in 2016 counted 45 employees) and a number of partners that contribute to the development of the portal. The organization is illustrated in Fig. 13.2.

The stakeholders (see the left box) contribute to sundhed.dk through participation in governance activities, projects, and by providing content such as information

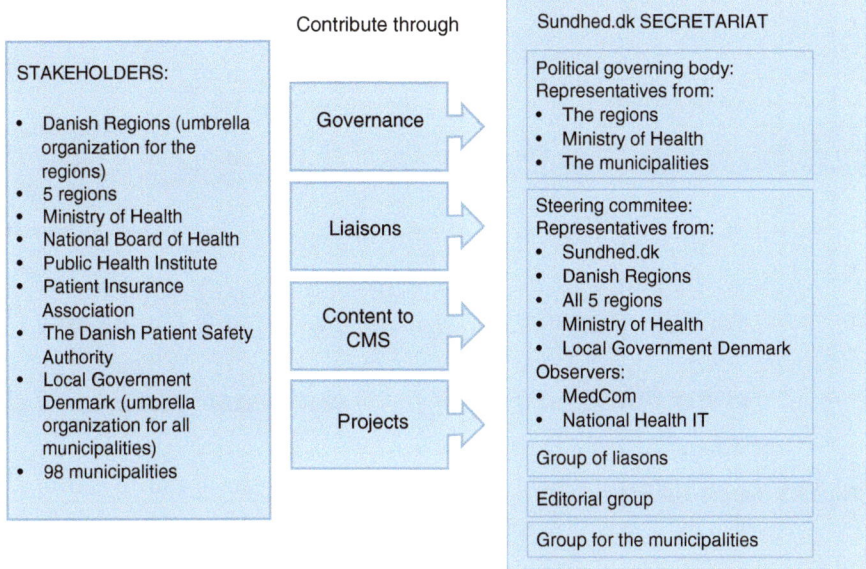

Fig. 13.2 Organization of sundhed.dk

about their activities, updated guidelines, etc. The secretariat in sundhed.dk (see the right box) is responsible for administration, marketing, maintenance, and daily running of the portal. The secretariat further comprises a team of assisting partners that take part in conceptualizing and developing new solutions. A political governing body with representatives from Danish Regions, the Ministry of Health, and the municipalities, as well as a steering committee with representatives from the main areas in healthcare are responsible for the overall strategy and prioritization of services and funds.

Health data and services provided through sundhed.dk is based on displaying already existing data from various sources. In some cases, data is being extracted from data sources such as hospital systems, GP systems, prescription databases, and lab systems to be presented through sundhed.dk's presentation layer. In other cases, services are "framed" to achieve sundhed.dk's 'look and feel' although the service is located and run somewhere else. Lastly, sundhed.dk also points or directs users to other existing services in the healthcare sphere, such as booking of appointments for GPs. Figure 13.3 illustrates the architecture of sundhed.dk.

Security is maintained with patient login by means of the national electronic identifier scheme, NemID. Health personnel can access patient data provided through sundhed.dk in their electronic medical records. Health personnel's access to patient data is restricted by ensuring there is an existing treatment relation between patient and health personnel and further that the patient approves health personnel access. Access to patient data by the health personnel is logged and the logs are available to the patient.

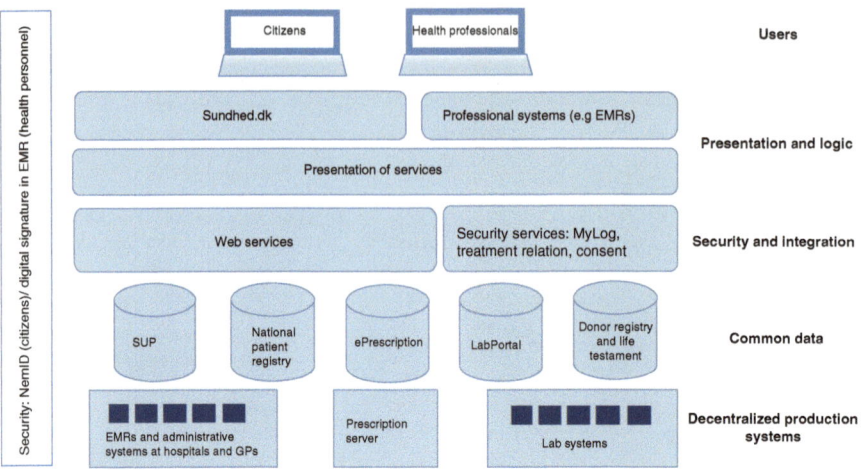

Fig. 13.3 Sundhed.dk architecture

13.4   Analysis: Three Modes of Capitalizing on the Installed Base

The introduction to sundhed.dk gives an indication of how the organization draws upon, recombines, and repurposes existing technical, legislative, and organizational resources and services. In this section, we detail how the organization of sundhed. dk has: (1) collated and assembled existing data resources, (2) repurposed and enhanced current data sources in the health sector, and (3) engaged multiple stakeholders to obtain its current position. The three modes of capitalizing on the installed base have corresponding opportunities and challenges that we present below.

13.4.1 Collate and Assemble Existing Data Resources

Sundhed.dk explicitly aims to provide access to health information, and several of their services involve a collation of pre-existing data sources: "*Our ambition is to collect data and to establish easy access to data*" (head of administration, sundhed. dk). One example of collated data is 'sundhedsjournalen,' where various data sources, such as lab results, prescriptions, and medical records from hospitals are displayed in one view for the citizen and health personnel. In 'sundhedsjournalen,' citizens can also access laboratory results, and they can register for organ donation, as well as set up their living will.

Another example of collated data is the functionality, whereby all healthcare providers are listed with details about opening hours, core services, email consultations, renewal of e-prescriptions, etc. Patients can get information about and overview of healthcare providers, and they can gain direct access to their websites through the portal.

A third example is the collection of quality-assured health information. The assembling of data sources enhances the value and usefulness of singular data sources in terms of providing easy access to as well as a contextualizing of information. For example, in the case of 'sundhedsjournalen,' data from one source is shown in relation to another. This means that a patient or health professional can see where a patient has been admitted, and at the same time, they can gain access to prescribed medications and discharge notes.

Displaying information to patients relies on laborious work conducted over several years to achieve extraction of data from multiple sources. A representative from one of the regions argued: "*Some of these services already existed such as the Landspatientregisteret [The National Patient Registry], so basically, in Denmark, we had an existing infrastructure that was useful when establishing sundhed.dk*". In addition, Denmark has a well-established IT infrastructure such as the common standard for health message exchange and the secure Danish healthcare network. This infrastructure has been a prerequisite for the success of sundhed.dk: "*In Denmark, we have a strong tradition of digitalization and many solutions were already established locally – let the thousand flowers bloom*" (representative, SSI[3]). In other words, the informant argued that, opposed to centrally directed development of digital services in the healthcare sector, local initiatives have been the source of many current information systems. For example, the e-record builds on a mature infrastructure that was the outcome of the project, initiated in 2000, called 'Standardized pull of patient data' (SUP). This database was built to make registered patient data in EPR systems, the Patient Administrative Systems (PAS), and other systems on currently and previously admitted patients available in other hospitals across the country. Initially, SUP provided a majority of hospitals and GPs across Denmark with the possibility of accessing electronic health records across counties. Extracts of patient data are transferred via a nationwide MedCom XML standard to a SUP database/Internet server, where an Internet browser provides access for healthcare professionals to view selected patient information and record data by searching on the patient's civil registry number (Aanestad and Jensen 2011; Jensen 2013). The head of administration at sundhed.dk explained: "*We have 'buttoned on' services and applications over time [...]. We had no ambition of developing something new... rather, we wanted to enable access and gather what already existed [...]. So, basically what we do is to develop a user interface that covers all existing solutions and then make data available from there*" (head of administration, sundhed.dk).

Collating and assembling already existing data sources provides easy access to a number of health services for citizens and healthcare professionals; however, it also comes with some challenges. For example, collecting and publishing quality-assured health information and information about the healthcare services requires comprehensive quality control: "*More and more quality requirements are being posed from our side [sundhed.dk]. At some point, the amount of editorial content on sundhed.dk was simply overwhelming and then we started talking about quality*" (head of administration, sundhed.dk).

---

[3] SSI stands for 'Statens Serum Institut', National Institute for Health Data and Disease Control.

Similarly, the organization of sundhed.dk needs to adhere to national regulations and procedures, including pre-existing legal frameworks concerning data ownership on how data is treated and how it can be displayed and accessed. The organization needs to take into account these regulations and therefore it engages in close collaboration with authorities when displaying these data. For example, displaying a collection of medical information to the patient is based on existing legislation on the right to view own health information, in which a person over the age of 15 has the right to see what is being written about him/her. Requesting a physical copy of one's record directly from the hospital requires that the medical staff perform an evaluation of what is disclosed to the patient to avoid distributing sensitive material. However, when making the records available to citizens through the e-health portal, this professional "filter" is no longer present. Through discussions with the health authorities, and interpretation of the existing law on information access, a 14-day delay has been implemented on availability of records to the patient (this delay has been further reduced to 3 days in 2015). This way, health staff can communicate and explain results to the patient before he or she accesses them online. Health personnel on the other hand can access the patient's data immediately.

13.4.2 Repurpose and Enhance Current Data Sources in the Health Sector

Part of the ambition of sundhed.dk is to create access to current healthcare data sources, not to *"reinvent the wheel"* (head of administration, sundhed.dk). Some of the first services on the portal provided access to existing registries. Several of the data sources, which are displayed through sundhed.dk, were originally intended for other purposes than citizen access.

For example, the central reimbursement registry mainly ensures that health providers are reimbursed for the services they provide to patients. The registry serves administrative and research purposes. Another registry is the National Patient Registry whereby a range of data is recorded about patients when they receive care as part of the specialist healthcare service. The data is used for several purposes; for health research, surveillance of diseases, activity monitoring at the hospital, and to estimate and review the total use of hospital services across counties and regions (representative, SSI). Through building on already existing data sources by giving a new user group access, new use of the data is enabled. Through sundhed.dk, patients can use the same data to get an overview of their treatments and movements around the health service.

Second, a gradual expansion of linking to new registers and systems has taken place, and in some instances, sundhed.dk has not only displayed the data, but also enhanced the underlying systems. One example is the donor register; in 1990, legislation was passed defining the legal criteria for being brain dead, which meant that donating organs, besides kidneys, could be performed. Consequently, a donor registry was established to keep track of potential donors. By 2005, an electronic sign-up option for the donor registry was created. This means that patients can now register whether they allow all or no organs to be donated, whether they want only some organs to be donated, or whether the decision is to be made of next of kin. Another example of enhancing an already existing system is the program for colon cancer screening, which all Danes between 50 and 74 years are offered. Through sundhed.dk, it is possible to opt out of this screening.

Third, sundhed.dk also utilizes and repurposes already familiar infrastructures for their users. For example, authentication that citizens are familiar with from banking and other public electronic service was introduced in 2009 (i.e., NemID). By exploiting an authentication method, which is available to and widely used by the Danish population, sundhed.dk is readily available to the Danes.

Although existing data sources, systems, and registries are repurposed through the e-health portal, the organization behind sundhed.dk avoids "data management" responsibilities. Rather, the solutions and data repositories which sundhed.dk links to or integrates with are themselves responsible for data management. For example, if the user has questions regarding data presented via sundhed.dk, the entities in the health service, which provided the health service and subsequently health data, are the point of contact. The role sundhed.dk has had in terms of being a public, authoritative site on health without having any form of responsibilities for the data displayed was *"new turf"* (head of administration, sundhed.dk). The fact that Danish health authorities have a long tradition of registering data and providing local health services challenges the repurposing and enhancing of existing data on the portal. For example, the partners have started to discuss and agree upon who owns what and how (representative, SSI).

Furthermore, the repurposing and enhancing of existing healthcare services has gradually changed the way in which partners perceive the organization behind the e-health portal. They have started to question the role of the portal and they voice their critique of sundhed.dk for not having ensured that its strategy is aligned with that of the partners. They question the overall direction of the portal: *"It seems that it is the jukebox principle that defines what services are developed. To us it is not clear what are the criteria for prioritizing services... the strategy is not clear and sometimes I wonder if the strategy is technically driven in the sense of 'we have this new thing' and then they build it without any overarching strategy"* (representative, the regions). For sundhed.dk, establishing a clear strategy is further challenged by the fact that there is not one common strategy for healthcare in Denmark: *"It gets really complicated when you have so many strategies in play – the Digitization Strategy and the Healthcare Digitization Strategy at a national level, the Healthcare IT Strategy at a regional level, and then the municipalities have their own strategy"* (head of administration, sundhed.dk). Whereas there is a common understanding of the overall vision of sundhed.dk, the existing ideas and strategies among the partners seem to be difficult to reconcile. In addition, partners question whether a regional strategy is more important compared to a national initiative. These concerns reflect the third mode of capitalizing on the installed base, which has to do with the engagement of multiple stakeholders, as we discuss next.

13.4.3 Engage Multiple Stakeholders

The governing bodies and financing partners of sundhed.dk consist of members from Denmark's five regions, the Danish Regions, the Municipal Organization, and the Ministry of Health. This broad representation of key actors gave legitimacy to the portal at an early stage: "*The purpose was to establish a common public healthcare portal [...] that vision was crucial, and then of course it was important that they managed to engage the most influential partners, such as Danish Regions, that primarily runs sundhed.dk, together with the municipalities and the Ministry of Health as partners*" (representative, The Ministry of Health). In addition, informants describe it as a clear advantage that the organization of the governing bodies resembles the way in which the remaining healthcare system is organized. For example, the relationship between the regions, the government, and GPs has been maintained through general agreements: "*The collaboration model we find in the Danish healthcare system is reflected in the organization of sundhed.dk. I believe that if we wouldn't have had this organization in place, it would have been very difficult to establish sundhed.dk*" (representative, the regions).

The initial phase of sundhed.dk can be characterized as a political showcase for regional collaboration with solid political unity and common ambition. The involved parties have largely gathered around the common ambition of having one access point to the healthcare services: "*At the outset, there was a clear vision, which was politically anchored in the Association of County Councils – one entrance point to healthcare services and cross-sectorial collaboration – it was a vision we all could agree upon*" (head of administration, sundhed.dk). In addition: "*We were told that if we could find a project that could strategically mark the 14 counties across, and not as silos, we would receive funding*" (representative, the regions). In the initial phase, there was little disagreement concerning what should be offered to citizens and healthcare providers. The political unity and broad collaboration of stakeholders was described as key reasons for the success of the portal.

While there was a clear political mandate and a broadly agreed-upon vision, the partners had different starting points in terms of already existing digital services. One of the initial challenges was to get everyone at the same level: "*It was a great opportunity to establish cross-sectorial collaboration, but this was also one of the biggest challenges [...] For example, not all regions had very advanced webpages*" (head of administration, sundhed.dk). In addition, it was a challenge to get everyone onboard: "*In the beginning, a lot of partners were happy about sundhed.dk and many believed in the overall vision. But if a region was working on a local project, it was difficult to get its buy-in. We spent much time in the beginning to go out locally and defend our existence. There was no choice for opting out. We basically told them that they themselves had decided that we should exist*" (head of administration, sundhed.dk). The engagement of multiple stakeholders did not come automatically but had to be enabled actively by the staff at sundhed.dk. It was important to engage actors, since sundhed.dk did not have any authoritative responsibility or obligations. The overall purpose was to make services available and to establish editorial access to more than 900 partners over time. The role of sundhed.dk was to engage and, at the same time, control the partners. This was considered a *"…difficult balancing act for sundhed.dk"* to get the regions and municipalities to engage and own the process while at the same time manage and coordinate the efforts (representative, the regions).

Building on the installed base of a core set of actors was in this case a double-edged sword, as one of the informants also stated; *"What is their [sundhed.dk] strength is also their weakness"* (representative, SSI). The informant here is referring to the broad alliance of partners, which gave the organization and e-health portal legitimacy, but also made it heavy and inflexible in the sense that many considerations were required for every decision. For example, the prioritization of tasks was described as a politicized decision-making process: *"It is very difficult to be sundhed.dk in terms of serving so many masters"* (representative, Ministry of Health). The head of administration in sundhed.dk further elaborated on the challenges in decision-making and prioritization processes: *"We cannot prioritize projects ourselves [internally in sundhed.dk]. We need to do that in collaboration with our partners. They have their own interests and local benchmarks and we don't have resources to financially support all their wishes"*. This situation put sundhed.dk in a certain bind. In addition, priorities seemed to shift after certain tasks had been initiated, thus making the daily development of new services cumbersome: *"You can risk that when the economical agreements are made, a politician will suddenly say 'Now we need more people to donate their organs, so in 2013 this should be registered on sundhed.dk'. This was not how it was earlier – we knew very well what we needed to do. Now our partners often want to lift their IT-strategies and projects via the portal"* (head of administration, sundhed.dk). Although it complicates development when having to accommodate all partners' needs and IT strategies, it is encouraged and part of sundhed.dk's overall mission.

Overall, there has been broad support from relevant players in the Danish healthcare arena, but at the same time, it has been challenging for the sundhed.dk organization to serve so many masters. As time passed, the majority of actors started to question what was in it for them. The regions, who financed 80% of sundhed.dk, wanted to see their requests being realized: *"When we pay for a service, we also assume that it will appear on the portal"* (representative, the regions). In particular in 2009, when sundhed.dk decided to do most development of services in-house as opposed to development by external consultants, it was a challenge for them to keep up with the pace of demands since *"the pipeline was getting too tight"* (head of administration, sundhed.dk). A representative from one of the regions, who argued that the production line was too limited with the consequence of delayed projects, confirmed this observation: *"… there has been a shift from being a client to being a vendor, and this has been a challenge for sundhed.dk. Mostly because the production line has become very narrow […] and there has been too many things that have been important for the regions, but we don't want to constantly discuss prioritizing those services that are included on sundhed.dk"* (representative, the regions). The request for the future was that the organization behind sundhed.dk would be able to develop projects in parallel.

In the next section, we conclude the chapter by discussing the findings and reflecting upon the future of sundhed.dk.

13.5   Discussion: Moving Forward

What makes the sundhed.dk case unique is the mobilization of a large number of stakeholders. Sundhed.dk has managed to cultivate a large network of alliances, which makes it successful and at the same time difficult for other countries to replicate. As we demonstrated in the analysis, the engagement of multiple stakeholders did not come automatically. Although the initiation of the portal came with a political mandate, sundhed.dk still had to engage actively the different stakeholders. It is fascinating to see how the collaboration among different stakeholders made it possible to integrate divergent priorities and strategies into one shared portal. This conclusion is in line with previous research (e.g., Aanestad and Jensen 2011), which shows that the realization of nation-wide information infrastructures for healthcare not only requires a gradual transition of the installed base; the development also needs to ensure the mobilization and organization of multiple stakeholders.

However, it was not only the active engagement of stakeholders, which made sundhed.dk a success. The installed base in the form of pre-existing technologies, regulatory frameworks, data resources, and organizational arrangements played a key role in the gradual evolution of sundhed.dk. The main reason for the current positioning of sundhed.dk was its ability to collate and assemble existing data resources, and also to repurpose and enhance current data sources in the health sector.

Taken together, these activities were important for sundhed.dk in order to capitalize on the installed base. At the same time, however, the organization now faces a number of challenges in staying relevant for its partners in the time ahead. While the portal was very visionary at the beginning, it could easily get behind regarding current trends in a fast moving sector of digital health services. Large leaps are being made in fields such as mobility and "quantified self," whereby patients provide data about themselves either manually or through sensors and this leads to high demands from society, and the younger generations specifically, on how services are offered digitally. Additionally, as new digital systems are being introduced in the health service in the regions in Denmark, sundhed.dk needs to be aligned with these changes. For example, at the time of writing, the regions in and around the capital are introducing EPIC as an all-encompassing suite for the tertiary health service (Jensen 2016), and sundhed.dk needs to link up with these new data sources and providers.

To stay relevant over time, sundhed.dk also needs to broaden its capacity to develop services at a pace that is needed for the involved partners. This could mean easing the possibility for external developers to create services and having a flexible governance structure and an agile development methodology. These measures should, at the same time, be balanced with measures to ensure that quality and professionalism are not compromised. These are issues that sundhed.dk are working on at the time of writing. A program, targeting the above-mentioned challenges, has led to a reorganization of sundhed.dk to ensure increased delivery capacity and stronger portfolio management. In the future, focus is on being proactive and assist the partners in developing and maturing new service concepts. According to sources at sundhed.dk, this work yields positive results.

Lastly, without any formal mandate, sundhed.dk has to keep a balance between being a receiving part, acting on their partners' wishes, while at the same time contributing to a clear direction within the Danish healthcare sector. This is the main premise of the organization behind sundhed.dk, which has led to the evolution of the e-health portal, but now needs to show the future direction of the portal.

References

Aanestad M, Jensen TB. Building nation-wide information infrastructures in healthcare through modular implementation strategies. J Strateg Inf Syst. 2011;20(2):161–75.

Danish Regions. IT brings the Danish health sector together. In: Danish Regions, M., Sundhed.dk, Digital Health, Local Government Denmark (Ed.). Copenhagen.2010.

Jensen TB. Design principles for achieving integrated healthcare information systems. Health Inform J. 2013;19(1):29–45.

Jensen TB. The Danish IT healthcare platform: real-time hospital management, In: Cases on IT Leadership: CIO Challenges for Innovation and Keeping the Lights on, Niels Bjørn-Andersen, editor. 2016. Samfundslitteratur: 217-236

Lynge E, Sandegaard JL, Rebolj M. The Danish national patient register. Scand J Publ Health. 2011;39(7 suppl):30–3.

NemID. Statistik om NemID, Digitaliseringsstyrelsen. 2014.

Pedersen, K. M., Andersen, J. S. and Søndergaard, J. General Practice and Primary Health Care in Denmark, Journal of American Board of Family Medicine 2012;25: 34–38.

Protti, D. and Johansen, I. Widespread Adoption of Information Technology in Primary CarePhysician Offices in Denmark: A Case Study, Issues in International Health Policy, TheCommonwealth Fund 2010: 1–14

Sundhed.dk. Recognition to sundhed.dk. https://www.sundhed.dk/borger/service/nyt-og-presse/presserum/pressemeddelelser/. 2014a. Accessed on the January 2017.

Sundhed.dk. Press Room. https://www.sundhed.dk/borger/service/om-sundheddk/om-organisationen/. 2014b. Accessed on January 2017.

Sundhed.dk. About the Organization. https://www.sundhed.dk/borger/service/om-sundheddk/om-organisationen/. 2016. Accessed on January 2017.

The Danish Government, Danish Regions and Local Government Denmark. National strategy for digitalization of the healthcare service. https://www.sundhed.dk/content/cms/6/3406_national-strategi-2008-2012.pdf. 2008. Accessed on November 2014.

The Danish Government, Danish Regions and Local government Denmark. Making e-Health work. National Strategy for Digitalization of the Danish Healthcare Sector 2013–2017, The Danish Government, Copenhagen. 2012.

Thorseng A, Jensen TB. Building national infrastructures for patient-centred digital services. In: 23rd European Conference on Information Systems (ECIS), Münster. 2015.

Open Access This chapter is distributed under the terms of the Creative Commons Attribution-NonCommercial 2.5 International License (http://creativecommons.org/licenses/by-nc/2.5/), which permits any noncommercial use, duplication, adaptation, distribution and reproduction in any medium or format, as long as you give appropriate credit to the original author(s) and the source, provide a link to the Creative Commons license and indicate if changes were made.

The images or other third party material in this chapter are included in the chapter's Creative Commons license, unless indicated otherwise in a credit line to the material. If material is not included in the chapter's Creative Commons license and your intended use is not permitted by statutory regulation or exceeds the permitted use, you will need to obtain permission directly from the copyright holder.

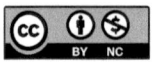

The Swedish Patient Portal and Its Relation to the National Reference Architecture and the Overall eHealth Infrastructure

14

Nina Sellberg and Johan Eltes

14.1 Introduction

This chapter presents the evolution of the Swedish patient portal and how it has co-evolved with the eHealth architecture and the overall national eHealth infrastructure. It focuses on the period from 2000 to 2015. The patient portal with related e-services give citizens access to for instance e-scheduling, e-pharmacy, e-referrals, telemedicine, access to personal health information, digital self-services around the clock, Internet-Psychiatry, Electronic Health Record (EHR) logs, e-services that visualize planned care procedures including upcoming encounters, pre-visit form submission, e-communication with their physician or nurse, and secure disclosure of their health data (generated in the public health care system) to third party vendor's apps and systems.

The case narratives illustrate the role a broadly and timely agreed upon national reference architecture has played during 8 years of distributed, yet harmonized development of a national eHealth infrastructure and the eHealth innovation made possible by that infrastructure. During these 8 years the installed base was organically expanded with new regulations, users, infrastructure components, portals and e-services, proving the importance of the infrastructure as a basis for innovation carried out and utilized by a broad range of stakeholders.

The remainder of the chapter is structured as follows: in the next section the Swedish healthcare model is presented, thereafter an overview of the core components building the Swedish eHealth architecture is illustrated. This section is followed by our narrative of the Swedish case. Next we analyze and discuss the core activities and actors that have evolved the installed base supporting innovation and

N. Sellberg (✉) • J. Eltes
LIME, Karolinska Institutet, Tomtebodavägen 18A, 171 65 Solna, Sweden
e-mail: nina.sellberg@ki-information.se; johan.eltes@ki.se

© The Author(s) 2017
M. Aanestad et al. (eds.), *Information Infrastructures within European Health Care*, Health Informatics, DOI 10.1007/978-3-319-51020-0_14

225

entrepreneurship. Our findings support the argument that infrastructure evolvement comes out of the complex interplay between many different actors intertwined in step-by-step cultivation. In Sweden the infrastructure evolvement is done through the governance of a reference architecture endorsed by all entities contributing to the installed base. The installed base has evolved through the strategy of extending existing components, through complementing the installed base with new components and through the substitution of existing components with new ones. We also see a reference architecture as a vision-carrying foundation for many years of bottom-up, middle-out, top-down and yet harmonized, infrastructure evolution. More specifically, a shared, well understood and purposeful reference architecture may even be a contributing factor in reducing the probability and implication of "political" games.

Method
Data were collected as an action research study conducted from 2009 to 2015. Nina Sellberg was the R&D manager at the department of eHealth, Stockholm County Council (largest eHealth department in Sweden) between 2010 and 2014 and CTO at 1177 Vårdguiden between 2014 and 2015, with the responsibility of the national citizen platform. She was also appointed project manager of the My Care Pathways project, between 2011 and 2015 and appointed project leader of the development of the New Patient Overview Service implemented in all county councils and municipalities in Sweden from December 2015. Johan Eltes was consulting as head of architecture of My Care Pathways between 2011 and 2013. He was consulting architect at Inera AB between 2006 and 2013 for the development and management of the national reference architecture. He is deputy CTO at Inera AB since 2014, with the responsibility of the national interoperability profiles and the national reference architecture. Data collection included information gathering (a) from central stakeholders at Inera AB, My Healthcare Contacts, and project developers and vendors and, (b) from documents on national eHealth strategies, project management documents, the system specifications and IT architecture documents.

14.2   Swedish Healthcare

14.2.1 Overview of the Swedish Healthcare Model

The responsibility for health and medical care in Sweden is shared by the central government, county councils and municipalities. The Health and Medical Service Act regulates the responsibilities of county councils and municipalities, and gives local governments more freedom in this area. The role of the central government is to establish principles and guidelines, and to set the political agenda for health and medical care. It does this through laws and ordinances or by reaching agreements with the Swedish Association of Local Authorities and Regions (SALAR), which represents the county councils and municipalities. Sweden is divided into 290 municipalities and 20 county councils. There is no hierarchical relation (chain of command) across state, county councils and municipalities. The patients have free choice of hospitals, but General Practitioners (GPs) serve as gatekeepers for referrals to hospitals or specialists. The councils' and municipalities' autonomy is strong, and they make their own ICT investments. Costs for healthcare of Sweden's gross domestic product (GDP) is fairly stable and on par with most other European countries. They represent in 2016 about 9.5 % of GDP (OECD 2014, WHO). The bulk of health and medical costs in Sweden are paid for by county council and municipal taxes. Contributions from the national government are another source of funding, while patient fees cover only a small percentage of costs.

14.2.2 Rationale for Developing the Swedish eHealth Architecture

The rationale for the development of the Swedish eHealth architecture was firstly the National IT Strategy that was taken forward in 2005. This was a work initiated by the Swedish Government with the intention to support (1) Citizens', patients' and families' access to readily available and comprehensive information on health in general and on their own health, (2) Professionals' access to information across organizational boundaries using effective and interoperable IT integration platforms that ensure patient safety and facilitate health professionals' daily work, and (3) Healthcare decision makers' access to relevant information enabling them to monitor and follow up patient safety, quality of care and healthcare performance.

The second rationale for developing the Swedish eHealth architecture was the National EHealth Strategy for Accessible and Secure Information in Health care, 2010. This work was also initiated by the Swedish Government with the intention to support: (1) Citizens, patients, clients and family members with access to quality-assured information on health also including access to clinical documentation from their previous efforts and treatments. Citizens should be offered innovative e-services for the exercise of participation and self-determination on their own terms, (2) Professionals with innovative and integrated decision support systems facilitating their daily work. Access to information across organizational boundaries should build the basis for the decision support systems, and (3) Healthcare decision makers with innovative tools and authority systems to continuously monitor the quality and performance of activities in order to optimize resource allocation. The focus was chosen to secure individual's integrity in the follow-up and management of work.

The third rationale for evolving the Swedish eHealth architecture was the National Action Plan for eHealth, 2009–2012 and further evolved along the subsequent national action plan for eHealth, 2013–2018. The national action plans were agreed upon by the Swedish public care buyers – the 21 county councils. The county councils organize the national coordination of the action plans through the company Inera AB, which is owned by the county councils[1]. The action plans were set up to

---

[1] Inera AB was formerly known as Center for eHealth.

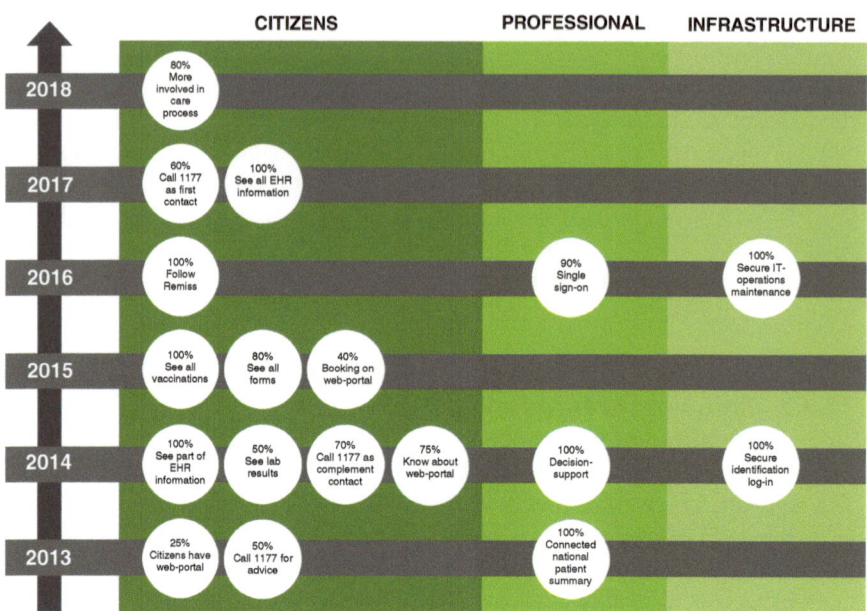

Fig. 14.1 Visualization of the National Action Plan for eHealth, 2013–2018

reach a set of goals: (1) that citizens shall both be able to access all clinical information about themselves and actively participate in their care. This shall result in increased patient empowerment, active participation with smarter eHealth services and collaboration across organizational boundaries – Care Anywhere, (2) professionals with smarter eHealth services and access to all relevant medical information about a patient across organizational boundaries, and (3) infrastructure in place with secured operational maintenance and identification log-in.

The first and second strategies intended to change people's mindset, promoting a vision of eHealth use. The third strategy is different from the first and second ones as it is not promoting an abstract vision but rather a very clear action plan demanding all county councils to get on board the eHealth train, with a clear structure of what should be done when. This led to a process where a number of national services and solutions were planned and implemented on a larger national scale. The third strategy is followed up in a different way compared to the first two strategies. It is followed up by statistical documentation of eHealth goal fulfilment (see Fig. 14.1), whilst the first two strategies were followed by early adopter success stories.

14.2.3 Core Components in the Swedish eHealth Architecture

This section presents the core components of the Swedish eHealth architecture (see also Fig. 14.2). Our account of the architecture is a snapshot from 2015. The presentation of these components aims to help the readers to follow the case narratives

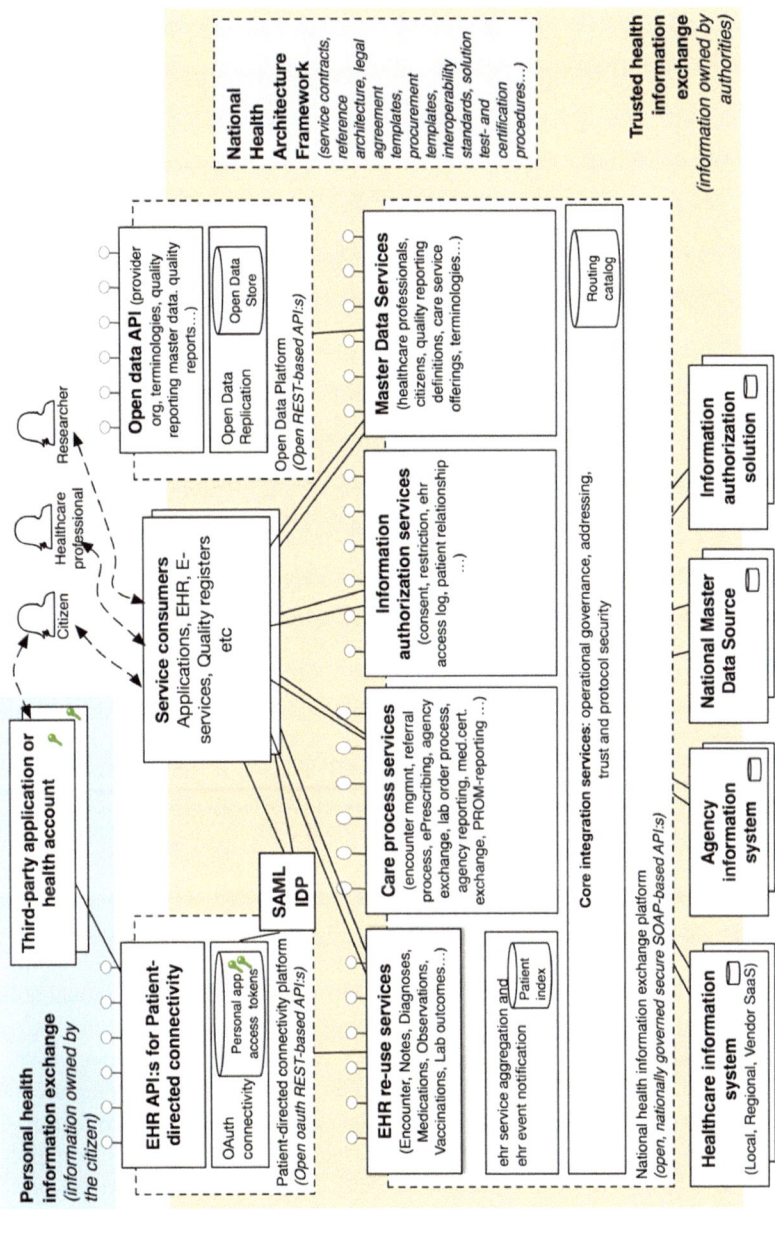

Fig. 14.2 Simplified illustration of the Swedish eHealth Architecture. Examples of missing parts are: Health innovation framework, citizen, care and academic portal

presented. The narrative outlines events of importance to the trajectory of the case study, but is confined to the events that are significant to the e-services of the case study. As a consequence, it doesn't list events related to national eHealth development in areas such as cross-provider referral processes, medical certificate exchange, e-prescription processes, quality indicators, analysis of healthcare-associated infections and birth certificates.

The National Reference Architecture Framework was the first component of the Swedish eHealth architecture to be nationally applied by Inera AB and its owners (the 21 county councils). It has been in operation since 2007. The reference architecture defines a set of architecture principles, architecture patterns and guiding examples that govern nationally as well as regionally funded projects that contribute to the evolution of the Swedish ecosystem of connected eHealth. The reference architecture states six architecture principles: (1) A set of architecture principles govern eHealth projects. (2) The principle of information security, (3) The principle of national functional scope, (4) The principle of loose coupling, (5) The principle of organic/local evolution/contribution to the national ecosystem (6) The principle of federation. It is referred to the installed base as an ecosystem. The fifth architecture principle encourages local and regional organizations to initiate development of missing core components to the Swedish eHealth infrastructure. Thus, many core components have been developed and implemented by regional projects that were neither steered nor funded nationally. Over time they were linked or canonized to the national eHealth architecture, either as a new, an updated or a replaced component. New components are able to be linked when the shared reference architecture framework has been applied during the development work regardless if it has been conducted on a local, regional or national level.

Local, regional and national parties have cooperated, in a case by case way, in evolving the installed base in a successful way through the shared use of the national reference architectural framework. Of course a county council like Stockholm has contributed more than others due to its size and financial capability. When national prioritizations have not been aligned with local and regional needs, a group of county councils, municipalities and solution vendors have been able to join forces to develop solutions on their own for more local and regional use. The principles of national functional scope, secures that the solution can be applied on a national scale in the future. As time passes by, county councils, municipalities and solution vendors continuously negotiate to bring their local or regional solution to a national level, sharing the solution with all publicly funded care in Sweden. Therefore, the core components in the Swedish eHealth infrastructure are owned by various parties although shared through the Swedish eHealth Architecture and coordinated by Inera AB. Examples of such components are clinical APIs (Application Programming Interfaces for access to medical record information), care process services, core integration services, application frameworks and a patient-directed connectivity platform. Whether local and regional component will develop into national components or not depends on how they align with the national action plans for eHealth and the national reference architecture. In practice, there is ongoing collaboration and knowledge exchange between local, regional and national projects over time. Inera AB has implemented a national program office in order to formalize a process for supporting local and regional initiatives with a national ambition. There is currently a dispute between Inera AB and some regions whether ownership (IPR etc.) has to be transferred to Inera in order to get national funding as part of national canonization of a regional solution. This fact may affect the power balance between national, regional and local projects. The Swedish healthcare system evolves through a combination of centralized and decentralized models for ICT innovation (bottom-up, middle-out and top-down). The reference architecture framework is a centralized joint effort of all county councils and municipalities while the ICT development work occurs locally, regionally and nationally.

The second component developed was the national health information exchange (HIE) platform. The concept of a national health information exchange platform is defined by the national reference architecture. It defines a set of strategic service-oriented integration patterns along with a set of platform capabilities required for systematic and manageable instantiation of these patterns. The patterns aim at supporting technical and semantic connectivity requirements while still supporting regional and local evolution of the installed base (primarily the regional ongoing consolidation of health information systems). The patterns are information aggregation, service virtualization and protocol adaption. The protocol adaption pattern is however only applied at the national level when protocol adaption is not possible at the local or regional level. The overarching idea is to represent all local and regional EHR solutions as a single virtual, national EHR system in terms of an API and management via Inera AB. The API is utilized by national, regional and local API clients. The HIE platform makes it possible for an API client to access information and invoke transactions on all EHR systems in Sweden through a single connection point (the HIE platform) and a single API.

The Swedish reference architecture does not rely upon central storage of EHRs. The architecture is service oriented. All transactions and information requests are processed by the source system of the care provider in real-time. Technical and semantic interoperability depends on agreed integration profiles. These are labeled "service contracts" in compliance with OASIS Reference Model. The national HIE platform depends on a couple of utility services: a patient index to support information aggregation and a service routing registry to support a virtual service contract endpoint to resolve the logical address (e.g. an id of a healthcare provider) into the web service end-point address of the regional or local EHR system supporting that logical address (i.e. a healthcare provider). The national HIE platform was first released into production in 2010 by Inera AB. Inera AB has maintained the national health information exchange platform since its release. In October 2015, the monthly service invocation rate was 280,000,000, scattered across 180 national service contracts (integration profiles) supported by 4,500 endpoints (local and regional health information system installations). Roughly 2,000 of the clinical endpoints were connected during 2015, as part of the migration from the legacy EHR viewer (built on a closed/dedicated connectivity architecture) to a new version built to utilize the national HIE platform.

The third category of components developed was national service contracts. A service contract defines the requirements of a service-oriented communication end-point in terms of technical protocol, message formats (request and response messages) and functional and nonfunctional requirements of the interacting parties. The EHRs of the Swedish health care providers implement service-oriented communication end-points in line with these service contracts. The service contracts are based on OASIS WS-I Basic Profile 1.1 for technical interoperability. The messages of the clinical service contracts are designed according to the HL7 green CDA methodology. Security of message transfer between connected nodes is achieved at the transport level, by standardizing on https and mutual authentication (TLS). Message-based security is not used in the national technical interoperability profiles. The portfolio of national service contracts is governed by Inera AB. The service contract portfolio contains about 200 released service contracts (interoperability profiles). They have been developed, verified and applied in production scenarios since 2009. About 25 % of the released service contracts have been developed by Stockholm county council and thereafter handed over to Inera for governance and maintenance. The financing of this development has either been made directly by Stockholm county council or by external funding that Stockholm has applied for. Sometimes the external funding has been channeled through Inera due to administrative reasons although the application has been made by Stockholm county council.

The exchange of healthcare provider information across the HIE platform is regulated through commercial and data control agreements between county councils and Inera AB. The HIE platform and its management has become a hub for both information exchange and data control agreements.

Service contracts comprise API requirements for security, functionality and message structure. This means that beside APIs with code, service contracts contain for instance SLA requirements, e.g. response time, uptime, load, speed and recovery time. Over the period 2009–2011 service contracts were developed to support interoperability domains of scheduling, listing, security and drugs. Hereafter the focus has been on facilitating reuse of clinical data stored in local and regional health information systems. By the end of 2010, 95 % of hospital care and primary care centers were connected in line with the preferred care provider service contracts. Appointment scheduling expanded in a slower process. By the end of 2015, about 50 EHR end point systems support the service contracts for appointment scheduling. In Stockholm county council there are more than 1,500 Electronic Health Record (EHR) systems installed. However, one of the EHR systems holds about 80 % of the clinical data in Stockholm county council.

The ministry of Social Affairs promoted the interconnections of healthcare provider's systems to clinical service contracts by means of economic incentives and support. At the end of 2015 100 % of the county council's healthcare providers will be connected to the subset of clinical service contracts (facilitating reuse of clinical data) of most interest to the patient and the healthcare professionals. These are the service contracts covering medication history (ordination, prescription and administration of medications), clinical notes, care contacts, diagnosis and laboratory order outcome. In all there are 21 clinical service contracts covering reuse of all patient related clinical data in an EHR system.

The service contracts cover several areas of information exchange: (1) Re-use of medical records from the complete health care system: Clinical notes, medication history, structured observations, referral outcomes, imaging outcomes, laboratory order outcomes, referral status, immunization history, alert information, ECG outcomes, maternity medical records, care encounters and care plans (2) Care provider/ Governmental agency information exchange: e-prescriptions, medical certificates; (3) National Master data Catalogues (unique citizen social security numbers, unique medical professional and healthcare provider identities; and (4) National agencies (Social Insurance (illness certificates) and Ministry of Social Affairs (code systems)).

All healthcare providers work with their preferred EHR systems and work processes in a heterogeneous environment where they can exchange information across organizational boundaries with partners that are supported by completely different EHR systems and work processes. Everyone has access to the information in its own installed technology base and in its own existing work processes. In this way the multiplicity and heterogeneity can remain whilst access to information across organizational boundaries is secured.

14.2.4 Core Components Developed by Stockholm County Council

In addition to the three components described above, four other core components were developed in parallel by Stockholm county council. They are offered on a national level by Stockholm county council. This means that maintenance is not yet funded by all county councils through Inera and is not yet governed by Inera. It is instead funded and governed by Stockholm county council through a parallel business model with connected county councils, however, negotiations are ongoing regarding ownership and funding in order to have a single coordinated funding and governance structure. The handover of components between local, regional and national levels are conveyed according a complicated organizational arrangement. It had reached a point where it was unclear if de facto-national infrastructure components developed by Stockholm County Council would be canonized into national governance at Inera AB. Meanwhile Stockholm county council has – for future development of nationally applicable solutions – decided to initiate development through the Inera program office. However, since Inera has limited resources to govern initiatives, the board of the 21 county councils has to prioritize which regional projects to govern. In that respect the ecosystem evolution seems threatened by new elements of centralization in conflict with the architecture principle of organic/local evolution/contribution to the national ecosystem.

The fourth component is the Application Framework. This is a generic name for application frameworks supporting development targeted at healthcare, researchers and citizens. The application frameworks consist of downloadable open source code framework and API documentation for simplified development of solutions that depend on web browser and mobile app client access to the HIE platform. Applications require login via strong authentication. Through the application framework, various systems and e-services can reuse for example single-sign-on and context-managing functions. Simplified access to the endpoints of the HIE platform are managed by the Application framework, e.g. ADL, Imaging Outcome, Diagnosis, Care Documentation, ECG, Functional Status, Prescribed Medication, Laboratory Outcome, Care Contacts, Maternity Medical History, Care Plan, Alerts, Medication History, Vaccinations, Care services, Other Examinations, Medication, Form service.

The fifth component is the Application Innovation Portal (HIP – Health Innovation Platform). It is a web-based one-stop-shop for developers of eHealth solutions that want to utilize national and regional infrastructures. The aim of the Health Innovation Platform is to provide information and access to service development kits (SDK) of various infrastructure components, including the application frameworks. The information includes methods, guidelines and complete code samples for service development – in both traditional environment and for mobile solutions for developers and designers. Through the Innovation Platform, developers both within and outside health care get up-to-date and streamlined one-stop-shop access to resources they need to create solutions that access data from medical record systems and other sources in a simple and secure manner according to national rules for access to patient data. The Innovation Platform holds development Kits targeted for the innovation of citizen, healthcare and research services. In short, the Innovation Platform is the software developer's user interface to innovation resources that boost application development.

The sixth component is the Open Data Platform, a storage- and API platform for open access to data that is made available in line with the European Public Sector Information directive. Open data is made available to support innovation but it is also the means to provide APIs to non-personal healthcare master data required by e-services. This includes care provider master data, such as organizational structure, contact information, opening hours and care offering. Other examples include terminology and quality indicator master data. This offloads the national HIE platform from handling data that is publically accessible. Open data do not contain personal information and thus places no demands on secure access. The Open Data Platform is implemented in a highly scalable cloud infrastructure. Data kept in the Open Data Platform is synchronized (double stored) from the sources and made available via APIs that follow today's best practice ("RESTFul"). APIs are described on the Application innovation portal.

The seventh component is the Patient-directed Connectivity Platform. This is a platform that offers patients the ability to share EHR information services and applications, and has been part of the national infrastructure since 2014. Social media has evolved far beyond e-services supplied by healthcare information owners. We can see how social services like Twitter, Google, LinkedIn, Runkeeper and Facebook have moved beyond e-services by offering its users the ability to control how information from the user's account is shared with other services and applications. Information and functions are made available through APIs. Facebook and many other social media services offer its users a dual interface: applications (e.g. the Facebook web application and the Facebook iOS application) and a user-controlled API. The Swedish county councils have a strategy to mirror this duality: The National Patient Portal offer a citizen/patient-controlled API in addition to patient e-services (detailed in the next section). The citizen/patient-controlled API is secured by the OAuth protocol. The use of the OAuth protocol makes sure that the patient is in control of which data is accessible by which app that connects to the Patient-directed Connectivity Platform. Only the patient/citizen can grant a third-party application access to EHR data through the Patient-directed Connectivity Platform. Technically, the platform obtains EHR data "on demand" from the source EHR, via the national HIE platform services. In other words, the patient-controlled API is an infrastructure layered on top of the HIE platform. This is a property it shares with patient e-services. The e-services however – do not depend on user/patient authorization to be able to access the information. They are part of the trusted network and information access of these e-services are – unlike the third party apps – under the responsibility and data control of the county councils.

From a legal perspective, the information is owned by the patient as soon as it leaves this infrastructure component and enters a patient-directed (and authorized) endpoint (third-party application). An organization that offers such an application to its users, must obtain the user's consent to be able to store or process personal data on behalf of the user. This applies even if the organization is a care provider, since the data – although sourced from an EHR – has become a possession of the user during its journey from the EHR to the app.

14.3   The Development and Evolution of the Swedish Patient Directed Infrastructure

In the beginning of 2000 Stockholm County Council started a patient portal and a personal health record project. The aim was to enable patients to communicate with their physician or nurse and to refill medications. The long term objective was to achieve patient centered safe and high quality care and prevention. In parallel the Association of County Councils in Sweden took the initiative to establish a public eHealth portal. This was extended in 2006 by the Association of County Councils to also include a patient portal project to offer patient-initiated refill of medications. How these different regional and national projects aligned into one gateway for Swedish citizen's national patient portal and personal health record will be described in this section (see also Fig. 14.3. for the overall timeline). This is the first phase of the evolution into a Patient Directed infrastructure.

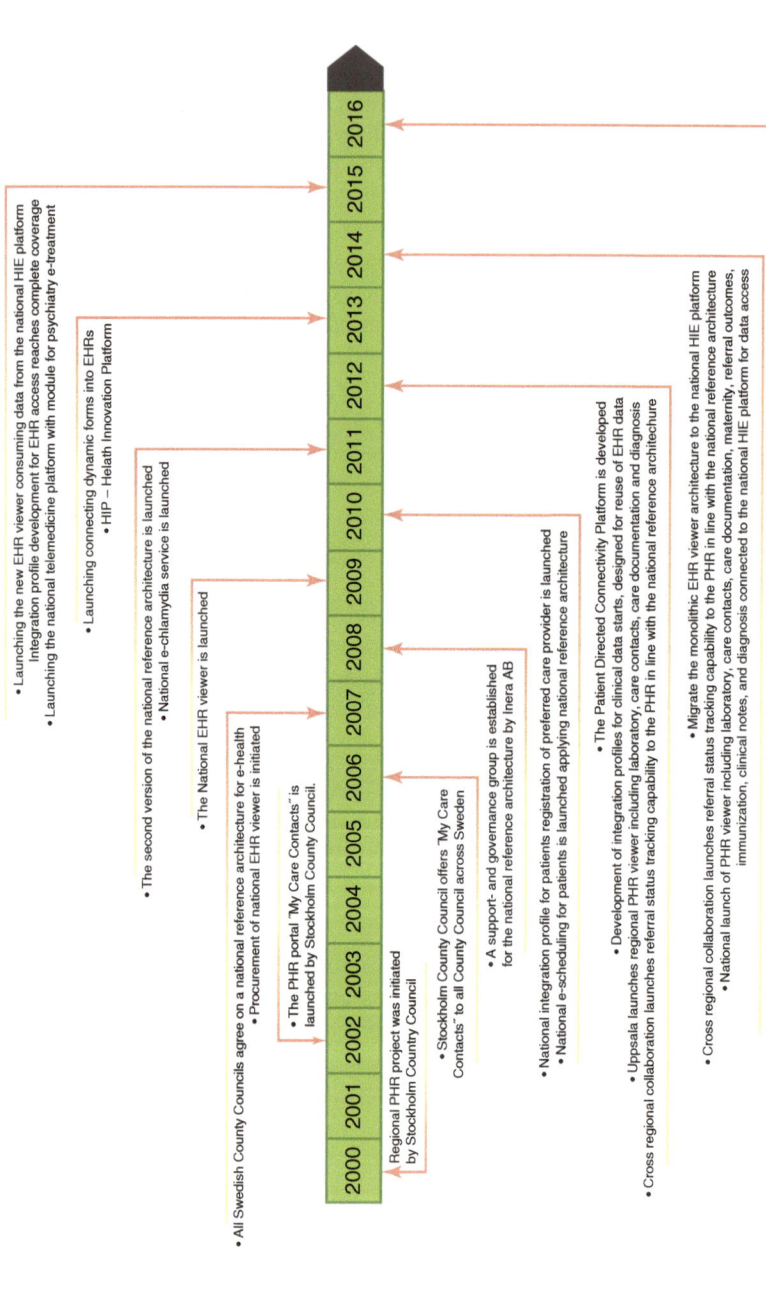

Fig. 14.3. Timeline of Swedish eHealth Architecture development

14.3.1   Phase 1: Development of My Healthcare Contacts and Public Web

In the spring of 2000 the Stockholm County Council Executive Board decided to start the project Healthcare Guide. The stated aim for Healthcare Guide was to provide a "secure message feature" between patients and healthcare providers, and this was compared to the increasing use of Internet banks. The secure messaging could be used to share information, send inquiries, communicate and inform patients. It created a digital channel for individual care by offering a network of information and services that promoted the responsibility and participation of citizens in matters of their own health (preventive actions management and self-care); allowed digital interaction between citizens and the health system, providers and professionals; provided information on health care quality in different care areas in particular related to common diseases. Technically the creation of the public web portal started with the requirement on the platform to support x.509 certificates which was the standard for Swedish eID. The digital channel for individual care got the name My Healthcare Contacts after an internal Stockholm County Council name contest. The new platform was managed and owned by Stockholm County Council. In the spring of 2002, the development of My Healthcare Contacts began together with six healthcare centers (four Stockholm county council owned and two privately owned). During the fall 2002, the first pilots were launched with a limited number of forms such as Schedule Appointment, Renew Prescription and Cancel/Reschedule Appointment. There was a high demand for prescription services since it was often difficult to reach healthcare centers by phone. Consultation and prescription over the phone is a medical practice in Sweden. The rollout involved the cooperation and engagement of several local health providers and professionals who worked close to citizens and patients; information and communication campaigns to the public. There was never a conflict with professionals regarding My Healthcare Contacts. A reason for this may be that the e-services offered did not entail profound changes in the role and relationships between doctors and patients, and between doctors themselves. Instead early on results showed increased work processes effectiveness and less need for accessing healthcare centers by phone for renewal of prescriptions or bookings. As the awareness and use of My Healthcare Contacts increased in Stockholm county council the interest in the solution was also increasing from various other county councils. A negotiation process started which resulted in agreements between Stockholm county council and other councils e.g. Västmanland, Skåne and Halland. Through the agreements signed in 2011 all remaining councils join the cooperative development of My Healthcare Contacts led by Stockholm county council.

At that time Inera (which was then named "Sjukvårdsrådgivningen AB"), was offering public national medical related advice to patients – as searchable text on the web and through a phone service operated by healthcare professionals. My Healthcare Contacts (also including a public web site) and Sjukvårdsrådgivningen had become equally large sites by 2010. However, My Healthcare Contacts offered more services than the national site, e.g. Find Care Unit and Compare Queue Time.

A new national project called Healthcare Online started in 2006, where Sjukvårdsrådgivningen wanted to create a national patient service where both the public web and the personal part would be built into a single portal platform. The public procurement that Sjukvårdsrådgivningen had conducted wasn't able to deliver, and the agreement with the vendor was terminated in the end of 2008.

At the same time, in 2008, Stockholm county council had continued its work to modernize their public site by switching to a supplier who already worked with agile practices and high delivery capability. Meanwhile, the national use of "My Healthcare Contacts" grew as an independent and relatively modular service, by means that its governance was not funded by national finances. Interestingly, by that time Stockholm county council was outperformed by another county council in terms of the number of care units connected to My Healthcare Contacts. Gradually it became obvious that the technical platform would need to be replaced as it got obsolete, but the question was how. Some felt that the entire application should be rewritten. But in the end it was decided not to shift platform. Instead, the strategy was to keep the technical platform for message handling and complement and link it to other more modern and open technology platforms for new functionality and new services. Said and done, My Healthcare Contacts got a new interface with responsive design for adaptation to mobile devices in 2012.

When Sjukvårdsrådgivningen had terminated their agreement with their preferred partner in 2008, the manager at Stockholm county council got a request to collaborate with the national Healthcare Online project. The result from the negotiations was that Stockholm provided a copy of the public web sites code to Sjukvårdsrådgivningen. The site got a new name 1177.se, and was now maintained by Sjukvårdsrådgivningen and not Stockholm. At this time Sjukvårdsrådgivningen was transformed into Inera. Inera was assigned to work with infrastructure including national HIE platforms.

In 2007, CareLink – a national eHealth standardization body owned by the county councils – released the first version of a national reference architecture for eHealth. In 2007 a new national eHealth program office was formed in which counties interacted and cooperated in an organized manner. This national program office function was called CeHis – Center for eHealth. A subsection of CeHis established an architecture governance unit to secure reference architecture conformance across the national eHealth projects coordinated by CeHis. The responsibility of the reference architecture development was transferred from CareLink to this unit. A new version of the reference architecture was released in 2011. The major highlights of the new version of the reference architecture were related to patient empowerment. The result of this work was for example six architecture principles and a set of supporting architectural patterns. It also contributed guiding examples for a list of prioritized eHealth scenarios. Stockholm county council and to some extent Inera initiated projects to establish the the national infrastructure capabilities outlined by the national reference architecture. Stockholm county council funded the majority of these capabilities. After capabilities had been developed and piloted by Stockholm county council they were handed over to Inera for maintenance. Inera receives collective financing from the county councils for this maintenance work. The uptake of the reference architecture among county councils, national projects and vendors on the market increased gradually with the increased awareness of its value to the eHealth ecosystem. In 2013 CeHis was incorporated into Inera AB. The architecture unit of former CeHis was reborn as the department of architecture of Inera AB.

In 2012 Stockholm got the national responsibility for citizen services including both the public web site and the secure digital channel My Healthcare Contacts. In 2014 My Healthcare Contacts was extended with a patient EHR viewer. This work has been funded by both regional and national program offices for development and maintenance. The purpose was to give citizens and patients digital access to the health records of the complete installed base of EHR systems. This was a prioritized goal of the national eHealth action plan for 2013–2018. The primary information data sets to be shared with patients were care contacts, care documentation, vaccinations, referral and lab results, maternity care and diagnosis. Since all parts of the national eHealth architecture are de facto developed there is a mixture of national and non-national budgets supporting its operation and maintenance. The positive outcomes of this mixture point to the key role of organic evolution for the Swedish eHealth ecosystem. The pre-requisites of an organically grown national eHealth ecosystem are captured in one of the architecture principles of the national reference architecture. This principle (i.e. allowing organic development by county councils without relying to central directions by Inera) has been fundamental for the controlled – yet organic – evolution of the national infrastructure. If this development was not opened for many stakeholders the national installed infrastructure would have taken much longer time to develop. In this way many different actor networks in parallel developed the national infrastructure. Sometimes, the principle of organic development contributed to unexpected parallel development of competing solutions. Uppsala County Council and Stockholm County Council developed competing patient EHR viewer applications- both with national ambitions. At the end of 2015 the Uppsala solution had reached a significantly larger user base. Stockholm county council then decided to decommission the "My Care Pathways" viewer eService in favor of the Uppsala patient EHR viewer. This meant that the frontend of My Care Pathways solution was decommissioned but the backend, which had become a central part of the national HIE platform for EHR access, was utilized. One frontend eService that uses this backend is Uppsala Count Council's patient EHR system. For Swedish county councils to switch from one frontend (viewer eService) to another based on the same backend only requires administration of access rights.

14.3.2 Phase 2: Establishing and Developing the Patient Directed Connectivity Platform

This section describes how the development and modernization of My Care Contacts was conducted. It started with a presentation of an idea of a Patient Directed Connectivity Platform in late 2011. Work behind the idea was funded by Vinnova, the innovation agency in Sweden. One of the goals of the modernization project was to open up the portal architecture of My Healthcare Contacts to allow e-services to be developed and deployed outside of the portal platform itself. This should be accomplished in a way that independently deployed e-services would bring the same user experience as that of an e-service developed and deployed using the tools and infrastructure of the core portal product of My Healthcare Contacts. This would allow for regional development of national e-services using the development and deployment infrastructure of choice. The concept was labeled "The virtual portal architecture". The virtual portal architecture is aligned with the 4th national reference architectural principle "Integrations shall be loosely mapped and re-usable for many purposes" and is thus part of the national eHealth architecture.

The modernization project had a substantial budget. It was critical to expand the pace in development of patient e-services beyond what was possible with the portal infrastructure which was available at the time and its vendor lock-in. However, the platform modernization didn't really happen – at least not in the intended sense. Instead, focus shifted from strategic goals of vendor neutrality and increase of e-service delivery capabilities into the following main priorities:

– A new look-and-feel with support for mobile devices through responsive design
– Development of new e-services
– Governance and policy framework for hosting e-services from multiple sources

The idea of providing patient-controlled APIs along with e-services was scoped out due to resource constraints. The modernization project started in late 2010 and finished in midst of 2012. My Care Pathways was set up in 2011 with a high ambition to create several of the national service contracts, an open architecture for e-service as well as third party connectivity. In this aspect, the new project picked up where the prior modernization project was stopped: among other deliveries it delivered a virtual portal architecture proof-of-concept and a Patient Directed Connectivity Platform. All infrastructure deliveries were aligned with the national reference architecture, catering for future national uptake. This was achieved by tight collaboration with architects of the national program office at Inera. This project delivered both several back-end infrastructure components e.g. the open data API platform, Patient-Directed Connectivity Platform, Application Innovation Portal, Application Framework, Care Process Services and Questionnaire engine and front-end web services and APPs, e.g. national Form service, Survey tool, Notices, Referral status and My Care Pathways.

The Patient Directed Connectivity Platform was developed during 3 months starting in December 2011 with its first live demo on the national eHealth fair in April 2012. The demo third party application was a utility application that re-published appointments as live, subscribable webcal links. The vendor of the utility application offered the patient a live view of appointments directly in the private native calendar application of any mobile device:

Because several appointment/encounter modules of local and regional health information systems were connected to the HIE platform, the Patient Directed Connectivity Platform just had to connect to the appointment scheduling API of the

HIE platform as client in order to access patient's appointments within all connected health information systems. The Patient Directed Connectivity Platform then re-publishes the SOAP APIs as OAuth-secured REST APIs. The third party demo application acts as a client to the OAuth-protected API of the Patient Directed Connectivity Platform. The developers of the third party application used the Application Innovation Portal to learn about and explore the appointment API of the Patient Directed Connectivity Platform. They also utilized the open data platform API to get access to health care organization master data so that they could display opening hours and contact information of the appointed facility. More e-services and apps are being developed. More importantly there has been a cultural shift where apps are requested by both caregivers, patients and researchers, whereas it before was not considered as safe. Now the focus is what app is needed and how fast and easy can it be designed through the use of the Application Innovation Portal.

Although every relevant piece of the installed base were connected using the national HIE platform and applicable service contracts, information wouldn't be accessible by the third party application unless (a) each care provider authorizes the Patient Directed Connectivity Platform access to appointment records and (b) the patient uses the patient portal to grant the utility application access to a personal copy of appointment information serviced by the Patient Directed Connectivity Platform.

Both of these requirements have proven to be challenging. The public care providers generally don't seem to prioritize patient-controlled information access to the same extent as private care providers.

Regarding "b" the national organization holding the policy for connecting applications needs to find a balance between a thriving marketplace and trusting information owners. Several options are discussed for boosting the care provider's willingness to support the concept of patient-directed connectivity:

–   Third-party/care provider match-making forums
–   Providing the patient means to digitally request information sharing capabilities from her care provider (as a feature of the patient portal)
–   Public quality indicators that allows public ranking of healthcare facilities based on the amount of data that is available for sharing with third-party applications

If the trust problem is solved a number of new possibilities to create value on patients copy of EHR data are foreseen.

A number of workshops and conference presentations have been performed over 4 years of time to inform about the new possibilities. But the main efforts were targeted at the developer community. Public care providers still show very little awareness of the concept and thus do not actively grant the patient directed connectivity platform access to the EHR data through their existing national HIE platform connections.

There is however an agreement between the Ministry of EHealth and the 21 county councils to support the infrastructure as soon as the nationally procured Personal Health Account is launched. The purpose of the agreement is that the PHR will connect to the patient directed connectivity platform. The patients will then be able to direct EHR connectivity to their account of the PHR service. In order for information to actually be available for transfer to the PHR, each care provider need to authorize the patient directed connectivity platform EHR access. Once this has happened, the same EHR information will be available for other third party applications as will (in addition to the national PHR).

Examples on information sets accessible by users of My Care Pathways include: clinical notes, healthcare contacts/appointment, prenatal care records, vaccinations, referral statuses, laboratory results, advice and support related to specific diagnoses, information about health care guarantee (referrals), child health information, living habits. Similar information sets were provided by the service delivered by the Uppsala project.

In 2013 Inera contacted Stockholm county council to negotiate a takeover of the e-service My Care Pathways. Inera wanted to combine this service with the solution provided by the Uppsala county council project. Due to contractual agreement with the financier of My Care Pathways this was not possible as there was commitment on commercialization outside of Sweden. However, Uppsala came to an agreement with Inera.

During the same time My Healthcare Contacts put forward the idea of developing a new national EHR viewer for all care givers in county councils and municipalities in Sweden. It was forwarded through Inera. The idea was granted and the development initiated. My Healthcare Contacts could give this offer due to the work conducted with My Care Pathways. Said and done, the new national EHR viewer for healthcare professionals, accessing information across organizational borders, was designed and internally tested over a period of 6 months. It was thereafter externally tested and verified for 1 year. In the end the e-service My Care Pathways for patients and citizens and the national EHR viewer for caregivers shared to 80% the same program code. The 15th of December 2015 the new National EHR viewer for healthcare professional was implemented in all county councils and municipalities. The implementation was a cooperation between My Healthcare Contacts at Stockholm County Council and Inera. It was a success project where all parties shared the same vision, aims, working structure and process, no second agendas were applied. During the rollout of the new national EHR viewer for healthcare professional, a new national test process was applied. From the implementation of the new national EHR viewer , the 15th of December, there has in average been 80,000 request for information daily. Its development was smooth, quick and successful and was an example of the installed infrastructures' flexibility, scaling and reusability. Over this period only one web application error has been reported. Never has it been so quiet around the implementation of a new national e-service with 5,000 connected EHR systems. When the trains run on time this does not generate any headlines in the media. This illustrates the meaning of aligned interests, appropriate test procedures, coming to agreements and following it up with a full commitment. At the same period Stockholm county council through negotiations with Inera decided to decommission and stop the My Care Pathways solution in favor of the Uppsala one. In return the assignment of developing a new platform for My Healthcare Contacts is being negotiated. The results of the negotiations are not finished.

14.4   Discussion: Cultivation of the Patient Portal and the Overall Installed eHealth Ecosystem

Analyzing the trajectory of the co-evolution of the Swedish patient portal, the eHealth Architecture and the overall eHealth infrastructure we can state that much work has been done within personal health informatics and clinical informatics as well as on integrating these two. In Sweden it is understood that in order to achieve patient centered safe and high quality care these two need to be integrated in an overall SOA architecture. Many different e-services have been developed e.g. e-services that give citizens access to for instance e-scheduling, e-pharmacy, access to personal health information, e-communication with their physician or nurse, and secure disclosure to their health data (generated in the public health-care system). These services have evolved by the replacement of old components, by complementing existing components and by building new ones. There are today many developments with further extensions of the existing eHealth Architecture. These projects are not restricted to one particular functionality but rather to manifold e.g. focusing on national interoperability issues between clinical information, patient care connectivity services whereas patient's own measurement are integrated with clinical information through apps and services linked to the EHR.

As has been described in this case, important parts of developing the national information infrastructure were security, safety and confidentiality issues, which are important since the question of trust is a key factor in the establishment of new digital tools. Security, safety and confidentiality is not only involving patients but also all Swedish County Councils and their care providers in an intertwined two-way information infrastructure that is evolving in a step-by-step process extending the installed base over time according to user, also including safety, needs. An important issue to elaborate on, when Sweden has come so far, is the security of the information infrastructure that can handle high volumes of national clinical data visualized through personalized health services.

New components can be linked as the shared reference architecture framework has been applied during the development work regardless of whether they has been developed on a local, regional or national level. Evolving the installed base local, regional and national parties have cooperated in a successful way through the shared use of the national reference architectural framework.

Various strategies and projects and activities have played different roles depending upon their character and timing. Many projects have cultivated the way individuals think about the design, interoperability and innovation of eHealth. Although some e-services did not reach a national implementation they still made an impact on the development of other e-services and infrastructure components. The importance of choosing the relevant marketing and implementation channel is crucial for the spread and usage of e-services. These examples illustrate that factors of quality, costs and functionality are of minor importance. The examples also illustrates that if a strategy has reached a maturity among its stakeholders and if implementation channels are chosen by influence and power anything can work.

In Sweden the eHealth projects have undergone a transformation from being cultural to structural and process oriented when they share the same backend. Overall, the foundation of Swedish eHealth development work is based on complicated organizational arrangements. The national reference architecture has shown itself to be an important stability actor in this work, i.e. something that actors can fall back on and agree on in their discussions. The National reference architecture constitute here a direction of what is correct, even though it is open to interpretation.

To allow different actors to individually or jointly contribute to the applied SOA architecture has led to a distributed development work. The challenges have primarily been related to power factors, i.e. negotiations between different parties at different levels. The county directors' role and responsibility to steer and control Inera's work have been more or less exerted over the years. This has of course led to a direct impact on Inera's prioritization work. In all, steering has become weaker over time.

One conclusion to draw is that if there is a national reference architecture in place, it is something that increases the likelihood of the parties to agree in negotiations. If they have a commitment to fulfill agreements is another issue. Much needs to be matched for the parties shall agree, cooperate, get involved and together successfully reach a goal.

Our findings support the argument that infrastructure evolvement come out of the complex interplay between many different actors intertwined in step-by-step cultivation. In Sweden the infrastructure evolvement is done through the governance of a reference architecture endorsed by all entities contributing to the installed base.

References

OECD, OECD Health Statistics 2014, How does Sweden compare? Available at: http://www.oecd.org/els/health-systems/Briefing-Note-SWEDEN-2014.pdf.
WHO, http://www.who.int/countries/swe/en/.

Open Access This chapter is distributed under the terms of the Creative Commons Attribution-NonCommercial 2.5 International License (http://creativecommons.org/licenses/by-nc/2.5/), which permits any noncommercial use, duplication, adaptation, distribution and reproduction in any medium or format, as long as you give appropriate credit to the original author(s) and the source, provide a link to the Creative Commons license and indicate if changes were made.

The images or other third party material in this chapter are included in the chapter's Creative Commons license, unless indicated otherwise in a credit line to the material. If material is not included in the chapter's Creative Commons license and your intended use is not permitted by statutory regulation or exceeds the permitted use, you will need to obtain permission directly from the copyright holder.

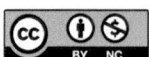

The Origins of a Healthcare e-Booking System in the Municipality of Bologna

15

Andrea Resca and Mauro Moruzzi

15.1   Introduction

In Italy, the introduction of the National Health Service (*Servizio Sanitario Nazionale* – SSN) in 1978, based on law 833/1978, provided municipalities with the opportunity to make substantial innovations in healthcare. Hospital-centred care was considered outdated. The aim was to dispense with a model based on hospital hubs on the one side and general practitioners (GPs) spread throughout the area on the other. The latter operated as gatekeepers to hospital services, and still do. The introduction of the SSN challenged a healthcare system that had developed largely independently from the characteristics of the socio-economic context. Hospitals, in alliance with the medical profession and the academic environment, determined services, or supply, that corresponded only partially to the demand from citizens and regions. The law outlined a framework for rebalancing this situation. Improving citizens' access to healthcare was an element of National Health Service reform, especially in the city of Bologna where long waiting lists, fragmented offerings and a lack of transparency characterized access to secondary care. The municipality of Bologna addressed these issues by creating booking centres supported by information technology enabling citizens to book services for secondary care. In Italy, and very probably Europe, this was the first instance of an information system connecting distributed booking offices at the city level. Since 1990, citizens have been able to use this e-booking service to access specialist ambulatory services, including visits and diagnostic activities.

A. Resca (✉)
LUISS Guido Carli University, Rome, Italy
e-mail: aresca@luiss.it

M. Moruzzi
CUP2000 s.p.a, Bologna, Italy
e-mail: mauro.moruzzi@cup2000.it

© The Author(s) 2017   245
M. Aanestad et al. (eds.), *Information Infrastructures within European Health Care*, Health Informatics, DOI 10.1007/978-3-319-51020-0_15

In this chapter, we analyze the origin of the e-booking service. The interpretative framework for investigating the advent of an e-booking service is provided by the concept of information infrastructure, focusing specifically on the role of the installed base (Hanseth and Lyytinen 2010; Hanseth et al. 1996). The concept of installed base includes both standing elements and systems already in place and existing institutional and organizational components (Bongsug and Lanzara 2006; Ciborra and Hanseth 2000). We study how the installed base was involved in the realization of this innovative service.

The literature suggests that the installed base can have both hindering and enabling effects on technical and institutional innovation (Lanzara 2009). The case in question represents an instance in which the existing installed base challenged the institutional and organizational innovation process. The healthcare system revealed itself as a trap from which it was difficult to escape (Lanzara 2009). In fact, a service like e-booking implied abandoning routines and practices that characterized paper-based booking. Alternative organizational arrangements had to be devised as the hospital and GP-centred model did not provide a supportive environment for this innovative form of access. Emphasis was put on the mobilization of installed base components related to political, organizational and technological resources originated outside healthcare. Our objective is to shed light on what led to innovative institutional arrangements and organizational routines and what capabilities were needed to challenge the established normative order and enable the creation of e-booking.

We begin with a brief overview of Italian healthcare. In the sections that follow we present the overall trajectory of the centralized booking system over the period 1990–2015 and subsequently present an investigation of the origins of the e-booking system. We focus on a period that starts in 1987 with the issue of the Health Plan by the municipality of Bologna and ends in 1993 when the innovative booking system went full speed. We end by presenting our analysis and discuss the mobilization of installed base resources for putting e-booking in place.

Method

This chapter is based on a longitudinal study on the evolution of an e-booking system. Following Yin (2009), this can be considered both a critical and a revelatory case study as it is, probably, the first example of a solution that supports citizens' access to healthcare in Europe and because of its capacity to develop both in scale and scope.

One of the authors had a leading role in the project and was a direct witness of its main phases, participating in meetings and boards at both the political and organizational level, with access to the related documentation. Data collection was integrated with semi-structured, in-depth interviews with the key players in the project. Twelve interviews were carried out between 2013 and 2015. Archival data were used as well as Italian publications related to this experience.

15.2 Italian Healthcare Overview

The National Health Service (*Servizio Sanitario Nazionale* – SSN) was introduced in Italy in 1978 (law 833/1978) and replaced the previous system of state insurance that had been founded after the Second World War. The aim was to create an efficient and uniform health system covering the entire population, irrespective of income or contributions, employment or pre-existing health conditions. The SSN provides free or low-cost healthcare to all residents (including those from other EU countries) and emergency care to visitors, irrespective of their nationality.

The proposed healthcare model outlined an alternative to the previous hospital-centred model, by creating a network of health facilities addressing the needs of the different socio-economic contexts. The aim was to create a network of health facilities able to respond to the characteristics of the different regions, which meant local government, specifically the municipalities, acquired a leading role. Healthcare based on the medical profession, academic medical science and technological development revolving around hospitals was challenged by a vision that put citizens and their living and working conditions at the centre – or, more accurately, proposed the *decentralization* of service provision, initiated by the establishment of local health facilities. However, results were questionable and the dwindling role of hospitals was not fully covered by the provision of appropriate continuity-of-care services as well as prevention, treatment and rehabilitation programmes. Families with members suffering from mental illnesses, chronic diseases and the non-self-sufficient elderly bore the burden of this situation (Moruzzi 2009).

Local health units (*Unità Sanitaria Locale* – USL) were in charge of the transformation of the healthcare model. These were local authorities and Bologna, a city with about 400,000 inhabitants, had three USLs. The national level allocated resources to regions that, in turn, supported USLs financially. Regions were also in charge of healthcare planning. However, USL management was in the hands of the municipalities. As the government level closest to citizens, they appointed USL management committees that represented local communities and spoke for them. The intention was to monitor closely healthcare provision to citizens.

At the beginning of the 1990s, this governance system went into crisis due to four main factors: the financial instability of the municipalities; the involvement of management committee members in political corruption scandals; the rise of neo-liberal policies at European level during the 1980s; and the expensive and fragmented organization of healthcare services (Moruzzi 2014).

Laws 502/1992 and 517/1993 reorganized healthcare and were dubbed the "counter-reform" of law 833/1978. USLs were transformed into local state-run companies (*Azienda Sanitaria Locale* – ASL) and big hospitals acquired a new status, University Hospital Company (*Azienda Ospedaliero Universitaria* – AOU). These organizations centralized control with three leadership positions (managing director, health director, administrative director). Management committees nominated by the municipalities were ousted and the region became the appointing authority. Social health districts, led by the municipalities, were introduced to represent local requirements and to promote integration with social services but their influence on healthcare has been limited.

A consequence of this reform was that traditional hospital-centred healthcare, governed by the medical profession and typical of the pre-National Health Service era, did not re-emerge. However, regional and corporate bureaucracy was imposed once the USL management committees were abolished. The most significant implication of this was that it proved impossible to integrate healthcare and social assistance in accordance with the 1978 legal schedule. Finally, healthcare in Italy is still governed by regulatory structures at both regional and unit level that emphasize political and bureaucratic control rather than the development of medical activities.

15.3   The Evolution of a Centralized Booking System: 1990–2015

Since 22 January 1990, every citizen of the municipality of Bologna in need of a specialist appointment or a medical examination has been able to access a dedicated centre and book an appointment through an e-booking system that pools the services available at city hospitals and health centres. A number of booking centres spread across the city was one of the main objectives of the 1987 Municipal Health Plan to deal with long waiting lists and the difficulties citizens encountered in accessing health services. At the end of the first year of operation, 264,048 users contacted e-booking centres for a total of 610,498 transactions.

In the years since, the centralized booking service has developed in both scale and scope. Table 15.1 outlines the phases that have characterized this evolution.

Pharmacies became involved shortly after the inauguration of the service, due to their network presence and the possibility of offering widespread access points to healthcare. As private businesses, they were not used to collaborate with public institutions, like the municipality of Bologna, for improving healthcare. Significant resistance had to be overcome, as e-booking was not considered an appropriate service to be provided to pharmacies and related competences were not available. However, it was clear that pharmacies did have a role to play in healthcare and after an initial experimental period, the large majority joined the project, representing a solution to offering a wider range of services. However, at first (1996) booking activity was limited to restricted services and it was only after several years that the same range was made available to both pharmacies and booking centres.

In 1990, citizens living outside the boundaries of the municipality of Bologna accessed secondary healthcare using paper-based procedures supplied in each health facility. Things changed in 1999 when the centralized e-booking service was enlarged to cover the entire area. At that point, further 600,000 people, making a total of about 1 million, were able to take advantage of e-booking centres. By the second half of the 1990s, the booking system, which had been designed in a pre-internet era, was considered outdated and inadequate for extending scale and scope. In 1999 a tender for its substitution was issued and the new e-booking system went

Table 15.1 Key milestones in the evolution of the centralized booking system for health services in Bologna

Year	Central e-booking system: scale	Central e-booking system: scope
1990	Every citizen has access to 25 e-booking centres (inc. hospitals, health centres and department store) throughout Bologna to book specialist appointments or medical examinations provided at municipal level	
1996	E-booking possible at pharmacies but only some medical examinations available. Number of centres reduced to 19	
1999	E-booking centres spread throughout the metropolitan area (Bologna and 50 municipalities in the province)	Able to book services provided by "*intramoenia*", accredited health facilities and private healthcare
2000	The software system is substituted following a competitive tender	Call centre introduced as an additional channel for booking. The range of services available is limited and will be extended in subsequent years
2003	Pharmacies provide the same services as e-booking centres	A website for changes and cancellations to bookings launched; only some services available for e-booking
2006		Electronic waiting lists introduced
2010	Ferrara is included in the e-booking system	
2012		Citizens able to book services from their own electronic personal health record (only services not subject to GP referral)
2013	Launch of the regional e-booking website	
2014	Modena and Reggio Emilia included in the e-booking system	Both the e-booking website and the electronic personal health record offer the possibility to book services subject to GP referral

into operation the following year. At first, the services provided were limited to the public healthcare. Later, the aim was to make available the full range of health services, including those supplied by the *intramoenia* (intramurale) regime (private practice confined to public facilities), accredited health facilities and private healthcare.

A call centre was established in 2000. This was an additional channel for managing appointments and medical examinations. In 2003 the booking website was launched. After this point, citizens did not need to turn to a booking centre, a pharmacy or a call centre to access healthcare. However, only changes to bookings, cancellations and a restricted number of services were made available online.

In 2006, electronic waiting lists were introduced. When a service provided by public healthcare did not meet citizens' needs, their position in these lists could be changed. This meant they were continuously monitored and were offered alternative opportunities that emerged in the meantime. The figures (2006) illustrate the extent of e-booking: 3,100,000 users per year; 13,000,000 operations per year; a catalogue of 1920 services available; 6600 specialists. All of this was facilitated by 136 counters in hospitals and health centres; 236 counters in pharmacies; a call centre with 28 dedicated telephone lines; and a website.

In recent years, other provinces in the Emilia Romagna region – Ferrara (2010), Modena (2014) and Reggio Emilia (2014) – have all decided to adopt the e-booking system used in Bologna. The e-booking service was a good fit with two other projects promoted by the region and central government: electronic personal health records and e-prescriptions. Since 2012, all citizens in Emilia Romagna had been able to access an electronic folder containing documents related to their care, provided by healthcare facilities and the patients themselves. The functions of the electronic personal health record included e-booking, which was limited to services not subject to GP referral, such as gynecology, ophthalmology and prevention. In 2014 e-prescriptions were also included in this category of services. In 2013 the regional booking website was launched. Due to the integration of several booking services, it was possible to have access to the entire range of services available at regional level.

15.4   Early Stages: From Design to Deployment of an e-Booking System

15.4.1 Antecedents of an e-Booking System

In the transition period that followed the introduction of the National Health Service, the new role of primary care and abandoning hospital-centred healthcare created problems in secondary care. Specifically, in the city of Bologna they resulted in long waiting lists and difficulty in accessing the range of services offered by a large number of providers. In 1987, the municipality of Bologna, in charge of the supervision of USLs, decided to formulate a Health Plan to addressing the emerging situation in consequence of unsatisfactory results related to the implementation of healthcare reform. The Health Plan had three main objectives: (1) to increase investment in diagnostic and therapeutic technologies; (2) to promote a campaign supporting health self-protection; (3) to improve citizens' access to healthcare.

The second half of the 1980s also saw the advent of informatics in the public sector. A large proportion of public administrations launched computerization plans to introduce automated procedures. Innovations, like e-booking systems, became objects of interest. In one of the city hospitals an automated registry of cancer cases was introduced, thanks to support from the University of Bologna. The collaboration between these two parties had produced a pilot of an e-booking system; it was presented to the city but without success. It was evident the project needed to scale-up to build a city-level system. So the collaboration was extended to the National Research Council and the state-owned ITALSIEL, at that time the largest software company in Italy.

15.4.2 Getting Ready for the Service Launch

Unlike today, neither central nor local governments were subject to financial pressures and the Ministry of Health decided to support the e-booking project proposed by the municipality of Bologna. Project design started at the beginning of 1989 and the system was expected to be ready by the end of the year. Within a few weeks, the architecture of the database was available and software development followed. At the same time, the service catalogue was compiled. Standardizing the terminology used to describe services was a fundamental concern: hospitals and health centres had different ways of identifying a radiology examination or an abdominal ultrasound on the basis of the practices they adopted. The catalogue also standardized guidelines for patients preparing for medical examinations. A software solution, supporting the use of synonyms, facilitated agreement about service descriptions and promoted the building of the service catalogue.

In 1989 the Single Booking Centre (*Centro Unificato di Prenotazione* – CUP) directorate was created within the Health Department of the municipality of Bologna. This was an inter-institutional office composed of personnel from the three USLs and led by the city councillor in charge of the department. This entity governed the entire project.

The decision not to assign the management of e-booking centres to USLs meant an alternative organizational unit, external to the healthcare sector, had to be created to take charge of them. SYNWARE was established in the spring of 1989 and staff selection (about 100 employees) began a few months later. In the autumn of that year, training courses introduced the basic elements of the healthcare system and the use of the software solution, even though it was not yet ready. At the beginning of the new year, staff were assigned to the 25 centres in hospitals, health centres and one department store.

15.4.3 Fine-Tuning the e-Booking Service

The service was launched at the end of January 1990. From the first days of operation, activity was surprisingly regular, considering that the system was finalized just days before the launch and both patients and clerks were unfamiliar with the service. An improvement process was launched simultaneously involving all the main protagonists: the Health Department, the three USLs, ITALSIEL and SYNWARE. The Health Department, specifically the CUP directorate, led this process and a number of actions were taken.

As far as ITALSIEL was concerned, a new phase for the evolution of the system was inaugurated. At first, only a limited range of specialist visits and diagnostic activities was available. More complicated diagnostic activities began to be offered in the 2 years following the launch of the service. Booking time was another issue that had to be faced during this period. It was possible to reduce booking time from an average of 18–20 to 8–10 min thanks to the optimization of user interfaces (command line interfaces) and the introduction of software tools that facilitated the retrieval of services.

SYNWARE was subject to continuous innovation of its organizational arrangements. At first, the position of primary contact was created in the most critical centres in the city. The primary contact was a point of reference for clerks and hospital/ health centre supervisors in case of problems raised during service provision. The introduction of this role was considered effective but insufficient and a further organizational solution was adopted. The area covered by the municipality was subdivided into five macro areas, each headed by a coordinator who played a pivotal role as the addressee of questions raised by all the centres and other actors involved in the service (Health Department, USLs, ITALSIEL). The five coordinators constituted a unit responsible for dealing with dysfunctionalities, staff assessments and technological and organizational resources to guarantee regularity of service provision. However, this solution was also considered inadequate and a primary contact was established in each centre. This supervisory role established a contact point for coordinators. A help desk was set up in each centre to deal with inaccurate prescriptions and provide information about the range of services provided.

Besides coordinating ITALSIEL and SYNWARE activities, the most delicate responsibility of the CUP directorate was negotiating with hospitals to obtain services that could be included in the e-booking system. Before the introduction of e- booking, each hospital managed the type and number of services provided to outpatients autonomously. With the advent of the e-booking project, control moved to the CUP directorate. This change involved lengthy negotiation with hospitals to increase the extent of services to be offered on the centralized booking system.

The CUP directorate also managed the updating of the service catalogue necessitated by the introduction of new services or modification of existing ones.

The launch of the service entailed another activity that was closely monitored by the CUP directorate: updating service schedules. There was a plurality of service providers (e.g. several radiology units for each health facility), so it was necessary to know the full extent of services available. Unexpected events also had to be managed. A union strike, participation in a conference or sick leave could interrupt service provision. In these cases, schedules needed to be updated, patients informed and new appointments offered.

15.5 Analysis: The Mobilization of Installed Base Resources for the Construction of an e-Booking Service

In this section we analyse the realization of an e-booking system in the municipality of Bologna from the installed base perspective (Hanseth and Monteiro 1997; Ciborra and Hanseth 2000). This entails looking at how an intricate web of technological and institutional resources (Bowker and Star 1999; Lanzara 2009; Star and Ruhleder 1996) was reconfigured to build this service. We focus on how political, organizational and technological resources were mobilized to move from paper-based booking in individual health facilities to a centralized e-booking system that could pool the health services available at city level.

15.5.1 The Mobilization of Political Resources

Political resources had to be mobilized for coordinating, negotiating and building consensus about the e-booking project. The Health Department, represented by a city councillor, was the main protagonist and played a leadership role in both the design and realization of the project. Like a large proportion of Bologna's city council, including the mayor, the city councillor was member of the local branch of the Italian Communist Party (PCI). However, the organization of healthcare was influenced not only by a state-centric perspective, typical of communist ideology, but also by the Europe-wide 1968 social movement. The experience of barefoot doctors in China, emphasizing the importance of local medicine, occupational health and de-hospitalization, also constituted an important point of reference. Unsurprisingly, some party members distrusted the role of technology in healthcare. The e-booking project was questioned closely and the subject of articulate debate within the party. To some degree, the Health Plan issued in 1987 mirrored this debate although in due course there was a rebalancing of policies towards a more important role for technology.

Healthcare policy was debated not only among political parties and social movements but also between stakeholders, including the medical profession, medical science and research activity in general. The activity of the city councillor in the Health Department was influenced not only by his membership of the political party governing the municipality but also by his involvement in local healthcare. In fact, he was supported by two leading medical figures, both "outsiders" due to lengthy periods spent in the US, where one studied oncology and the other innovative techniques in surgery. Both were advocates of the role technology could play in healthcare and so provided support for the city councillor. The councillor himself had been a student of a leading professor at the University of Bologna who had founded a new discipline, the sociology of healthcare, establishing a school that regrouped a significant number of researchers and students. Several members of the CUP directorate had studied under him. This professor has been a central figure in Bologna's political and cultural life, a councillor for more than a decade and one of the authors of the White Paper that outlined a profound transformation of the city administration. His support helped to legitimize the city councillor's position in health management.

The strength of this support drove a new vision of healthcare for the city. The aim was citizens' empowerment through provision of a means by which they could voice their needs and be taken into account. Pursuing this aim meant establishing new citizen/healthcare relationships, involving hospitals and health centres. The mediating role of the CUP directorate exemplified this new relationship. It shook up the prevailing normative order as the roles of the medical profession and healthcare institutions were reformulated.

Technology, specifically information technology, constituted the tool for establishing this new relationship. The number of services available, their type and timing became transparent for all providers. Healthcare access was standardized and no longer subject to the idiosyncrasies of providers. Equality in service access was guaranteed, preventing discriminatory practices. Finally, a simplified and time-saving e-booking process was made available to citizens.

Then a conflict erupted. Head physicians at the university and Bologna's largest hospital, with the support of medical organizations, opposed the intervention of a third party in mediating access to healthcare and threatened not to adopt the new booking system just weeks before the launch of the service. They maintained that it was too expensive and that services offered would be poor quality. It was an impasse. Only the intervention of the mayor, who convened all the parties and emphasized how the project would be beneficial for the city, succeeded in overcoming it. However, opposition did not disappear completely. Five years after the inauguration of the service there was a further attempt to stop it and 25 years later there are still disagreements between medical directors and the Emilia Romagna regional authority, which is now in charge of healthcare management.

To sum up, the e-booking project saw the light of day because several streams of support flowed into the local branch of the PCI and the mayor was committed to backing it. This powerful advocacy was able to resist opposition from USL boards of medical directors and head physicians. Financial resources were at stake and subject to the approval of municipal representative bodies. With such a complex project, only a small reduction in the budget would have put its development and implementation at risk. Again, the political context prevented this eventuality.

Looking at the role played by the installed base – specifically, political resources – for the realization of the e-booking project, it is clear that significant mobilization took place. Local government administrative and representative bodies, the majority party and USL top management were actively involved in both supporting and opposing the project. This is illustrated by the unusual protest from head physicians who threatened to stop the adoption of the booking system and the unorthodox meeting convened by the mayor to avert it. The traditional political arena for negotiation was abandoned or considered ineffective and new ways of building consensus were put in place involving the academic sector, which was usually external to the healthcare arena.

15.5.2 The Mobilization of Organizational Resources

The installed base was also involved in the mobilization of organizational resources. Several organizational arrangements were at stake in providing the operational context for e-booking. Traditional bureaucracies favoured it. Both the Health Department of the municipality of Bologna and USL, the bodies in charge of healthcare, were public bureaucracies. Each USL ran hospitals and health centres in a specific area, coordinating and monitoring the activities of GPs and paediatricians who were self-employed professionals. These public bodies were a type of in-house provider. Their mandate was to supply the medical needs of the people in their jurisdiction and as they were governed by executive committees nominated by municipalities they reflected each municipality's political bias. This is why the

Health Department of the municipality of Bologna was in charge of the e-booking project even though it did not have the professional competences and the organizational capabilities to manage booking centres. The department's institutional mission was healthcare policy implementation on the one hand, and policy monitoring and supervision on the other. A similar lack of competences and organizational capabilities also characterized USLs. Nevertheless, USLs were used to managing paper-based booking systems and so were the natural candidates for running booking centres. Nevertheless, a different decision was made. USLs, as public bodies, were subject to restrictions in workforce management typical of the public sector of that time. The relocation of personnel from one booking office to another, or the extensive use of part-time staff to deal with peak times and long office hours (7.30–18.30), were not possible in the public sector, only in the private sector. Staff training was also necessary. The public sector was heavily unionized and lengthy negotiations would be required to reach an agreement on training and changes to tasks. There were time constraints for the project and this option was not considered feasible. Finally, the three USLs were largely independent units and the service would involve personnel coming from three distinct organizations, creating coordination problems.

At this point, the decision to establish a new company was made. Bologna could be considered the capital of the cooperative movement and a large number of cooperatives were present in sectors like catering, mass distribution, logistics, building and construction. According to the International Alliance of Cooperatives, "a co-operative is an autonomous association of persons united voluntarily to meet their common economic, social, and cultural needs and aspirations through a jointly-owned and democratically-controlled enterprise. Co-operatives are based on the values of self-help, self-responsibility, democracy, equality, equity and solidarity (ICA 1995, p. 3–4)." The new company was part of a group of cooperatives in the software sector provided with technological and organizational capabilities developed in the cooperative environment, which shared the political orientation of the municipality of Bologna at that time. Turning to the cooperative movement meant establishing a link with a large business entity in the local context and promoting specific values in order to compete, in some sense, with traditional public bureaucratic organizations such as hospitals and health centres.

Against this background, SYNWARE was formed. Its activities were supported by weekly training sessions involving top management, five coordinators and on occasion the entire staff. The training content supported, among other things, the adoption of new software, the introduction of new laboratory examinations and the management of critical issues encountered in everyday practice. The weekly sessions were the context in which organizational solutions were conceived. From the detailed analysis of practices and the direct engagement of operators, it was possible to figure out how to improve service provision. The continuous solicitation of operators created an environment favourable to open debate of continuously emerging issues. This was considered the only way to deal with the innovative nature of the service and the lack of experience of those involved in its operation. From the launch of the service to its full implementation, the organizational structure of SYNWARE has not changed significantly, apart from the coordination figures. It has maintained its relatively simple structure, as it was felt that introducing further organizational units would have obstructed the integration of the different components, which was the principal aim of the organization.

A couple of SYNWARE and ITALSIEL managers collaborated actively with the CUP directorate established at the Health Department and led by the city councillor responsible for healthcare. The directorate was regarded as the driver and control tower of the entire e-booking project and requests for services from SYNWARE, USLs or ITALSIEL were relayed to it. Any decision made at the directorate level was passed on to the party or parties involved, which activated their organizational structures accordingly.

A number of actions were in the direct remit of the CUP directorate. One of these was the building of the service catalogue. Even though this involved the establishment of work groups, led by an expert in a medical specialism and an expert in administrative procedures, both physicians, these groups were supervised by the directorate. Activities related to the catalogue building were mainly conducted in the first phase of the project. However, the process was reintroduced when new services were added or existing services changed. Schedule management and the monitoring and management of information about the services available required close collaboration between the directorate and hospitals and health centres. Each facility was responsible for communicating updated information about the services it offered. Building the service catalogue was a long and arduous process.

The CUP directorate was considered an alien presence in an environment that had always been controlled by medical science and its elite. The directorate struggled with leading physicians for control of health services. Taking only partial control of service provision constituted a significant change to established practice and was met with a hostile response from the medical profession. Power distance was a factor in this context. The profession dragged its feet when it was necessary to establish a dialogue with the directorate as it was not sufficiently legitimized in the healthcare environment.

With the advent of the new service, booking management changed considerably. Traditional public bureaucracies now had the room to innovate organizational arrangements, indicating that the installed base, insofar as it was related to organizational resources, was mobilized radically. When hindering effects prevailed, resources available outside the healthcare domain were mobilized in preference to resources present in hospitals and health centres. The existence of these external resources was fundamental to the project, as demonstrated by the involvement of the cooperative movement in running booking centres and the active role played by ITALSIEL and SYNWARE within the directorate. Now areas that had traditionally been run by the public sector saw the participation of private players. The establishment of the directorate itself was a clear example of this. The close partnership with USLs was supported by forms of coordination and control that differed significantly from those of typical bureaucracies.

15.5.3 The Mobilization of Technological Resources

During the 1980s, a computerization scheme was launched throughout the Italian public administration system and subsequently in healthcare. However, it was not able to support the e-booking system and developers had recourse to resources external to the healthcare domain – ultimately the largest Italian software company of the time became involved. Only companies of that size and experience had to capability to build systems on this scale. ITALSIEL, with branches throughout the country, had been the software provider for the whole public sector and the Italian banking system, which was largely controlled by the state at that time. Informatica Friuli Venezia Giulia (IFVG), one of these branches, developed software solutions for healthcare and was involved in designing the architecture of the centralized booking system. Two solutions were proposed by the IFVG top management, one based on the ORACLE database and the other on the dBase database. The possibility of using a product like ORACLE Forms to create screens to interact with the ORACLE database sealed the decision to select the former, which was perceived as more stable and performative. The Ministry of Health approved the solution other than the Health Department coordinated by the National Research Council and the University of Bologna. The system was expected to extend throughout the country once adopted by an important city like Bologna. Being a so-called prime mover in this business would create the conditions to achieve a competitive advantage over other software providers.

Given the size and the innovative functions of the project, the architecture proposed by IFVG was evaluated at ITALSIEL headquarters in Rome. The adoption of the ORACLE database was confirmed but not the software designed to interact with it and the COBOL programming language was selected instead. Back in the 1980s, all large projects turned to this language as it provided the most robust solutions in high complex cases. While IFVG did not fully agree with this decision, on the grounds that other and more innovative solutions could have been found, the decision was considered rational for a number of reasons. First, there were time constraints. The centralized booking system had to be deployable within 6 months and there were not sufficient competences related to specific programming languages for ORACLE databases at IFVG or ITALSIEL headquarters. Second, a large number of COBOL software components that could interact with an ORACLE database were available. The challenge was to group them together to provide interfaces connecting the database and related functions. Finally, the system performance achieved was judged satisfactory, due to the experience acquired in the COBOL environment.

Going live with the e-booking service heralded a new phase in the evolution of the system, as it was necessary to accommodate the needs of nationwide health facilities that required new services or existing services to be reformulated. The aim was to offer the most complicated diagnostic activities – those involving multiple operators and sequential steps – in the 2 years following the launch of the service. The role of staff at booking centres was fundamental to a well functioning system. At the time, automated booking processes were limited and skilled staff with expertise in using the system played a decisive role in providing an appropriate service. Another issue was GPs' handwriting: a statistical analysis of those whose prescriptions were most often rejected by operators due to their illegibility was introduced.

The identification of citizens at booking centres was enabled by a magnetic card containing personal details. Delivering a novel tool to more than 400,000 inhabitants of Bologna carried a high risk of its misuse. However, at that time polling cards were delivered to households by traffic police officers (municipal employees) and in 1990 local elections were held. The e-booking cards were delivered along with polling cards by the police, who emphasized their importance and how they were to be used. The card soon became a symbol of an innovative solution for accessing healthcare through digital technology.

The partnership with ITALSIEL confirmed the importance of the installed base in terms of technological resources. Adoption of the COBOL programming language was contingent on the presence of existing software components that were mobilized to interact with the ORACLE database. Finally, the mobilization of technological resources was necessary for the introduction of the magnetic identification card and the role of the police determined its correct use.

15.6 Discussion

The origins of the e-booking system raises questions about the role of the installed base and its constraining and enabling effects. A healthcare model characterized by a polarization between hospitals on the one hand, and GPs on the other did not provide a supportive environment for creating innovative solutions to accessing healthcare. Hospitals and health centres conceived as professional bureaucracies (Mintzberg 1979; Lam 2000) operate according to standardized and bureaucratic methods of coordination and control in a context where individual expertise and professional bodies both held relevant roles. Even though routines and practices are governed by protocol, personal judgement and peer consultation were important in these organizations. Within professional bureaucracies, such as universities, schools, hospitals and courts, supervision and control are assigned not only to hierarchical superiors but also to external professional associations. These establish regulations and guidelines and are the custodians of the profession, determining appropriate and non-appropriate behaviours. It is understandable that the introduction of an innovative, IT-based system of access to healthcare would meet opposition within a healthcare model governed by professional bureaucracies and medical associations.

It was necessary to mobilize political, organizational and technological resources that could counter this situation. Political activity led the way in coordination, negotiation and building consensus. The municipality of Bologna and the Health Department were conscious of citizens' dissatisfaction with the long waiting lists, lack of transparency and inconvenience of accessing healthcare and formulated a response.

How was the mobilization of political, organizational and technological resources demonstrated? The role played by IT was decisive here. Information technology was conceived as the driver for delineating new ways of accessing healthcare. An innovative scenario for improving healthcare services was established and contrasted sharply with existing ones. Turning to IT inevitably implied an openness towards innovation and continuous updating of implemented solutions.

The constitution of a third party able to mediate between citizens and healthcare providers represented a further aspect of the mobilization process. The CUP directorate supported by SYNWARE provided the e-booking service, eliminating professional bureaucracies such as hospitals and health centres. The service provided by these bureaucracies was substituted by organizational arrangements within the socio-economic context of the Bologna area and exemplified by the cooperative movement.

The leading role of the Health Department and the CUP directorate contributed to the legitimization of service provision outside the healthcare sphere. It was demonstrated that alternative forms of service organization could replace established ones. Traditional healthcare responsibilities, such as service bookings, shifted to an entity supervised by the Health Department and subsequently by representatives of social and political movements. Citizen empowerment was an additional aim.

Finally, the opposition of vested interests, represented by medical associations and head physicians practicing in hospitals, was overcome due to the supporting role played by the local section of the Italian Communist Party and civil society in general. The figure of the mayor was emblematic here. His authority and the consensus he acquired in the city enabled the introduction of e-booking in healthcare.

References

Bowker GC, Star SL. Sorting things out: classification and its consequences. Cambridge, MA: MIT Press; 1999.

Chae B, Lanzara GF. Self-destructive dynamics in large-scale technochange and some ways of counteracting it. Inf Technol People. 2006;19(1):74–97.

Ciborra C, Hanseth O. Introduction. In: Ciborra C, editor. From control to drift: the dynamics of corporate information infrastructures. Oxford: Oxford University Press; 2000. p. 1–15.

Hanseth O, Lyytinen K. Design theory for dynamic complexity in information infrastructures: the case of building internet. J Inf Technol. 2010;25(1):1–19.

Hanseth O, Monteiro E. Inscribing behaviour in information infrastructure standards. Account Manag Inf Technol. 1997;7(4):183–211.

Hanseth O, Monteiro E, Hatling M. Developing information infrastructure: the tension between standardization and flexibility. Sci Technol Hum Values. 1996;21(4):407–26.

ICA. Cooperative principles for the 21st century: introduction. Rev Int Co-Operation. 1995;88(3):3–4.

Lam A. Tacit knowledge, organizational learning and societal institutions: an integrated framework. Organ Stud. 2000;21(3):487–513.

Lanzara GF. Building digital institutions: ICT and the rise of assemblages in government. In: Contini F, Lanzara GF, editors. ICT and innovation in the public sector. Houndmills: Palgrave MacMillan; 2009. p. 269–96.

Mintzberg H. The professional bureaucracy. Organization and governance in higher education. 1979. p. 50–70.

Moruzzi M. e-Health e fascicolo sanitario elettronico. Milan: Gruppo 24 Ore; 2009.

Moruzzi M. La sanità dematerializzita e il fascicolo sanitario elettronico. Roma: Il Pensiero Scientifico Editore; 2014.

Star SL, Ruhleder K. Steps toward an ecology of infrastructure: design and access for large information spaces. Inf Syst Res. 1996;7(1):111–34.

Yin R. Case study research: design and methods. Thousand Oaks: Sage; 2009.

Open Access This chapter is distributed under the terms of the Creative Commons Attribution-NonCommercial 2.5 International License (http://creativecommons.org/licenses/by-nc/2.5/), which permits any noncommercial use, duplication, adaptation, distribution and reproduction in any medium or format, as long as you give appropriate credit to the original author(s) and the source, provide a link to the Creative Commons license and indicate if changes were made.

The images or other third party material in this chapter are included in the chapter's Creative Commons license, unless indicated otherwise in a credit line to the material. If material is not included in the chapter's Creative Commons license and your intended use is not permitted by statutory regulation or exceeds the permitted use, you will need to obtain permission directly from the copyright holder.

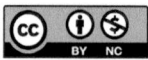

Index

© The Author(s) 2017
M. Aanestad et al. (eds.), *Information Infrastructures within European Health Care*, Health Informatics, DOI 10.1007/978-3-319-51020-0

261

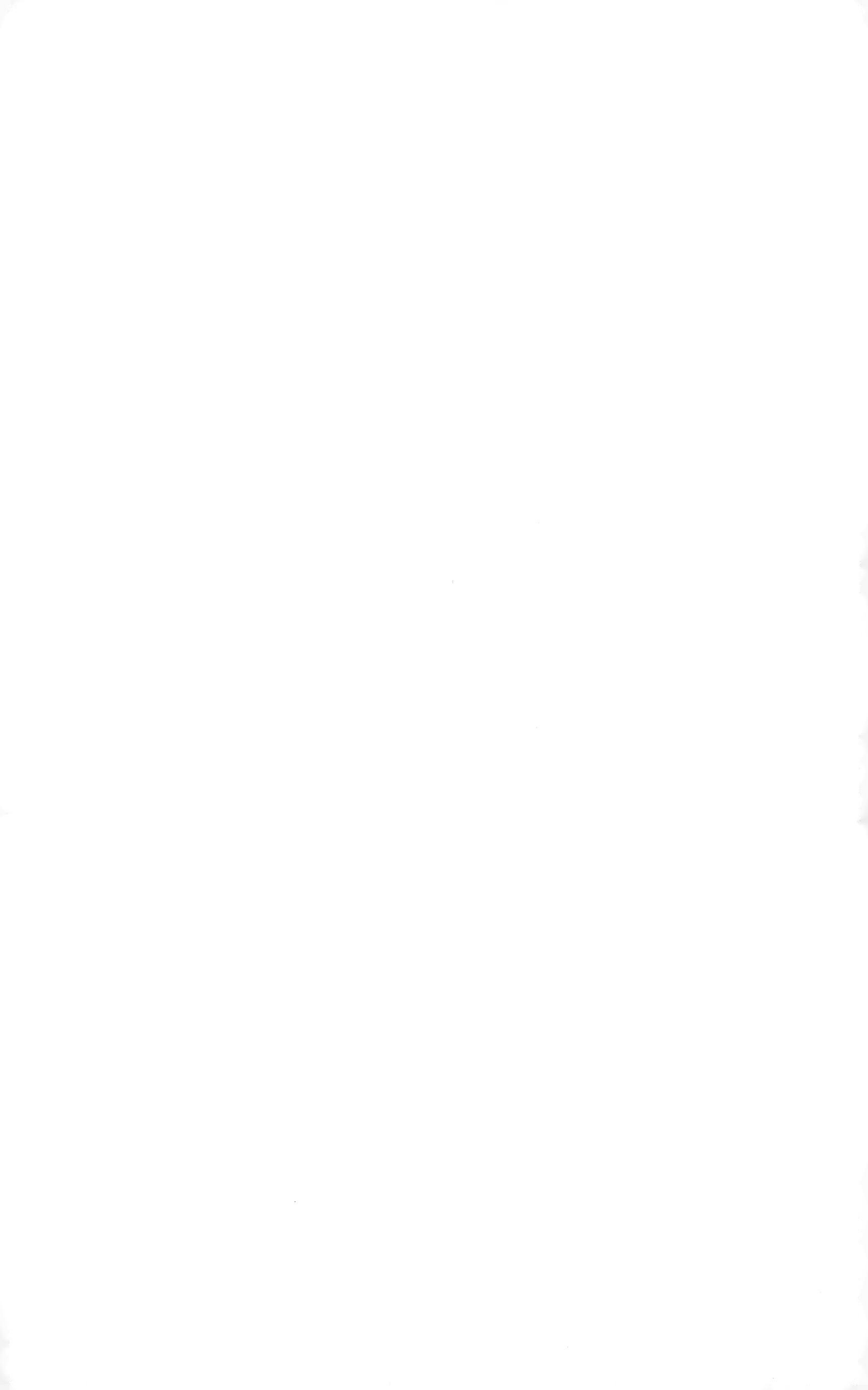